Chinese
Holistic Medicine

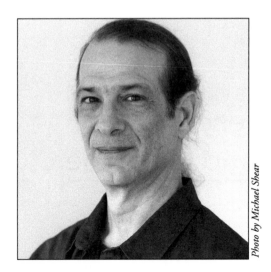

About the Author

Steven Cardoza earned a master of science degree in Traditional Chinese Medicine in 1994 from the American College of TCM, San Francisco. An alternative health provider since 1985 and a practicing Chinese medical physician (acupuncture, Chinese herbs, therapeutic bodywork, medical qigong, etc.) since 1995, he is nationally certified and licensed in California and Massachusetts. Steven holds numerous certifications in many styles of Qigong and Wu Taiji from living Daoist lineage holder Master B. K. Frantzis.

Chinese
Holistic Medicine

In Your Daily Life

Combine Acupressure, Herbal
Remedies & Qigong for Integrated
Natural Healing

Steven Cardoza, MS, LAc

Llewellyn Publications
Woodbury, Minnesota

First Edition
First Printing, 2017

Cover design by Ellen Lawson
Interior Illustrations by Mary Ann Zapalac

Llewellyn Publications is a registered trademark of Llewellyn Worldwide Ltd.

Library of Congress Cataloging-in-Publication Data
Names: Cardoza, Steven, author.
Title: Chinese holistic medicine in your daily life : combine acupressure,
    herbal remedies & qigong for integrated natural healing / Steven Cardoza,
    MS, LAc.
Description: First edition. | Woodbury, Minnesota : Llewellyn Publications,
    [2017] | Includes bibliographical references and index.
Identifiers: LCCN 2016045767 (print) | LCCN 2016046923 (ebook) | ISBN
    9780738749303 | ISBN 9780738750958 (ebook)
Subjects: LCSH: Medicine, Chinese. | Integrative medicine.
Classification: LCC R601 .C374 2017 (print) | LCC R601 (ebook) | DDC 610—dc23 LC record available at
    https://lccn.loc.gov/2016045767

Llewellyn Worldwide Ltd. does not participate in, endorse, or have any authority or responsibility concerning private business transactions between our authors and the public.

All mail addressed to the author is forwarded, but the publisher cannot, unless specifically instructed by the author, give out an address or phone number.

Any Internet references contained in this work are current at publication time, but the publisher cannot guarantee that a specific location will continue to be maintained. Please refer to the publisher's website for links to authors' websites and other sources.

Llewellyn Publications
A Division of Llewellyn Worldwide Ltd.
2143 Wooddale Drive
Woodbury, MN 55125-2989
www.llewellyn.com

Printed in the United States of America

Also by Steven Cardoza

Chinese Healing Exercises: A Personalized Practice for Health & Longevity

Acknowledgments

I'd like to extend my gratitude to all of the remarkable teachers and physicians I've been privileged to learn from over the years, whose wisdom and insights shaped my own healing and teaching abilities and whose contributions to my growth helped make this book possible.

Thanks to the faculty of the San Francisco College of Acupuncture in 1991:

- Robert Johns, a maverick who allowed me to attend his Advanced Classical Needling Techniques classes before I even knew how to properly locate a point.
- Richard Liao—in addition to providing comprehensive herbal instruction, his treatments cured me of three types of asthma simultaneously, strongly motivating me to learn Chinese herbology.
- John Yeh, MD, who first opened my eyes to the ways in which Western medical constructs and paradigms could be analyzed within the context of Chinese medicine.

Thanks to the faculty and staff of the American College of Traditional Chinese Medicine in 1991–1994 for their diligence and patience and for their passion and enthusiasm for sharing their knowledge of Chinese medicine. Those whose guidance remains most notable include Xingguo Fu, Denise Hsu, Daniel Jiao, Lifang Liang, Lee Wugofski, MD (Western medicine), and Baibing Zhu.

Thanks to all of the outstanding Qigong masters dedicated to imparting the deepest and most subtle aspects of Chinese healing and spirituality. Their teachings continue to influence and further my cultivation. Special thanks to three of the most personally significant, for generously permitting me to relay some of their inspired teachings in this book:

- Master B. K. Frantzis, Daoist lineage holder and my primary Qigong teacher since 1987.
- Deguang He, acupuncturist, herbalist, and medical Qigong physician.
- Grandmaster Hong Liu, Qigong master, healer, herbalist, and medical researcher.

A special thanks to Michael Shear for contributing the photographs that were used to create many of the illustrations found in this book.

Contents

Disclaimer   *xvii*

Introduction   *1*

    Some Conventions Used in This Book:

    Pinyin, Capitalizations, and Italics   3

Overview: An Integrated Approach to Natural Healing   *5*

    Branches of Chinese Medicine   6

    Acupuncture   6

    Herbal Medicine   7

    Qigong, Taiji, and Other Physical Therapies   7

    Dietetics   8

    Lifestyle   8

    Chinese Medicine Is Holistic   10

    Chinese Diagnosis and Western Diagnosis   12

    Integrating the Branches   13

    Integrated Practices in Western Medicine   16

Part 1: Foundational Theories in Chinese Medicine

Chapter 1: First Concept: Qi, The Energy of Life . . . 19

    Qualities and Functions within the Body   21

    Biological Energies Used in Western Medicine   22

Chapter 2: Second Concept: Meridians, The Pathways of Health . . . 25

    The Twelve Regular Meridians   27

    The Eight Extraordinary Meridians   29

    Meridians and Western Medicine   31

Chapter 3: Third Concept: Yin and Yang, Polarities, and Balance . . . 35

    Yin and Yang in the Natural World   37

    Four Primary Aspects of Yin and Yang Pairings   38

    Yin and Yang within the Body   41

    Western Correspondences to Yin and Yang   47

Chapter 4: Introduction to the Internal Organs . . . 51

Zangfu: The Internal Organs and Their Correspondences 51

Terminology 52

Chapter 5: Zang: The Yin Organs . . . 57

The Heart 57

The Lungs 61

The Liver 65

The Spleen 71

The Kidneys 75

Chapter 6: Fu: The Yang Organs . . . 87

The Stomach 88

The Small Intestine 89

The Gall Bladder 90

The Large Intestine 92

The Urinary Bladder 93

The Sanjiao 94

Chapter 7: Pathogenesis: The Origins of Disease . . . 99

The Causes of Disharmony 100

Overview of External Pathogenic Factors 101

Overview of Internal Pathogenic Factors 102

The Six External Pathogenic Factors 103

The Seven Emotions as Internal Pathogenic Factors 111

Miscellaneous Factors 115

Chapter 8: Introducing Patterns of Disharmony . . . 131

Many Patterns for One Disease; One Pattern for Many Diseases 131

The Lenses of Diagnosis 133

Criteria of TCM Pattern Identification 135

Eight Principle Considerations 136

Chapter 9: Selected Patterns of Disharmony . . . 139

1. Wind Cold Invading the Lungs 140

2. Heart Blood Deficiency 141

3. Liver Qi Stagnation 142

4. Spleen Qi Deficiency   144

5. Kidney Yang Deficiency   145

Part 2: Holistic Self-Care with Chinese Medicine

Chapter 10: Diagnosis: Finding the Root of the Problem . . . 151

Diagnostic Methods   151

Inquiry   152

Pulse Diagnosis   153

Tongue Diagnosis   157

Chapter 11: Tools and Practice of Chinese Medicine:
    Holism and Integration . . . 161

Acupuncture   161

Three Case Histories   164

Adjunctive Therapies   168

Western Perspectives on Acupuncture   169

Conditions Treated   170

Herbal Medicine   173

Physical Therapies   176

Diet and Lifestyle   180

Chapter 12: Acupressure Self-Care: Your Healing Hands . . . 183

Methods of Locating the Points   185

Acupressure Techniques   189

Selected Acupressure Points   192

Chapter 13: The Acupressure Points: Names, Locations,
    and Functions . . . 195

Lungs, Hand Taiyin   196

Large Intestine, Hand Yangming   200

Stomach, Foot Yangming   202

Spleen, Foot Taiyin   207

Heart, Hand Shaoyin   210

Small Intestine, Hand Taiyang   212

Urinary Bladder, Foot Taiyang   215

Kidney, Foot Shaoyin   219

Pericardium, Hand Jueyin   222

Sanjiao, Hand Shaoyang   224

Gall Bladder, Foot Shaoyang   226

Liver, Foot Jueyin   230

Du, Governing Vessel   232

Ren, Conception Vessel   235

Chapter 14: Chinese Herbs: Nature's Healing Allies . . . 239

Main Attributes of Chinese Herbs: Temperature and Taste   240

Directionality   241

Channels Entered   241

Categorizing Herbs   242

Herb Categories   243

Formula Basics   257

Chapter 15: Chinese Herbal Formulas . . . 259

Lungs: Common Cold with Variations   260

Lungs: Asthma, Emphysema, Bronchitis   263

Stomach/Spleen: Digestive Disorders   263

Heart: Insomnia, Anxiety   265

Liver: Detox, Stress   266

Kidneys: Low Energy, Urinary
and Sexual Dysfunction, Arthritis   268

Qi Tonics   269

Blood Tonics   270

Yang Tonics   271

Yin Tonics   272

Pain: General, Traumatic, Arthritis   273

Topicals for Pain   275

Chapter 16: Introduction to Qigong: Harnessing the Energy of Life . . . 277

Defining Qigong   277

The Basic Standing Posture: The Side Channel Stance   278

General Breathing Guidelines   281

Working with Your Qi   282

Practice Times   283

Length of Practice   284

Ending a Practice Session: Storing Qi in the Dantian   285

Final Practice Guidelines   286

Chapter 17: Qigong Practices for Each Organ . . . 289

Qigong for the Lungs and Large Intestines   289

Qigong for the Spleen and Stomach   299

Qigong for the Heart   305

Qigong for the Kidneys   316

Qigong for the Liver   323

Chapter 18: Prescriptions: Restore and Maintain Inner Harmony . . . 329

Abscesses   332

Allergies   333

Arthritis   333

Breathing Disorders   335

Common Cold or Flu   338

Digestive System Disorders   339

Dizziness   341

Dry Hair, Nails, and Skin   342

Eczema   342

Edema (Generalized)   343

Emotional Distress   344

Eye/Vision Problems   344

Fatigue   346

Fever   346

Gall Bladder, Inflammation and Stones   347

Headache   347

Heart Conditions   348

Hemorrhoids   349

Hepatitis, Enlarged Liver   349

Hernia   350

Herpes, Oral or Genital   351

Hives   351

High Blood Pressure   352
Immune Support   353
Insomnia   353
Men's Health   354
Motion Sickness   356
Pain, Joints and Limbs   356
Pain, General and Traumatic   358
Poor Memory   359
Urinary System Disorders   359
Women's Health/Gynecology   360
Wellness Self-Care Protocol   362

Concluding Remarks   365
Glossary of Western Drug Actions . . . 367
Appendix 1: Point Location by Body Region . . . 371
Appendix 2: Chapter Notes . . . 383
Bibliography . . . 389
Recommended Reading . . . 391
Index . . . 393

Disclaimer

This book is not intended as a substitute for medical advice from Chinese or Western physicians. It is not intended to diagnose, treat, or cure any medical condition. The reader assumes all responsibility for using any technique, herb, exercise, or dietary modification presented in this book. Consult your medical professional before beginning any new health or fitness regimen or if you have a medical condition.

Introduction

This book teaches both the theory and practice of natural healing methods used in China. Every branch of Chinese medicine is holistic, but there are numerous layers of holistic interconnection possible. In order to achieve the greatest synergy, they should be integrated according to the principles contained here. That's how these methods are used to best advantage in China, with some variations as you'll learn in Chapter 1 and throughout Part 2.

The book is presented in two distinct yet intimately entwined parts and follows the guidance of many wise teachers I've had the privilege to know over decades of study. Two core ideas were repeatedly encountered, and while some teachers worded them differently, the essential meanings were always the same.

The first core idea is "In order to learn any practice or discipline well, you need both a solid intellectual understanding and a strong foundation in its practical application." All agreed that the actual practice (Qigong, Taiji, healing exercises, acupressure) or application of the method (acupuncture, herbal medicine, food therapies) is the ultimate goal. Greater intellectual understanding can support greater practical ability, but it is only valuable as it serves to further that end. Otherwise, it may provide for some interesting conversations but will not tangibly improve your health and life.

The second core idea is "Mastery means mastering the basics." The basics are the root of both theory and practice. A broad, solid foundation provides the stability on which to build and grow. Even if you choose to not build more than a foundation, that will be your bedrock during any times of hardship.

1

Part 1, "Foundational Theories in Chinese Medicine," introduces the theoretical underpinnings of all Chinese medical science and philosophy. While not as detailed as a medical textbook, it is fairly extensive for two reasons. It provides the intellectual core necessary for understanding and accomplishment, and it thoroughly acquaints the Western reader with a different way of looking at the world, from a Chinese perspective. The concepts and practices taught throughout this book grow out of that cultural perspective, and if we are to learn to apply those practices in our daily life, some effort must be made to drop our own cultural preconceptions and see things with fresh eyes. The detail in Part 1 is intended to facilitate that perceptual shift.

The majority of Part 2, "Holistic Self-Care with Chinese Medicine," carefully teaches the practical basics of Chinese holistic self-care methods using principles learned in Part 1 and provides plenty of room to grow as you become more adept in each. Doing the practices regularly is most important and ultimately leads to mastery, giving you simple yet valuable and effective options for taking control of your health in a variety of natural and holistic ways. These are methods that you can use forever and that will greatly reduce the likelihood of needing to visit any physician, whether Chinese or Western.

There are times when an integrated natural healing approach might include professional medical help. The insights into Chinese medicine from Part 1 will prepare you well if you decide to seek such help. Part 2 opens with things you can expect when visiting a Chinese physician, beyond what many Westerners know, and introduces you to the diagnostics and treatments of Chinese medicine. This will help you have a more informed dialogue with your Chinese physician and establish realistic expectations and goals, making it most productive for you both.

Keep in mind that just as illness rarely happens overnight, healing won't happen overnight either. Daily practice is required to make healing changes in your life.

Readers who want to jump right into the practices in Part 2 can safely do so, but realize that by better understanding any practice, including its basic theory and the ways in which it works within a holistic system, you will have more freedom and flexibility when selecting practices that match your specific needs and health goals.

Some Conventions Used in This Book: Pinyin, Capitalizations, and Italics

Pinyin is the official standardized alphabetic transliteration system that has been in use in China since the early 1950s. It contains clues to the meaning and guidance in the correct pronunciation of Mandarin Chinese words not found in the older Wade-Giles spellings that may be more familiar to some readers. Pinyin is the intended transliteration system used here, except when quoting sources that may use older spellings. Some examples of pinyin, with Wade-Giles equivalents in parentheses, include Qi (Ch'i), Taiji (Tai Chi), Qigong (Ch'i Gung), and Jing (Ching).

Pinyin is a synthetic language, meaning that while each syllable is a discrete word, new words are made by joining those syllables/words into multisyllabic words. Common examples include Qigong ("energy" and "practice" or "cultivation") and Taijiquan ("supreme ultimate fist"). Some authors prefer to split those words into their component syllables, depicting them as Qi Gong and Tai Ji Quan. While this is not strictly correct, it does allow the reader to clearly see the syllables that make up those words. Throughout this book, when an unfamiliar Chinese word is first introduced its component syllables will also be shown in parentheses, allowing readers with some pinyin experience to easily see the syllables that make up the word and quickly understand its meaning. This will also help less experienced readers see the commonalities among words that may at first appear very different. Examples involving different qualities of Qi include Jingqi (Jing Qi), Yuanqi (Yuan Qi), Guqi (Gu Qi), and Waiqi (Wai Qi).

Among the many Chinese words you'll encounter, some will be more familiar—such as Qi, Yin, and Yang—while others like Tuina, Mingmen, or Dantian may appear strange to readers who are relatively new to these topics. They are not proper nouns, but all will be capitalized throughout the book to help readers recognize them as Chinese words. Their meanings are explained in the text.

Some English words are capitalized to distinguish them from their use as part of a Chinese medical designation. Most of the time those will be the names of organs (such as Spleen, Liver, or Kidneys) when referring to the holistic Organ System as described later, rather than to the organ as understood by Western medicine. Blood can have connotations outside of the English word meaning and will be capitalized when used in that way. Other English words will be capitalized when part of a principle designation, such as Yin-Yang theory, or when part of a Chinese medical pattern, such as Spleen Qi Deficiency. When not capitalized, they are used as commonly understood English words.

Last, the phrase "Chinese physician" is used to mean someone of any nationality who practices Chinese medicine, not necessarily a physician who is Chinese.

Overview

An Integrated Approach
to Natural Healing

With a rich and varied history spanning over five thousand years, Chinese medicine is perhaps both the oldest and most widespread form of medicine practiced in the world today. It is a dynamic, living system that continues to grow and evolve while remaining true to its ancient roots.

Many Westerners are interested in the different perspectives of Asian culture, its spiritual philosophies, and strikingly unusual health and medical practices. Some are fascinated by, while others are skeptical about, the promise of greater health that Chinese medicine can provide. Before that promise can be fully and accurately evaluated, a significant challenge must first be recognized and overcome.

Chinese medicine has rigorous, well-defined methodologies to preserve health and to diagnose, treat, and prevent illness, but its principles and paradigms are vastly different from those commonly followed in the West. It needs to be understood, accepted, and applied completely on its own terms, adhering to those intrinsic paradigms and principles. This takes an open mind, some effort, and a level of trust, since it will require learning new concepts, new terminology, and some new ways of thinking as well as stepping outside of the comfortable familiarity of Western medical conventions. Only then can it be used optimally, as it has been designed and practiced for millennia in China and in many other countries, to achieve its expected and sometimes nearly miraculous health benefits.

Branches of Chinese Medicine

- Acupuncture and adjunctive acupuncture modalities
- Chinese herbal medicine
- Qigong, Taiji, and other active physical therapies
- Tuina, acupressure and other passive physical therapies
- Dietetics
- Lifestyle considerations

Each branch of Chinese medicine is introduced here separately. Many Westerners may think of each branch as complete and separate from the others, but each is part of a cohesive whole. In order to most quickly and thoroughly restore a healthy balance when injured or ill, and to maintain or increase optimal health otherwise, all branches should be integrated. Throughout this book, we'll examine their interrelationships and provide ways for you to incorporate them into your daily life.

Almost everyone has heard of acupuncture, the branch that is most familiar in the Western world. It's been researched by Western science and has been reported on frequently in the popular media, leading many people to believe that acupuncture is the totality of Chinese medicine. Although the landscape is changing, for a time many Chinese medical colleges in the United States only taught acupuncture, contributing to that popular misconception. Of course, Chinese medicine is not just acupuncture, but rather a network of many complementary branches that work synergistically to produce the most desired therapeutic outcomes. While each will be examined in great detail throughout the book, the following is an introduction to the various branches. Any unfamiliar terminology is defined later within its related topic.

Acupuncture

Acupuncture involves the insertion of very fine, sterile needles of surgical quality into acupuncture points specific to each patient's individual needs. Those points are located along well-defined energetic pathways found throughout the body called "meridians" or "channels." Each meridian is associated with a primary organ, influencing its function. Many points on a single meridian also influence the functions of organs secondary to the primary organ being addressed.

Acupuncture's main strength is in moving *Qi* (the vital energy of life), stimulating its flow when it's weak, redirecting it to areas that are more in need while drawing it away from areas that are in excess, and opening up obstructions so it can flow freely. This improves the functionality of the treated Organ Systems, which include the associated meridians and the whole body by extension.

An acupuncturist may choose to use various adjunctive therapies to augment the benefits of the acupuncture treatment. The most commonly employed are electroacupuncture, moxibustion, and cupping. They are discussed in Chapter 12.

Herbal Medicine

Chinese herbal medicine is older than acupuncture and central to the practice of Chinese medicine. Although plant sources make up the largest part of its pharmacopoeia, substances from the animal and mineral kingdoms are also used.

With thousands of years of research and development, it's a highly refined and most elegant branch of Chinese medicine, taking into account more variables than are considered when employing acupuncture alone. Each herb belongs to one of over thirty categories, groupings of herbs indicating their overall qualities and main purpose. The unique therapeutic effects of each herb are defined by their taste, their temperature (Qi), and the channel(s) that the herb enters. These are discussed in Chapter 15. Also taken into account are the herb's effective range of dosages, functions, and clinical usage, herbs it may most typically be combined with, and cautions or contraindications in certain health conditions. Used this way, herbal medicine is very safe, is very effective, and produces no side effects.

Qigong, Taiji, and Other Physical Therapies

In the context of Chinese medicine and natural healing, physical therapies can mean that a patient passively receives a treatment, such as acupressure or *Tuina*, which are different types of Chinese medical massage therapies; bone-setting, which is a sort of Chinese chiropractic; or medical Qigong, an energy healing modality in which a Qigong doctor directs his own Qi to manipulate the Qi of a patient in a way very similar to acupuncture, frequently with little or no physical contact involved.

It can also mean the patient is taught to perform an active practice combining physical and energetic aspects of healing. Chinese healing exercises can be combined prescriptively to treat a wide range of health conditions. Most Qigongs have, or can be modified to have, a specific purpose that targets a particular organ, illness, imbalance, or disharmony. In its original long forms, Taiji is a more complex practice. However, it too can be modified, and many short forms have been created for targeted healing purposes when it may be best suited to address a patient's needs. In most cases, the patient is instructed to perform those practices daily to most effectively treat health challenges.

Dietetics

Foods have properties similar to herbs—including taste, temperature (Qi), and channels entered—so they may be used in a similar way. The therapeutic effects of foods are often weaker than those of herbs, but because we eat every day, foods have a cumulative effect over time on our overall health. Chinese medical professionals have analyzed the properties of foods, adhering to the same principles that are used in categorizing medicinal herbs, so a diet can be tailored to an individual like an herbal formula is prescribed. Certain foods may need to be added to your diet to help improve your health, and some foods should be avoided when facing specific health challenges, just as some pharmaceutical drugs may be contraindicated for some people or conditions.

While nutritional supplementation is not traditionally included in the practice of Chinese medicine, some practitioners in the West choose to include it as part of their therapeutic strategy. In that case, supplements need to be personalized, as herbs are. Apart from standard nutrition from carbohydrates, fats, and proteins and basic vitamin and mineral content, there are principles drawn from herbal medicine that determine the best diet and the most helpful supplements for any individual. As an obvious if simple example, someone who is underweight will have different dietary, caloric, and nutritional needs than someone who is overweight.

Lifestyle

Lifestyle factors need to be examined and improved to whatever extent may be possible if necessary. Many of these things are common sense, no matter what style of medicine you employ or what health practices you follow. There are simple changes you can make to support good health, like getting adequate fresh air, sunshine, exercise, and rest. Achieving or maintaining a healthy weight, improving the quality of relationships with family, friends, and colleagues, and having satisfying and meaningful work all reduce stress and contribute to better health. It's equally important to limit or eliminate factors that obviously contribute to poor health, such as smoking (including second-hand smoke) and the use of alcohol and recreational drugs. If actively dating, it's important to employ safe-sex practices. These relatively simple considerations are crucial for anyone interested in enjoying a long and healthy life.

Chinese medicine takes a few additional lifestyle factors into account, which may be less easy to understand at first glance. While briefly introduced in the following paragraphs, some are discussed in greater detail later in this book.

To achieve optimal health, it's necessary to maintain emotional balance. Every emotion we experience is appropriate when circumstances arise to elicit that emotional expression. This includes emotions we may not like or may interpret as negative, like anger, frustration, grief, or fear. Once the triggering circumstance is gone, we must be able to resolve the emotion and return to a state of equanimity and balance. Similarly, a prolonged or overly intense experience and expression of emotions we may regard as positive, like joy or exuberance, can be equally destabilizing and cause health problems over time.

Every emotion, whether interpreted as positive or negative, is linked with a particular internal organ, and the prolonged experience of any emotion will tax the related organ and diminish its functional energy, setting the stage for various diseases. A lifestyle that supports emotional balance, which can include the addition of practices that help regulate those emotions (meditation, Qigong, some types of yoga, aromatherapy, etc.), will promote health. We may not be able to control all the circumstances of our life, but we can learn to control our response to those circumstances. Emotions are discussed with their related organs in Chapters 5 and 6 and as pathological factors in Chapter 7.

Environmental factors, present both in your immediate living quarters and in your general geographical region, play a significant role in overall health. For example, a person may be either constitutionally Damp or may have a health condition that has created Damp within them. Damp is one pathogenic factor in Chinese medicine and can manifest as low energy or lethargy, excessive body fat, chronic diarrhea, or chronic sinus congestion with mucus or phlegm. A person with a Damp condition should not live in a damp environment. A basement apartment is a typical example of damp living quarters, and beachfront property, as appealing as it might otherwise be to some, is a damp geographical location. Those environments will worsen the health of someone suffering from a Damp condition or constitution.

Regulating work, sleep, and meal times are important for a couple of reasons. First, as the purely physical part of our being, the body likes regularity in the same way domesticated animals like the activities of their day to be regulated. The body will function a bit better when it has set expectations that are met. Less energy is expended as daily rhythms are established. Second, when regulated in the healthiest ways according to the principles of Chinese medicine, activities will be aligned with natural biological rhythms as the Qi of individual related organs achieves prominence at its respective hours of the day.

As a final lifestyle consideration, it's recommended that sexual activity be regulated, particularly in men, and especially as men get older. The stereotype of a man needing to sleep immediately after having sex demonstrates that more energy has been lost than what can be accounted for from the basic physical activity of sex. If a man has frequent unregulated (here, that primarily means ejaculatory) sex, he expends a great deal of life energy and will age faster, while experiencing the various declines of health that accompany typical aging. Women fare much better during sex and often experience a net gain of energy. They can lose more life energy during pregnancy and childbirth, especially when bearing many children close together.

Chinese Medicine Is Holistic

Most people have heard the word "holism" and have some understanding of the concept because some familiar medical practices are holistic to varying degrees. Homeopathy, naturopathy, osteopathy, and chiropractic are all types of holistic medicine. But what does that mean, and how does that differ from conventional Western medicine?

Chinese medicine is holistic, viewing the whole person as a unique individual and not just a collection of symptoms to be treated. On a physical level, it has its methodologies for observing and assessing the interconnections and interplay among all organs and body tissues, the way the health of one organ may influence the functioning of all the others and everything else in the body. No one body part exists in isolation from the whole body. Diagnostic information is gleaned through all the senses: listening to the quality of the voice and breathing; viewing the tongue, skin, hair, eyes, and nails; smelling body scents; touching the pulses, the skin, and the abdomen; and classically, physicians would sometimes taste the patient's urine, though this is no longer practiced today. Further, the Chinese idea of holism includes the influence of emotional, mental, and possibly spiritual states and the quality of interpersonal relationships. As we've seen, dietary and lifestyle factors are also taken into account.

At deeper and subtler levels, Chinese medicine examines the holistic interrelationships beyond what is present within the body. It looks at environmental factors, our unique interactions and interface with the immediate environment, the energetics of diurnal and seasonal cycles, and celestial events in relation to overall health and well-being. Physicians who are Qigong masters might read the Qi that emanates from a patient, outside the surface of their body, as well as the Qi flowing within the body.

The words "holistic" and "holism" have the same root as the word "whole." In fact, it's fairly common to see them spelled "wholistic" and "wholism." As the name implies, any holistic medical practice looks at the whole person (using the criteria relevant to the particular holistic practice) to determine what is out of balance and what body system or systems have been impacted to create the underlying cause of their disharmony or disease. The holistic practice then uses that information to help restore the person to whole health. By treating the whole person rather than the disease, the body's own natural healing abilities are supported, the body regains a healthy balance, and the symptoms as well as the underlying causes are resolved. If a person is fully restored to a state of harmonious functional balance, the predisposition toward the recurrence of an otherwise chronic condition may at the very least be safely and effectively managed, likely greatly reduced, and often completely eliminated. This includes but is not limited to the Western biological concept of homeostasis.

Homeostasis is the tendency of physiological systems to maintain an internal stability, including psychological equilibrium, usually through various internal feedback controls, against any external stimulus or change that might disturb normal physiological functions or conditions. It helps maintain a constant internal environment, including the optimal functioning of all the internal organs, sense organs, and skin; a constant, stable body temperature; appropriate pH; and so on. This regulation of various metabolic processes arises from the body's innate natural intelligence. In most people, and under most circumstances, it is beyond conscious control, but it can easily be supported by applying the holistic principles presented in this book.

In contrast to holism, conventional Western medicine, often called "allopathic," is more accurately a reductionist practice, looking for the smallest physiological or biological unit believed to be responsible for a disease condition. Once found, it can be surgically altered or removed, or drugs may be administered to kill a pathogen, dull the perception of pain, reduce an inflammation, or supply a missing biochemical ingredient, while the body attempts to heal itself and restore homeostasis.

Neither system is inherently better or worse than the other, but each has its primary strengths and weaknesses. Understanding those may make one or the other better suited to treat an individual's particular health needs or be better aligned with an individual's way of life. It's also possible to effectively combine both approaches, as discussed later in the text.

Generally speaking, holistic approaches are better at dealing with chronic conditions and often give the person a better chance of recovering from the condition rather than just managing the symptoms. Under the care of a holistic physician, a patient's imbalance may be observed and never allowed to progress to a disease state or surgical situation, such as the removal of a gall bladder, uterus, or prostate. For example, an inflamed appendix can be treated so that it never approaches rupturing and returns to its normal, healthy state.

Western medicine is better at addressing acute, emergency situations, using what is sometimes referred to as "heroic medicine." Some examples are complicated or compound fractures, surgical emergencies, gunshot wounds, other massive trauma, or a faltering or stopped heart. In these cases, holistic procedures, at least as they are legally allowed to be practiced in the United States, are often too slow to save a person's life or to rapidly relieve excruciating pain.

Chinese Diagnosis and Western Diagnosis

Chinese medicine is holistic, taking the state of the whole person—body, mind, emotions, and spirit—into account instead of just the apparent disease. Western biomedical diagnosis is often of limited help in determining a patient's condition from a Chinese medical perspective, since the biomedically defined disease is just one collection of symptoms among many that may define the particular pattern(s) of disharmony affecting the person. Accordingly, ten people with the same Western diagnosis may be treated in ten different ways with Chinese medicine. Conversely, ten people with very different Western diagnoses may be treated identically with Chinese medicine, if the underlying cause, the pattern of disharmony, is determined to be the same according to Chinese diagnostics. This is often a significant point of confusion, and even consternation, for Western patients who decide to seek help from Chinese medicine. They can be concerned that their "real" diagnosis—that is, the Western, technologically derived diagnosis—is being ignored or overlooked and that the care of their health is being relegated to some primitive, careless, or naive superstition. This is an example of one of the ways a Western perspective must shift and grow if one wants to benefit from Chinese medicine in the fullest way possible.

Integrating the Branches

Like virtually every aspect of Chinese medicine and associated medical and spiritual philosophies, there are many perspectives, sometimes conflicting or contradictory, regarding integration. China is a very large country, and some regions have ways of doing things quite differently from other regions. Similarly, in different periods of Chinese history, some methods of medical practice were officially favored over others, based largely upon the preference of the contemporary emperor. All of those historic and geographical preferences still exist and are practiced, to a greater or lesser degree, throughout China today.

Ideally all of the branches of Chinese medicine introduced above should be employed in a unified and integrated way to bring about the fastest and most complete restoration of health. "Unified and integrated" means either that a single physician makes a diagnosis and treatment plan and applies and/or provides instruction on all the required treatment modalities or two or more practitioners agree upon the diagnosis and treatment plan, with each implementing the component of that treatment in which they may specialize.

Acupuncture and Chinese herbal medicine have their unique strengths and work together powerfully to restore or maintain optimal health. Although each can address the whole body, acupuncture's focus is more on the functional, energetic, Qi, and Yang aspects, while herbal medicine, also very good at addressing those same aspects, is better than acupuncture at addressing the structural, substance, blood/body fluids, Jing, and Yin aspects. This is because herbal medicine directly adds something tangible and substantive to the body. This can be most useful in building up a body after a debilitating illness or injury, increasing the production of blood and healthy body tissue. It also helps generate other body fluids that may be used to lubricate dry, arthritic joints, boost or balance hormone production, soften tight, achy muscles, or strengthen and heal bones.

Any branch of Chinese medicine can be very effective when used alone, as it frequently is even in China. When acupuncture might be the first treatment of choice, a typical treatment plan involves giving the patient an acupuncture treatment each day or every other day for ten treatments, which constitutes one course of treatment. After a five-day break, another course of treatment is made, and that may be repeated up to three or four times. If the patient isn't substantially better after three or four courses of treatment, then herbal medicine may be tried. It is usually administered by a different physician, who may make a different diagnosis and consequently create a different treatment plan. This is a sequential use of acupuncture and then herbs: it is not an integrated approach, but it has its adherents and is effective in many cases.

In most Chinese hospitals, patients will more typically be treated with acupuncture and take herbs simultaneously. The physician will first examine the patient and make a diagnosis. If trained and experienced in both acupuncture and herbal medicine, as most of the best doctors are, they will give the patient the acupuncture treatment and then write up an herbal prescription that the patient will get filled at the on-site pharmacy, in much the same way as a Western doctor will prescribe a pharmaceutical drug. This is the simplest and most common integrated method, in which the acupuncture treatment and herbal formula mutually support each other based on the diagnosis made by a single physician.

Depending on the condition being treated, a patient may receive a Tuina treatment, either instead of or in addition to an acupuncture treatment. While Tuina may have a superficial resemblance to a conventional spa type of massage, it has many specific therapeutic variables and techniques, following exactly the same principles that underlie every other branch of Chinese medicine. Accordingly, a Tuina practitioner will give a treatment in keeping with the diagnosis made by the primary physician.

China has a huge population, and like the United States it has an overburdened medical system. In the early 1990s, one of my Qigong teachers told me that in the most crowded regions, except in cases of an emergency or immediately life-threatening condition, once a patient has received a treatment and gotten their herbal prescription, they would be given a punch-card and told to attend Taiji or Qigong classes with a specified master instructor. The instructor would punch the card for each lesson attended. After a certain number of lessons, usually ranging between five and ten, the patient would then be allowed to receive their next treatment at the hospital. This is another way that an integrated treatment approach is used, while helping to relieve an overwhelming patient load. The patient is required to take personal responsibility for their health by being actively engaged in their self-care through learning a Qigong practice suited to their medical diagnosis, which supports and enhances the acupuncture and herbal treatments.

In all cases, patients are instructed about healthy modifications to their diet and lifestyle in accordance with their particular needs, based upon their diagnosis. This becomes the most complete type of integrated practice, in which acupuncture, herbs, physical therapies (Qigong or Taiji in these examples), diet, and lifestyle are all addressed with a single, unified purpose.

Another aspect of integration involves the use of Chinese and Western medicine combined in ways that follow the principles of Chinese medicine as closely as possible. In China, Chinese and Western medicine are practiced equally in most large hospitals, and this may be a truer form of complementary medicine than is found in the United States and other Western countries, where Chinese medicine is often treated as a subsidiary adjunct to Western medicine. That has placed China in the unique position of being able to evaluate the relative effectiveness of Chinese and Western medicine side by side in treating the same conditions.

While I was still a student in Chinese medical college, one of my teachers told me he did half of his clinical internship at a hospital in China that specialized in cancer treatment. There, they found that the five-year survival rate, the gold standard used to determine the effectiveness of any cancer treatment, from treatments using only Chinese medicine was virtually equal to those using only Western medicine. But when practiced together, in a unified, integrated manner, the five-year survival rate more than doubled. Unfortunately, it will be some time before we see that type of integration and the spectacular results it can yield in most Western countries. That is because while contemporary Chinese doctors fully understand Western medicine and can perform all surgical procedures and apply radiation and chemotherapy, Western doctors do not similarly understand the use of Chinese herbs and acupuncture and do not even have a working concept of Qi, which is integral to the practice of every aspect of Chinese medicine.

Integrated Practices in Western Medicine

While not applied holistically, the concept of integrated health care should be familiar to most people, as it is a staple of Western medicine, and unified according to its own criteria. Western medicine includes surgery, pharmacology, radiology, nuclear medicine, orthopedics, physical therapy, and other branches that are frequently used together to achieve the best therapeutic outcome.

Radiology may be used as the primary diagnostic method, often in preparation for surgery. The surgical procedure often simultaneously makes use of pharmacology in the forms of anesthesia to render the patient unconscious, analgesics to reduce pain, and antibiotics to reduce the risk of peri- and postoperative infection. Postoperatively, pharmacology may be the modality of choice. Antibiotics and analgesics may be continued, anti-inflammatories may be added, and other pharmaceutical substances may be recommended to speed recovery or provide the patient with needed enzymes, nutrition, hormones, or other drugs. Physical therapy might be included to more fully restore functionality and strength. For general diet and lifestyle considerations, a physician may recommend that you get more rest, exercise, lose weight, drink more water, or eliminate salt or junk foods from your diet.

Many people still don't expect that same integration in Chinese medical practices, due to the previously mentioned emphasis that the popular media has placed on acupuncture. This book dispels that misconception and will provide you with both a new, more complete understanding and many integrated tools and practices you can incorporate into your daily life.

PART 1

Foundational Theories In Chinese Medicine

The paradigms of Chinese medicine are substantially different from those of Western medicine. The best way to begin to understand those differences is by examining the foundational concepts that underlie them. While each concept is equally important and all are mutually supportive, arising as an interdependent whole, the sequence in which they are presented here allows each to build on the one that came before, and this may be the easiest way to learn about them.

Chapter 1

First Concept: Qi, the Energy of Life

The single greatest foundational concept to examine is that of Qi, since it has no exact counterpart in Western medicine nor in the Western worldview. The most ubiquitous single English word translation of Qi is "energy." This is a useful introductory interpretation, and with a more complete understanding of the concept, it becomes a convenient convention with which to refer to Qi. However, it needs significant amplification for a full, authentic understanding, enabling one to know and utilize Qi and to eventually directly access it for the betterment of health.

In his seminal book *The Web That Has No Weaver*, Ted Kaptchuk states, "The idea of Qi is fundamental to Chinese medical thinking, yet no one English word or phrase can adequately capture its meaning. ... We can perhaps think of Qi as matter on the verge of becoming energy, or energy at the point of materializing."[1]

In the broadest universal sense, not limited to medical practice or thinking, Qi is simultaneously both the material foundation (substance) of everything in existence and the motive force (energy) driving all activity, animate and inanimate alike. This might be a difficult idea to grasp, but it is very similar to the way physics describes the properties of light. Light is a discrete particle, a photon (substance), and a wave (energy). While most people may think of light as belonging entirely in the realm of the inanimate energy, medical scientists working in the field of biophysics know that

---

1. Ted Kaptchuk, *The Web That Has No Weaver: Understanding Chinese Medicine* (Chicago: Congdon and Weed, 1983), 35.

our DNA emits biophotons, packets of light energy that inform and direct every aspect of our physical being from a genetic level. In this way, within our body light may be viewed as the bridge between energy and matter and between the inanimate and animate, as it is incorporated into our core biology with no intervention from any external technological source.

Any reference to Qi in this book is primarily focused on how it exists and manifests within the body. It is important to have an understanding of Qi as it exists in the greater environment too. We perpetually interface with environmental Qi, so it exerts a strong influence on health, whether or not we are aware of it. That gives us a more complete idea of how it impacts our wellness, both in the health-supporting ways taught in this book and in the ways in which environmental Qi can support or adversely affect our health and give rise to various illnesses. For human beings to experience true health at every level—physical, emotional, mental, and spiritual—it's crucial to harmonize our life with our environment. Environmental energies are always a factor in determining health from the perspective of Chinese medicine. That concept is examined in more detail in Chapter 7.

The simplest translation of Qi as it relates to the physical body is usually "life force" or "vital life energy." These phrases contain all the meaning we need—an accurate general interpretation when using the word "Qi" as it manifests in the living body. The single Chinese character for Qi can also mean "air," "breath," or "breathing." While "air" and "breath" are not the same as the totality of Qi that is life energy, those interpretations support the connection between Qi and life (see Appendix 2, Note 1.1). In a very real way, Qi is life, and we could not live without it in the same way we could not live without air or breath. Qi is what warms and animates us, protects against illness, provides the functionality of all our organs and physiological systems, and sparks our awareness and intellect. Where there is abundant Qi, there is health. The infirmities of old age are all due to the decline in Qi, and when Qi runs out, death ensues.

The common Chinese medicine principle *Bu tong ze tong, tong ze bu tong* translates to "no free flow, pain; free flow, no pain." This simply means that any kind of pain is an indication of an obstruction in the normal flow of Qi, and with the free flow of Qi, there is no pain. This phrase is often also taken to mean that where there is a free flow of Qi, there is no disease of almost any sort, since Qi obstruction is at the root of many diseases, and that the presence of abundant, normal Qi is required for good health and all healing. If Qi is obstructed in any one part, or many parts, of the body, there is a corresponding deficiency of Qi in other parts of the body. This is exactly analogous to damming a river. Where the dam is built, the river water is effectively obstructed. Beyond the dam, there is little or no water.

Qualities and Functions within the Body

The Chinese character for the word Qi (**Figure 1.1**) depicts a bowl of rice, with steam issuing up from the rice. This pictogram contains a wealth of information. In Chinese medicine and in other facets of Chinese scientific, philosophical, and spiritual thought, it's understood that Qi is both the motive force and the material foundation, the most elemental substance in the universe, as previously introduced.

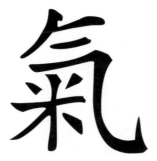

Figure 1.1 (Qi)

The rice in the character is a solid substance. As a staple food, it is nutritious and represents the material foundation of life and, by extension, the material foundation of everything in existence. In our body, Qi exists on a continuum from coarse and dense to light and fine, and the rice in the character represents the coarser manifestations of Qi. The rising steam is much less substantial and represents the energetic qualities of Qi. It is warm, in motion, and contains a functional energy enabling it to do work. Steam has been used to warm rooms, keeping people comfortable and safe from environmental adversity. It's been used to cleanse and detoxify the body, in sweat lodges and steam rooms, to promote better health. It has powered engines to help mankind accomplish varied tasks. It provides one of the simplest and healthiest ways to cook foods, maintaining the nutritional value of the food while transforming it and making it easier to digest. The steam can be viewed as the deeper, finer essential quality of the rice, not normally perceptible in its raw, uncooked state. Similarly, the Qi within us is not normally perceptible to an untrained eye.

There are many different types of Qi catalogued in Chinese literature that are relevant to the life and the health of a human being. Despite these apparent differences, it should be understood that they are all just different manifestations of what is essentially one Qi.

The Classic of Difficulties (a historically and foundationally important Chinese medical text) states, "Qi is the root of a human being."[2] This idea is further expanded in *Simple Questions* (the first of two texts contained within the ancient foundational Chinese medical canon, the *Huangdi Neijing*): "The union of the Qi of Heaven and Earth is called a human being."[3] From this we can see that Qi is an energy that manifests on both physical (Earth) and spiritual (Heaven) levels. A human being is a very complex organism, existing on many levels simultaneously—even secularly, we can consider just the physical, emotional, and mental levels—so it should also be understood that the Qi within a body also exists in various states simultaneously, that it is always changing and in motion. It may be very active, light, and fine in some areas, and very dense and substantive in other areas. Its functions can be both very general and very specific at the same time, and it can change its form based upon its physical location and the immediate functional needs within the body. As Qi condenses to coarser substance, it can transform into physical structure or cause physical structures to alter, gather, or aggregate. This can be either healthful, as in the case of tissue repair and regeneration, or pathological, as in the case of tumor formation, cysts, or nodularities.

Biological Energies Used in Western Medicine

A part of what Qi is can be thought of as the totality of all energies known to Western medical science. Some of these include the bioelectrical energy generated by the sinoatrial node that causes our heartbeat, as measured by electrocardiograms (ECG or EKG); the electrical energy of the brain, as measured by electroencephalograms (EEG); thermal energies, as measured by thermometers and thermal imaging and as indicated by daily caloric requirements/expenditures, which are calculated by basal metabolic

---

2. Giovanni Maciocia, *The Foundations of Chinese Medicine: A Comprehensive Text for Acupuncturists and Herbalists* (London: Churchill Livingstone, 1989), 37.

3. Ibid.

rate (BMR); and the electrical impulses that are transmitted through nerves that relay sensory information and cause muscles to contract. Sonically, we know about speech and audible body sounds that are often considered embarrassing, but sound is not thought of as an energy generated by the body in the way that the various bioelectrical energies above are. Yet some body sounds are useful diagnostically (in checking lung, heart, and intestinal sounds), and sound is used as a therapeutic energy. Physical therapists use ultrasound to facilitate tissue regeneration (see Appendix 2, Note 1.2). Sonograms are used for medical imaging. In other imaging technologies such as magnetic resonance imaging (MRI), a magnetic field is used to excite magnetically sensitive parts of our body, typically the positively charged proton in the nucleus of hydrogen atoms that are part of every water molecule that make up most of our body. The MRI-generated magnetic field is made to oscillate, or vibrate, at specific resonant frequencies that cause the excited proton to emit radio frequency signals that are then interpreted by the MRI receiver coil.

Just from these few examples we can see that Western medical science utilizes the energies of electricity, magnetism, radio frequency emission, sound, and heat, all of which have biological correspondences. We have already seen how light, in the form of biophotons, has a place in Western medical understanding. Qi encompasses all of those and more subtle energies yet to be understood and applied conventionally.

Qi is itself a holistic energy, as it is the unified totality of all of the above energies, and more, into a single, discrete entity. Qi manifests in many different ways, but it is one thing.

Chapter 2

Second Concept: Meridians, the Pathways of Health

The second foundational concept to understand is that of meridians, the nonphysical vessels through which Qi flows within the body (see Appendix 2, Note 2.1).

There are twelve regular meridians, divided into six bilateral Hand and six bilateral Foot meridians. Each meridian has its own set of acupoints that may be needled for specific therapeutic purposes. The Pericardium meridian has the fewest number of points, nine, while the Urinary Bladder has the most, sixty-seven.

They all have vertical trajectories, meaning they are more or less perpendicular to the ground when you are standing up. The Hand meridian end points, either the first or last point on any given meridian, are found at or very near the tips of the fingers, while the Foot meridian end points are found at or very near the tips of the toes. The Foot meridians do not travel directly into the arms, and the Hand meridians do not travel directly into the legs. Both do necessarily enter the torso, since each communicates with its associated internal organ. The Hand and Foot Yang meridians traverse the external part of the head and have points that may be needled there. They end inside the brain. The Hand and Foot Yin meridians also end in the brain, but they are entirely internal to the head and have no points able to be needled there. Yin-Yang theory will be discussed in detail in the next chapter.

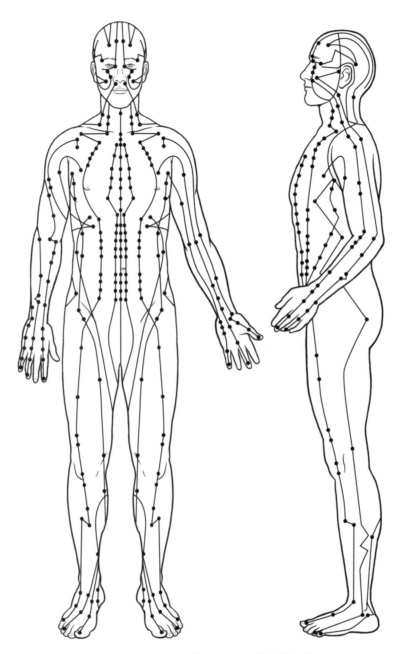

Figure 2.1 (Acupuncture Meridians)

The twelve regular meridians are bilateral. Each meridian enters and communicates with its associated organ, which gives the meridian its name.

The Twelve Regular Meridians

Common Meridian Name	*Yin/Yang Type*	*Chinese Meridian Designation*
Lung Meridian	Hand Yin	Hand Taiyin
Large Intestine Meridian	Hand Yang	Hand Yangming
Stomach Meridian	Foot Yang	Foot Yangming
Spleen Meridian	Foot Yin	Foot Taiyin
Heart Meridian	Hand Yin	Hand Shaoyin
Small Intestine Meridian	Hand Yang	Hand Taiyang
Urinary Bladder Meridian	Foot Yang	Foot Taiyang
Kidney Meridian	Foot Yin	Foot Shaoyin
Pericardium Meridian	Hand Yin	Hand Jueyin
Sanjiao Meridian	Hand Yang	Hand Shaoyang
Gall Bladder Meridian	Foot Yang	Foot Shaoyang
Liver Meridian	Foot Yin	Foot Jueyin

The names in the left column are the common meridian names. You can see how they are named exactly for their associated organ. The center column supplies the basic designation, showing whether the meridian is a Hand or Foot, Yin or Yang meridian. The right column provides a more specific Chinese designation for each meridian, and additionally indicates the meridian's relative depth. Yang meridians are more superficial, and Yin meridians are deeper, so the most superficial is the Yangming, and the deepest is the Jueyin. (Note that there is not universal agreement about meridian depth. Some sources say the Taiyang meridian is the most superficial.) Shaoyang is considered to be "half external, half internal," since it is at the most medium depth.

This is also a type of flow chart, depicting the order in which Qi flows through the meridian system, beginning with the Hand Taiyin and ending with the Foot Jueyin, which then cycles back to Hand Taiyin. The last point on the Liver Foot Jueyin meridian, Liver 14, is called *Qimen*, which translates to "Cycle Gate," to indicate this very function. It has been calculated that it takes Qi approximately twenty minutes to travel through the entire meridian system and return to its starting point. This is why a typical acupuncture treatment lasts approximately twenty minutes or multiples of twenty minutes. Note there are therapeutic reasons why a treatment may last longer or shorter than twenty minutes.

The last bit of information to consider in the meridians chart is that each meridian/Organ System appears as a part of a Yin-Yang organ pair. The Lungs and Large Intestine are a Yin-Yang organ pair, as are the Liver and Gall Bladder, and all the other organ pairs in between. Yin-Yang organ pairs have a strong interrelationship and a unique affinity for each other, and what affects one will most readily influence the other. There are special acupuncture points, called *Luo Xue*, or connecting points, that directly connect the Qi of a Yin organ to its paired Yang organ and the Qi of the Yang organ to its paired Yin organ.

The Qi that flows through the meridians is called *Jingluoqi* (Jing-Luo Qi), which simply means "vessels and collaterals Qi." "Vessels" is yet another name for meridians and channels. Collaterals are fine horizontal meridians that form an energetic mesh throughout the body and are a main way through which the Qi of the regular meridians interconnect. Collaterals do not contain acupuncture points. *Zhenqi* (Zhen Qi) or *Zhengqi* (Zheng Qi), "normal Qi" or "upright Qi," is another name for the Qi that flows through meridians. Zhenqi also exists throughout the body, outside of the meridian system, so Jingluo is the name most used to differentiate Qi within the vessels. Jingluoqi is the Qi that is directly influenced by a standard acupuncture treatment and is the Qi that's primarily accessed in any meridian-based medical Qigong.

Jingluoqi manifests in ways that are related yet different from the Qi of its associated organ. So it's entirely possible for there to be a problem with the Lung Jingluo meridian Qi, but the Lung organs may be functioning normally. Since there's a strong connection between the meridian and organ Qi, a problem in one, left uncorrected, will eventually result in a problem in the other. This may be understood easiest when considering that with acupuncture, the Qi of the organ is accessed through its associated meridian.

In other words, an organ is never intentionally directly punctured by an acupuncture needle, only its meridian, and that's what ultimately effects change within the organ.

The Eight Extraordinary Meridians

In addition to the twelve regular meridians, there are eight extra or extraordinary meridians. Some texts refer to them as "psychic" meridians, because their effects can be extremely profound and tap into deeper, subtler aspects of being. In a standard medical context, they have more conventionally practical applications, and they may be especially beneficial in instances of emotional, psychological and constitutional issues.

In clinical practice, the two most common Extraordinary Vessels are the *Du Mai,* or "Governing Vessel," and the *Ren Mai,* or "Conception Vessel." The Du runs up the centerline of the back of the body and influences all the Yang meridians and the entirety of the body's Yang Qi, and the Ren runs up the front centerline of the body and influences all the Yin meridians and the entirety of the body's Yin Qi. The lower portions of Du and Ren meridians connect near the perineum, and the upper portions connect where the tip of the tongue touches the roof of the mouth, just behind the upper teeth. Each has its own acupoints that can be needled.

The next most commonly used of the Extraordinary Vessels is the Daimai (Dai Mai), or "Girdling Vessel." This is the only meridian that has a horizontal trajectory around the body. It intersects the lower Dantian (the main energy center of the body, located two to three inches below the navel), rising slightly to travel over the iliac crest (the tops of the sides of the pelvis bone) and then running straight back to cross the spine at the height of the lower border of the second lumbar vertebra. (See **Figure 2.2** on next page.) As its name implies, it "girds," or binds and stabilizes, all the vertical meridians, aiding in their intercommunication. While it has no discrete acupoints of its own, it can be needled more or less directly through intersecting points on other meridians, primarily the Gall Bladder meridian. Because of its connections with all of the vertical meridians, it has a wide range of influence, but it is most commonly used in treating gynecological and reproductive disorders.

The remaining five Extraordinary Vessels include the *Yin Wei* (Yin Linking), the *Yang Wei* (Yang Linking), the *Yin Qiao* (Yin Heel), *Yang Qiao* (Yang Linking), and the *Chong Mai* (Penetrating Vessel). None of these has its own discrete acupoints, but they may be treated through intersecting points on other meridians.

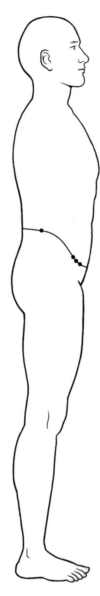

Figure 2.2 (The Daimai)

The Yin and Yang vessels are complementary pairs with related balancing functions. The Qiao vessels end in the eyes and influence whether the eyes want to remain open and wakeful or closed and sleepy. They also influence the muscles of the legs and may be used to treat flaccid (very loose) or hypertonic (very tight) muscles on the Yin or Yang surfaces of the legs, respectively. The wei vessels connect, or link, all the Yin meridians and Yang meridians, respectively. Accordingly, they have a wide range of applications and provide a great deal of flexibility in treatment options. For example, since the Du meridian influences all the Yang meridians, and the Yang Wei has points of intersection on the Du meridian, select Yang Wei intersecting points can enhance the effect of Du points in any given treatment.

The Chong Mai has a number of distinct pathways within the body but generally runs along the centerline of the body, close to the Ren and Kidney meridians in the front, and along the lower portion of the Du in the back. It also has a wide range of treatment applications, but since it grows out of the Kidneys and has a special affinity for the Ren, it can be used very effectively when combined with Kidney and Ren points. Among other possibilities, this is useful in treating gynecological, reproductive, and digestive disorders and is very beneficial in cases of constitutional weakness.

Meridians and Western Medicine

Since meridians are nonphysical and exist only to transport Qi, it's easy to understand why they are not contained in the Western medical paradigm. That does not mean there are no Western correspondences or verifications, only that when there is any Western medical interpretation considered at all, it is understandably biased toward a Western mindset.

For example, the lower portion of the Gall Bladder meridian (and the small portion of the Urinary Bladder meridian that is present at the sacrum) lies over regions of the sciatic nerve. When acupuncture is used to relieve sciatic nerve pain, the Western interpretation usually invokes gate control theory, also known as nerve gate theory, which states that a nerve can only effectively transmit one signal at a time, so the stimulus from the acupuncture needle overrides the preexisting pain stimulus of sciatic neuralgia, dulling the patient's perception of the sciatic pain. There are at least two problems with that interpretation, though.

First, no nerve is ever intentionally needled during an acupuncture treatment. A meridian is not the same thing as a nerve, even when they exist in close proximity. Second, the acupuncture needle may induce some sensation, but an acupuncture needle is so thin that the sensation produced by directly stimulating the nerve would not be able to overwhelm the much greater sensation of sciatic nerve pain.

Similarly, the portion of the Stomach meridian that runs through the cheek and jaw overlays the lymph vessels and portions of the trigeminal nerve in that same region of the face. The effects of the facial Stomach meridian points are clearly not mediated by the lymph system, and the same criteria cited for the sciatic nerve apply here for the trigeminal nerve.

Qi has already been discussed as the material foundation for everything in existence, which includes everything in the body. The meridians are vessels that contain and transmit Qi. Chinese medical thought includes the idea that the presence of energy, Qi, precedes all material manifestation, and from that point of view, the meridians helped form the physical structures they overlay. Therefore, effecting a change in the Gall Bladder meridian can easily influence the sciatic nerve, and effecting a change in the Stomach meridian can influence the functioning of the local lymph system and the trigeminal nerve. This is exactly the reverse of the Western medical view, when acupuncture is considered to be therapeutically effective at all.

A commonly cited reference of scientific proof of the existence of meridians discusses the injection of a radioactive dye into acupuncture points and the observation of the dye's progression along established acupuncture meridian pathways that have no other known physical, anatomical counterpart. In 1985, French scientist Pierre de Vernejoul at the University of Paris conducted this definitive experiment.[4] He injected the radioactive marker technetium-99m into subjects at classic acupuncture points. Using gamma camera imaging, he tracked the subsequent movement of the isotope, which showed that the tracer followed the linear trajectory of traditional meridian lines, traveling a distance of thirty centimeters in four to six minutes. (It should be noted here that the physical substance, while traveling relatively quickly and exactly following the acupuncture meridians, traveled more slowly than the Qi that moved it along.) As a control, he made a number of random injections into the skin, not at acupuncture points, and injected the tracer directly into veins and lymphatic channels

---

4. Pierre de Vernejoul, Pierre Albarède, and Jean Claude Darras, "Nuclear Medicine and Acupuncture Message Transmission," *The Journal of Nuclear Medicine* 33, no. 3 (March 1, 1992): 409–12.

as well. There was no significant migration of the tracer at sites other than acupuncture points.

One of the most groundbreaking Western researchers in bioelectricity, taking into account both Western and Eastern perspectives, is Dr. Robert O. Becker. In his first book (coauthored with Gary Selden), *The Body Electric: Electromagnetism and the Foundation of Life*,[5] he reports an experiment he conducted in the late 1970s with biophysicist Dr. Maria Reichmanis, in which they used thirty-six electrodes to measure the electrical conductivity of acupuncture points along the traditional pathways of the Large Intestine and Pericardium meridians. They predicted they would find lower electrical resistance, greater electrical conductivity, and a direct current (DC) power source detectable at each acupuncture point. Becker had earlier found the DC system of the human body, which gets more negative at the fingers and toes and becomes more positive in the torso and head. This is an objective, scientific correspondence to the Yin (negative) and Yang (positive) flows within the acupuncture meridians. Becker and Reichmanis found their exact predicted changes at half of all the acupoints tested, with the same points showing up as active on all people tested. They also found that the meridians were conducting current and its polarities, with the acupuncture points being positive relative to the surrounding tissue, and that each point exhibited a distinctive surrounding field. Finally, they found a fifteen-minute rhythm to the current's strength at the active points.

The Large Intestine (Hand Yangming) and Pericardium (Hand Jueyin) meridians are found on the arms, easily accessible for research purposes. Although not stipulated in the report, that's probably the reason they selected those particular meridians. Similar findings would reasonably be expected along any meridians selected. Although the electrical changes were found on half the points examined, the researchers posited that the other half may have had weaker fields or emitted a different type of energy than they were looking for. Another likely possibility, which is only conjecture because the particular active points were not disclosed in the report, is that the unresponsive points may have been deeper within the body. The researchers were specifically looking at superficial skin resistance and electrical changes.

---

5. Robert O. Becker and Gary Selden, *The Body Electric: Electromagnetism and the Foundation of Life* (New York: Quill, 1985), 235–36.

The directionality of electrical flow found by Becker and Reichmanis is an important corroboration of the directionality of meridian Qi flow, as each meridian has its own directional trajectory, and the electrical polarities imply the corresponding polarities of Yin and Yang. Finally, the fifteen-minute cyclical rhythm of current strength is an intriguing correlation with the long-held understanding that Qi flows through the entire network of acupuncture meridians in approximately twenty minutes, with some time variability based on room and seasonal temperature—warmer equaling a faster transit time—and the relative health and makeup of the individual. An acupuncture treatment commonly lasts for twenty minutes or multiples of twenty minutes for this reason, with treatments being shorter in warmer weather or for particular therapeutic purposes. Some alternate needling practices, such as *Bagua* needling techniques based on the *Yijing* (I Ching), require a twenty-eight-minute treatment time, approximately twice the fifteen-minute period noted by Becker.

Many similar Western studies have been conducted and published in the intervening years, and it's likely that trend will continue, especially as Western technology becomes better able to detect increasingly more subtle biological energies. The studies by de Vernejoul and by Becker and Reichmanis remain among the most compelling to date.

Chapter 3

Third Concept:
Yin and Yang, Polarities, and Balance

Yin and Yang might be the most familiar of these concepts in the Western world, at least superficially, since it is represented by the popular *Taiji* ("supreme ultimate") symbol, colloquially known as the Yin Yang symbol, or simply "the Yin Yang" (**Figure 3.1**). Its most striking features include its black (Yin) and white (Yang) halves, representing the complementary balancing opposites that underlie all related phenomena; the small dot of black Yin existing within the large white Yang region, with the corresponding small white dot of Yang within the larger Yin region, demonstrating that everything contains the seed of its opposite and that there is nothing that is purely Yin or Yang; and the curved line that both separates and unifies the opposing halves.

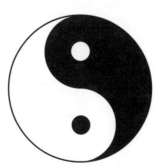

Figure 3.1 (Taiji Symbol)

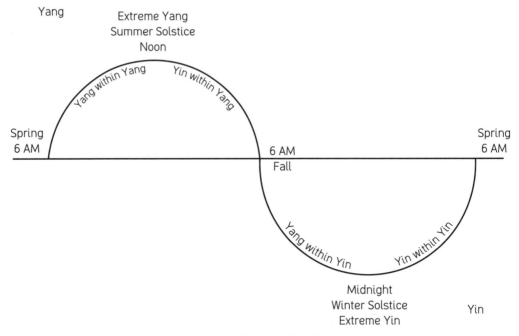

Figure 3.2 (Yin Yang Sine Wave)

The basic principle of Yin and Yang is that of the dynamic balance, the equilibrium, that exists throughout the natural world. That dynamism is indicated by the curved line between the opposing halves of the Taiji mandala. If you were to lay it on its side, you would see that it forms a familiar sine wave centered on the horizontal axis (**Figure 3.2**). It implies fluid, dynamic movement between alternating states, with the peak being most Yang (or positive) and the trough being most Yin (or negative). Yin and Yang are therefore not static and lifeless, which could be represented by a straight line between the two. The symbol indicates process, change, and the way things evolve over time through the interplay of equal opposites, which are intrinsic to all Yin and Yang pairs.

From the holistic perspective, this means that no one thing can exist in complete isolation: it always exits in relation to its balancing, complementary, polar counterpart (the holistic microcosm) and ultimately in relation to the universe as a whole (the holistic macrocosm). The part can only exist in relation to the whole. One of the earliest schools of thought devoted to the study of Yin and Yang was sometimes referred to as the Naturalist School, since it strove to understand and then use nature's laws for the betterment of humanity, by learning to live in harmony with those principles, the holistic approach. This is in direct contrast to the prevailing trend of Western science to control and manipulate nature.

Yin and Yang in the Natural World

All natural events and states of being can be observed and evaluated through the perspective of Yin and Yang, but they don't refer to any objective, material things. As stated in one of the most widely used contemporary texts about Chinese medicine, *Chinese Acupuncture and Moxibustion*, "It is, rather, a theoretical method for observing and analyzing phenomena. ... [It is] a philosophical conceptualization, a means to generalize the two opposite principles which may be observed in all related phenomena within the natural world."[6]

After the Taiji mandala, the most direct way to begin to understand the attributes of Yin and Yang is by considering the Chinese characters for both, as we did for Qi. The character for Yin depicts the shady side of a hill, while the character for Yang depicts the sunny side. So the Yang side of the hill displays many of the qualities associated with Yang—being sunny, bright, and warm—while the Yin side displays the complementary Yin qualities—shady, dark, and cool.

Similarly, in Chapter 5 of the ancient Chinese medical text, *Plain Questions*, it is stated that "Water and Fire are symbols of Yin and Yang."[7] They are iconic representations that graphically symbolize some of the qualities of Yin and Yang, all the balanced complementary and contrasting polarities that exist. For those completely new to these concepts, please note that as useful as the symbols of Water and Fire are, and all the attributes of Water and Fire are contained within Yin and Yang, not all the attributes of Yin and Yang can be contained within the representative Water and Fire. Similarly, not every attribute of Yang is directly equatable with every other attribute of Yang. Fire is Yang and is also bright and hot, two other Yang qualities, so you can say that both Yang and fire are bright and hot. But male is a Yang quality, and its paired Yin counterpart is female.

---

6. Deng Liangyue et al., *Chinese Acupuncture and Moxibustion* (Beijing, Foreign Languages Press, 1987), 11.
7. Ibid.

It would not be strictly correct to say that males are hot and bright, and females are cold and dark.

As on the shady side of the hill, where water is generated as moisture condenses on rock and dew readily forms on plants, water is cool and dark. It also displays other Yin qualities, such as stillness and a downward and inward directionality, as it tends to gather, pool, and is readily absorbed by dry earth. Like the sunny side of the hill, fire is hot and bright and possesses the additional Yang qualities of activity and an upward, outward directionality.

There are four primary aspects applicable to all Yin and Yang pairings, and these occur in their every manifestation, both in the outer world and within the body.

Four Primary Aspects of Yin and Yang Pairings

1. The Opposition of Yin and Yang
2. The Interdependence of Yin and Yang
3. The Mutual Consuming/Supporting Relationship of Yin and Yang
4. The Intertransformation of Yin and Yang.

Another aspect, sometimes cited as the fifth aspect, is the Infinite Divisibility of Yin and Yang. This is a way of saying that Yin and Yang are completely relative terms and not independent absolutes. Anything seen as Yang can always be further divided into Yin and Yang parts; anything Yin can be further divided into Yang and Yin parts. Whether or not we consider that as a fifth primary aspect, it is undeniably an attribute of Yin and Yang.

In the natural world, we readily see these aspects as interrelated and arising simultaneously. An example for one aspect may readily illustrate another equally well. Let's examine just a few Yin-Yang pairs to see how that occurs.

Yin-Yang Pairs	
Yang	**Yin**
Positive	Negative
Day	Night
Summer	Winter

Yin-Yang Pairs, cont.	
Hot	Cold
Light	Dark
Activity	Rest

The Opposition of Yin and Yang refers to them being polar opposites, and the qualities of one half balances or opposes the qualities of the other. We've seen how, when laying the Taiji symbol on its side, the resulting sine wave is positive at its peak and negative at its trough, but it is not static. The positive and negative aspects oppose and balance each other. Only at the absolute extremities do we see something that seems purely positive or purely negative, purely Yang or purely Yin. Even there, it is in transition; it does not remain at either extremity. This is a most obvious manifestation of the cyclic process of harmonious change brought about by such opposition.

Conceptually, we cannot have the existence of one half without its balancing counterpart. In addition to the examples given above, other Yang-Yin pairs include up and down, expanding and contracting, outside and inside, above and below, heaven and earth, male and female. One half of a pair is meaningless without its opposite.

In practical application, the opposing qualities of Fire and Water are commonly used in daily life. Water is used to put out unwanted or dangerous fires. When washing clothes, water is used to cleanse them, but they are then also Yin—cold and wet. The hot attribute of Fire, either from the very Yang sun or the electric clothes drier, is applied to them until they are warm and dry. The Yang characteristics of day and of summer are similar. They are both hot and light relative to their respective Yin counterparts, night and winter, which are cold and dark. The extremes of a day are comparable to the peak and trough of the sine wave, noon and midnight, respectively. As in the sine wave, day cycles into night, and night back into day. This is a manifestation of their interdependence. As with the Opposition of Yin and Yang, you cannot have one without the other.

When we look at the Mutual Consuming/Supporting Relationship between Yin and Yang, we again have to take into account their polarity or opposition and their interdependence. This is because the consumption and support depend on the ability of Yin and Yang to exert beneficial controls on each other, as only interdependent polarities can. Analyzing the diurnal cycle from a Yin-Yang perspective, noon is "Extreme Yang." As the daytime wanes and moves toward night, it is still Yang time, but Yin grows. This is called "Yin within Yang," as Yin begins to consume Yang. Dusk is a time of balance, when neither Yin nor Yang predominate, and is comparable to the sine wave crossing the horizontal axis, when it is neither positive nor negative. After dusk, night is entered and Yin continues to grow. This period of time is called "Yin within Yin." Nighttime peaks at midnight, "Extreme Yin." After midnight, it is still nighttime, Yin time, but moving toward daytime, and Yang begins to grow, or consume Yin. This is called "Yang within Yin." At dawn, neither Yin nor Yang predominates, and there is an instant of pure balance as the sine wave crosses the horizontal axis once more. As the sun rises to bring forth the daytime, Yang once more grows toward its noontime peak. This is called "Yang within Yang." At noon, Yang peaks, and the cycle begins again. This same cycle exists on a longer twelve-month scale when analyzing seasonal transitions, with midsummer being Extreme Yang and midwinter being Extreme Yin, most precisely on the summer and winter solstices. **Figure 3.2** provides a graphic representation of these cycles.

The above example also introduces the Infinite Divisibility or complete relativity of Yin and Yang. Dusk is more Yang than midnight but more Yin than noon. Three in the afternoon is a Yang time, but as Yin grows within Yang, it is more Yin than eleven in the morning, a Yang within Yang time that is very close to noon.

The Mutually Consuming/Supporting Relationship of Yin and Yang goes along with the Interdependence of Yin and Yang and may be best understood when we consider that the concept of Yin and Yang is first and foremost about balance, a healthy equilibrium. If daytime existed unabated, without the balancing influence of night-time, there would be too much heat without cooling, too much activity without rest, too much Fire without Water. This would damage all plant and animal life. If the supportive, balancing Yin qualities were not introduced to control the excessive Yang, before long all life on the planet would end. Conversely, if nighttime continued un-abated without the balancing support of day, the cold would become oppressive, there would be too much rest without activity, there would be no sunlight allowing plants to photosynthesize, and all life on the planet would end.

Keeping with the previous natural world examples, we've seen the Intertransforma-tion of Yin and Yang as day, summer, warmth, and light transform to night, winter, cold, and dark, and back again. Intertransformation is also implied by the small black dot of Yin within the white Yang half of the Taiji symbol and the small white dot of Yang within the black Yin half. The fact that Yin and Yang are not absolutes, each containing the seed of the other, allows for that seed to grow and eventually transform one into the other. Even at high noon, the most Yang time of any day, on the hottest, brightest day imaginable, you can still find shadows, small patches of cooler darkness—the Yin aspect within the Yang. Likewise, at darkest midnight, the most Yin time, you can still see the twinkle of stars in the sky, the light of Yang within the Yin.

Yin and Yang within the Body

The principles and attributes of Yin and Yang within the body are identical to those in the natural external world. The examples will differ, and the consequences of imbalance may manifest differently as appropriate to the physiology of a body.

One of the main principles that is foundational to all of Chinese medicine, regardless of style or school of thought, is called the Eight Principles. It uses Yin and Yang as a broad-stroke diagnostic tool in order to determine the primary nature of a pathology. While examining the Eight Principles, we'll introduce some basic diagnostics that relate to them.

The Eight Principles	
Yin	**Yang**
Interior	Exterior
Cold	Hot
Deficiency	Excess

Putting Yin and Yang at the top of the list serves both as a heading for the six principles that follow and as an umbrella to cover all other Yin and Yang imbalances that may exist when differentiating pathological syndromes. In general, a preponderance of Yin will make a person feel withdrawn (interior), cool or cold (a pale complexion or frank pallor is a common manifestation), and lethargic or sleepy (deficient). A preponderance of Yang will make a person boisterous or aggressive (exterior), warm or hot (a red face is a common manifestation), and very energetic or agitated (excessive).

The Interior and Exterior pairing has to do with location and is relevant to both the natural state of the body and to the nature and progression of a pathology. While all organs are internal, Yin organs are naturally deeper, more interior, while Yang organs are more superficial, since each communicates with the external world through the mouth, anus, and urethra.

Related to Interior and Exterior, the relatively synonymous pairing of Deep and Superficial may make some examples more clear. The skin and muscles are superficial, on the exterior portion of the body, relative to all the internal organs. Yang is naturally protective, and these superficial body tissues protect the more delicate, deep, internal structures from external pathogens and physical harm. Skin is the level at which *Weiqi* (Wei Qi), "defensive Qi," circulates, protecting the body from external pathogens. In Western terms, the skin is the acid mantle that protects against bacteria, viruses, and other pathogens as part of the first line of immune-system defense. Muscles are hard relative to the soft internal organs, as are the more superficial bones of the ribs and vertebrae, and are protective against physical injuries.

Pathologies that appear on the skin or primarily affect the exterior portions of the body, like eyes and nose, are exterior. Generally, they are early-stage imbalances and not very severe at that point. Both the common cold, caused by an external pathogen (whether environmental, according to Chinese thought, or germs, according to Western medical germ theory), and a poison ivy rash, caused by physical contact with an external irritant, are examples. Deeper yet still relatively external pathologies may affect the muscles, tendons, ligaments, superficial blood vessels and nerves, or meridians. Internal pathologies may occur when an external pathogen progresses deeper into the body, or they may arise from an internal imbalance due to constitution, prolonged emotional states, poor nutrition, parasites, or poisoning or as a side effect of a pharmaceutical drug. They will affect the internal organs, deep blood vessels and nerves, blood, brain, spinal cord, and bones. Note that many deep pathologies will cause secondary changes to superficial body parts such as skin and eyes and may appear similar to exterior pathologies. Other diagnostic criteria will distinguish between them.

Some schools of Chinese medical thought once attempted to analyze all disharmony (disease) through its relative depth within the body and designed the Four Level diagnosis. Those four levels include *Wei* (protective and most superficial), *Qi* (the level of meridian Qi, deeper), *Ying* (nutritive Qi, deeper still), and *Xue* (Blood level, the deepest and most severe). A common cold exists superficially at the Wei level or sometimes at the Qi level if it's a very bad cold. Graphic examples of Xue-level conditions include biomedically defined diseases such as hemophilia, tuberculosis (at the point at which the patient begins coughing blood), and hemorrhagic fevers. Four Level diagnosis is rarely if ever used exclusively these days, but it is still relevant in helping to determine the relative depth of a pathology along the continuum of Interior and Exterior, which strongly influences treatment choices.

The next pairing of principles, Cold and Hot, seems easier to understand from a diagnostic perspective. We've already seen that both day and summer are Yang, and are warm or hot relative to night and winter, which are Yin and cool or cold. So a person who is habitually cold or feels chilly easily might be more constitutionally Yin, while a person who is habitually hot or likes to avoid warm environments might be constitutionally Yang. An imbalance that creates a feeling of cool or cold, producing chills, might be a Yin pathology, while one which produces a fever might be a Yang pathology.

In the simplest textbook-perfect scenarios, the above examples would be exactly true, but I've purposely used the words "seem" and "might" as equivocations because this is one area where things can get tricky due to the relativity of Yin and Yang. That trickiness becomes easier to understand when we introduce the principles of Deficiency and Excess. In a perfectly balanced, healthy body, Yin and Yang exist in equal, if dynamic, proportions. We see that represented on the next page in **Figure 3.3** by Yin and Yang appearing "topped off" in equal measure at the horizontal line of complete balance. In the conditions of a preponderance of Yin or preponderance of Yang described earlier, either the Yin or the Yang column would grow upward of the horizontal axis, into the positive, or excess, regions. Then, Excess Yin would produce Cold symptoms, and Excess Yang would produce Hot symptoms. In these cases, an excess of Yang will create a deficiency of Yin, as Yang consumes Yin in the way heat will dry up a puddle. An excess of Yin will cause a deficiency of Yang, Yin Consuming Yang, as water can douse a flame.

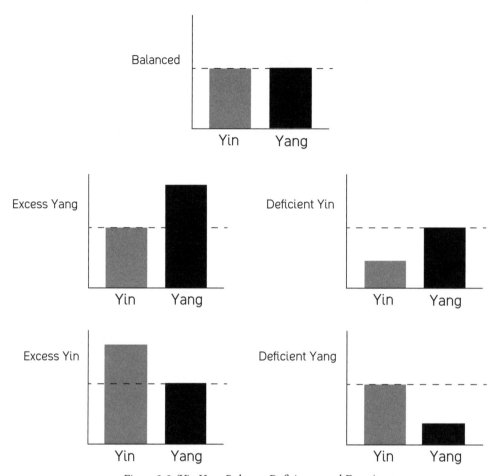

Figure 3.3 (Yin Yang Balance, Deficiency, and Excess)

It's just as possible, though, for there to be a deficiency of Yin or Yang. In the case of Deficient Yin, the Yin column would shrink below the dotted horizontal line and into the deficient region. Then, even though Yang would not be in excess and might stay exactly at the dotted horizontal line, it would be greater than Yin and produce feelings of Heat. This is an example of Deficiency Heat, since Yang would not be in excess. Conversely, Yin may stay at a normal, balanced level, but Yang may shrink below the dotted line, leading to feelings of Cold. This is an example of Deficiency Cold, since Yin would not be in excess. Whether due to Deficiency or Excess, the feelings of Cold or Heat are due to Yin and Yang being out of balance.

We've learned that daytime is Yang and nighttime is Yin. Here we can consider that a truly Yang condition of Excess Heat is likely to get worse during the daytime, Yang time, and a little better at night, Yin time. This is because as the Yang energy naturally increases during the daytime, its warmth would add to the warmth of the Yang pathology, making it feel worse, while the cooling energy of Yin, which flourishes at night, would balance some of the excess heat, so it would feel a little better. The converse is true for a Yin condition.

In the case of Deficiency Heat, the opposite occurs. If Yin energy is weak or deficient, leading to Deficiency Heat, the Heat symptoms would worsen at night. This is because the Yin energy is too weak to flourish during nighttime, Yin time, so its cooling influence would not be able to balance the warming energy of Yang, which would flourish unabated.

Deficiency and Excess can occur apart from overt associations with Heat and Cold, of course. "Deficiency" means a reduced functional energy and lowered capacity of any organ or physiological process. "Excess" means an abnormally high level of functional energy of any organ or physiologic process. It may occur along with an obstruction, since Qi, Blood, or body fluids can build up and become an Excess accumulation if they are obstructed from their normal patterns of flow.

When discussing the body, some other useful Yin-Yang pairings include below and above, front and back, Blood and Qi.

The lower part of the body (below the waist) and the front of the body are both more Yin, while the upper body (above the waist) and back of the body are more Yang. Leaving aside any diagnostic considerations for now, let's look at some of the factors that make this so. To see this most clearly, we need to introduce two related ideas.

The first is that Heaven, or anything celestial, is more Yang relative to the Earth, which is more Yin. Heaven and Earth is a Yang-Yin pairing. The second is that Chinese anatomical position, the position in which a person stands to accurately display the energetic aspect of anatomy, is in a hands-up position, or the stereotypical "I surrender" position, with arms extended above the head with palms facing forward. In this position, the head is naturally nearer to the sky, more Yang, while the feet are naturally closer to the earth, more Yin. The backs of the hands and arms face rearward, more Yang, while the palms and front of the arms face forward, more Yin.

Next, let's consider the external trajectory of the meridians themselves and see how that further ties in with Heaven and Earth and with Chinese anatomical position. All of the Hand Yang meridians begin at the fingertips (just outside the corner of the nail beds), travel down the back (Yang side) of the arms, and end in the head. All of the Foot Yang meridians begin in the head. Two of the three travel down the back (Yang side) of the torso. The Stomach meridian is the exception, the Yang within the Yin, and travels down the front of the torso. (While being a Yang organ, one of the main functions of the Stomach is a Yin one, that of supplying nourishment to the rest of the body. Its appearance on the Yin surface of the body is accordingly not very surprising nor truly anomalous.) The Gall Bladder (Foot Shaoyang) meridian zigzags a bit between Yin and Yang at the side of the torso, but stays primarily Yang. All travel down the backs and outsides (Yang sides) of the legs and end at the toes, at the corner of nail beds. In both the Hand and Foot Yang meridians, this is a downward flow of Qi, from Heaven to Earth.

All the Hand Yin meridians begin in the front of the torso, travel up the front (Yin side) of the arms and hands, and end at the fingertips, just outside the corner of the nail beds. All the Foot Yin Meridians begin at the tips of the toes at the corner of nail beds (the exception being the Kidney meridian, which begins on the sole near the ball of the foot), travel up the front and inside (Yin side) of the legs, up through the front of the torso, and end at the front of the torso. The Spleen meridian ends at the border between the front and back of the chest, behind the Gall Bladder (Shaoyang) meridian, and is the closest a Yin meridian gets to being the Yin within the Yang. In both the Hand and Foot Yin meridians, this is an upward flow of Qi, from Earth to Heaven.

Keep in mind that Yin and Yang are polar energies. Yin Earth wants to flow toward Yang Heaven; Yang Heaven wants to flow toward Yin Earth. The human being is one conduit through which that can occur, mediated by the energetics of the body. This principle is used extensively in many Qigongs and is one way in which physical movement influences Qi flow.

As integral components of body substance (matter) and function (energy), Blood and Qi are an interesting Yin-Yang pair. Most simply, Blood is Yin and Qi is Yang. Blood is a liquid material that carries nutrients, oxygen, various chemical messengers, and the physical aspects of the immune system to every cell in the body. It also carts away cellular waste products for disposal or recycling. Being fluid, it can moisten and lubricate body tissues. Qi is the sum of all the functional energy in the body, is warming and energizing, and is involved in all activity, thought, perception, and emotional experience.

It may seem very clear that Blood is exclusively Yin and Qi is exclusively Yang until we remember that Qi is also the material foundation for everything in existence. Some Chinese medical texts refer to Blood as the material form of Qi. Qi itself can be divided into Yin Qi (which is cooling, calming, and nourishing) and Yang Qi (which is warming, exciting, and active). As a Yin-Yang pair, the line between Blood and Qi may get blurred at times, but each instance of that apparent blurring has valuable therapeutic, health-building reasons.

For the most part, for our purposes we will keep them distinct. The Chinese medical phrase "The Qi is the commander of the Blood; the Blood is the mother of the Qi" embodies their mutual support and interdependence while keeping them more clearly defined as separate Yin-Yang entities. "The Qi is the commander of the Blood" means that Qi is responsible for directing every aspect of Blood movement throughout the body. This includes things like the heart's stroke volume, the speed and directionality of blood flow, blood sufficiency, venous return, and so on. "The Blood is the mother of the Qi" means that within the body, Qi needs a material foundation out of which to grow. The Blood supplies that substrate. When the Blood is deficient in any way, the Qi will be weak. If there is no Blood, there can be no Qi.

Western Correspondences to Yin and Yang

Western science and medicine does not overtly employ Yin-Yang theory, but we can look at some Western ideas that exemplify those principles nonetheless. We've seen that in the Taiji symbol, there is a seed of the Yin within the Yang and a seed of the Yang within the Yin. Men are Yang, and women are Yin. The primary male hormone is testosterone, which prenatally determines the sex of the fetus and then from puberty onward causes the male secondary sex characteristics, including increased body hair, deepening of the voice, thickening of the skin, increased muscle growth, and thickening and strengthening of the bones. One of the primary female hormones is estrogen, which along with progesterone is responsible for the female secondary sex characteristics, including the development of breasts, increased percentage of body fat, and an increased vascularization of the skin. Yet women's bodies produce small amounts of testosterone in the ovaries and adrenal glands that contribute to the female sex drive as well as maintain bone and muscle mass. This is the Yang within Yin, the seed of Yang on the Yin side of the Taiji mandala.

Men's bodies also produce small amounts of estrogen, converted from circulating testosterone, and it can be produced in the liver and muscle cells. Fat cells produce estrogen in both men and women. From the Chinese perspective, fat is a very Yin substance, so it is not surprising that it generates a very Yin molecule, estrogen. The role of estrogen in men's health is not entirely clear, but aging men with moderate estrogen levels seem to have fewer heart problems and better bone density than men with very low or very high estrogen levels. (As with all things Yin and Yang, balance is the key!) This is the Yin within the Yang, the seed of Yin on the Yang side of the Taiji symbol.

Another example involves nerve conduction, the way nerve impulses are transmitted. In simplest terms, each nerve cell receives an impulse, or charged stimulus, from the nerve cell next to it. The cell in its resting state is polarized—off and Yin. When it receives an impulse from an adjacent nerve cell, it depolarizes and becomes active and Yang. It transmits the impulse to the next adjacent nerve cell and then returns to its polarized, resting Yin state. This rapid depolarization/polarization of adjacent nerve cells, the alternation between Yin and Yang states, is what allows the impulse to be transmitted along the length of nerve pathways and is what's responsible for virtually every move we make (both voluntary and involuntary, or autonomic), every sensory input we experience, and thought itself—just from the simple alternation of off and on, negative and positive, Yin and Yang.

When first encountering Yin-Yang theory, many Westerners believe that the two aspects or states of being, Yin and Yang, are too simple, too limiting to be of any real value in defining and regulating something as complex as human health and human biology, let alone being an operating principle underlying the totality of life and everything in the universe. But consider that in the realm of modern technology, all things digital rely on just two numbers, zero and one. These are the "digits" to which the term "digital" refers. Binary code underlies the operation of every computer and computer-controlled device. It's responsible for all the audio and video presentation on your computer and TV, literally everything on the Internet, all the music you hear on your MP3 player, all the data stored on CDs, DVDs, and hard drives, the diagnostic and other control mechanisms in your car, your cell phone communication and all satellite communication, all electronic financial transactions and security, and on and on.

Someone who is not a computer programmer may not know exactly what is being turned on and off, being placed in alternating states, by those zeros and ones. The hardware can change, and the complexity of manifestations and applications is accomplished in part by extremely long strings of zeros and ones, but at its essential level, that's all it is: the binary code of Yin and Yang.

Chapter 4

Introduction to the Internal Organs

Zangfu: The Internal Organs and Their Correspondences

Zangfu is the general term for all internal organs. The *Zang* organs are the Yin organs. As a category, they are the more solid organs, and their shared main physiological functions are the manufacture and storage of essential substances, including vital essences (*Jing*), Qi, Blood, and body fluids. The Zang organs include the Heart, Pericardium, Lungs, Spleen, Liver, and Kidneys.

The *Fu* organs are the Yang organs. As a category, they are more hollow, and their shared main physiological functions are the receiving and processing (digesting) of food and other nutrients and transmitting and excreting wastes. The Fu organs include the Small Intestine, Large Intestine, Stomach, Gall Bladder, Urinary Bladder, and Sanjiao/Triple Burner.

Additionally, there are Six Extraordinary Fu organs. They are the Gall Bladder (which is also a regular Fu organ), Brain, Marrow, Bones, Vessels, and Uterus.

Almost all of the Western medical understanding of the internal organs is contained within the Chinese view. When there are significant divergences, they will be pointed out. We'll primarily be looking at the organs from the expanded perspective of Chinese medicine, using the concepts of Qi, meridians, and Yin and Yang as have been previously discussed.

When practitioners of Chinese medicine refer to the Heart, for example, they are referring to the Heart Qi, the functions of its associated Heart meridian, various Heart

Yin and Yang qualities and attributes, and the physical organ itself. This is more accurately an Organ System or Organ Network, encompassing the total functionality of the Heart system in that context rather than just the physical heart organ.

Because of Chinese medicine's emphasis on functionality, some glands are not considered separate entities. The functions of those glands are subsumed by the function of a related organ, even though the physical structure is known to exist. So adrenal gland function is considered part of Kidney function, and pancreatic function is considered part of Spleen function. Some Chinese medical subsystems refer to the Spleen as the Spleen/Pancreas for this reason.

Terminology

In the discussion of Organ Systems, commonly used descriptive phrases need some explanation. These indicate the holistic nature of this type of medicine, as some phrases refer to things that do not at first seem to relate to the organ at all. They include the wider scope of influence each organ has on the body and a subtler range of functional interrelationship than is considered in allopathic medicine.

In this context, these words or phrases have a specific, consistent meaning, although there are differences in translation and interpretation and some translators and authors may use them interchangeably. The written Chinese language is character-based, and many characters have no absolute, universally agreed-upon interpretation. The interpretations presented below are very common and will be used here for the sake of a standard, uniform presentation.

The word "govern" indicates an association with the organ's main physiological function, and usually most closely correlates with the Western understanding of at least a part of the organ's function. "The Lungs govern respiration" is a very clear example. "Rule" and "dominate" are translations sometimes used instead of "govern."

The word "dominates" means "exerts a strong influence on," usually in terms of generating or maintaining the healthy functioning of a particular body tissue. Sometimes the word "control" is used interchangeably, but that can be confusing, as an organ can control many things but has only one affinity to a body tissue that it dominates. "The Spleen dominates the muscles" is an example.

Every internal organ has a functional relationship with a particular sense organ. The phrase used to indicate that relationship is "opens to," as in "The Liver opens to the eyes." Most of the sense organs literally are openings to the outer world. The eyes have pupils, the ears have the auditory canal, the nose has nostrils, and the mouth is an opening. In the absence of trauma or contact-related irritation, a problem with a sense organ, such as blurred vision or reduced hearing, almost always indicates a problem with its associated organ and figures into the diagnosis. This includes age-related sensory declines, as they are caused by a decline in the related organ function.

Although the word "control" can be used as a gentler-sounding alternative to "dominate" it is typically a more generic word, meaning one of the many functions of the organ being discussed. Very often, "control" is used after another descriptive word or phrase to amplify its meaning. In this example, it follows the phrase "opens to": "The Liver opens to the eyes, controls vision, and controls tears." Of primary concern is the Liver opening to the eyes. The control of vision and tears relates to the functions of the eyes, still mediated by the Liver.

All of the phrases or descriptive words explained to this point fall under the province of the physical and energetic aspects of the organs. Analysis of these aspects presented in the next chapter is headed "Physical and Energetic Aspects of (the related Organ)."

Every organ has a particular affinity for an emotion or a few related emotions. In Chinese medicine, the stated emotional correspondences reflect the pathological manifestation that occurs when the related organ is not functioning properly. Conversely, when an emotion lingers long beyond what would otherwise be a normal, healthy response to a life situation, it becomes a pathological factor and will damage the related organ, functionally or materially. This "two-way street" feature is an aspect of holism that pervades all of Chinese medicine—Qi and Blood influence each other, Yin and Yang influence each other, and so on—but nowhere is that more obvious for Westerners than it is regarding emotions.

There are also normal, healthy emotional attributes associated with an organ that is functioning well and in concert with all the other organs. While some of these attributes are things we might not ordinarily think of as emotions, they all have emotional connections and require a healthy emotional balance in order to manifest. They can be diminished by a predominance of their unhealthy emotional counterpart. For example, the Liver's positive attribute of fortitude, defined as possessing physical and emotional strength, can be diminished by prolonged depression. Other positive attributes, like the

Heart's healthy expressions of compassion and empathy, are more easily seen as qualities associated with the emotion love, another of its positive attributes. Accordingly, we'll refer to all of these as the healthy emotions associated with each organ.

Somewhat paradoxically, the healthy expression of emotions is seldom discussed in Chinese medical texts, which are most concerned with what happens when things go wrong. The healthy emotional correspondences are presented here for you as well, under the heading "Emotional Aspect of the (Organ)."

From a Confucian perspective, the virtues are similar to positive emotions. Each organ has a related virtue, which can help to heal any problem associated with that organ, and will otherwise strengthen and nourish that organ. You will find the Confucian virtues presented after each organ's healthy emotional correspondence.

The word "houses" refers to an organ's association with a nonphysical, intangible attribute. "The Heart houses the mind" and "The Kidneys house willpower" are examples. Sometimes the word "stores" is used interchangeably with "houses." Most often, "stores" is used to refer to a physical essence that is stored in a Yin organ, as opposed to the intangible attribute indicated by "houses."

For the reader who might prefer to keep spirituality out of the discussion of medicine, these qualities can be easily and accurately thought of as addressing a psychological aspect of health. Accordingly, they are discussed under the heading "Psychospiritual Aspects of the (Organ)" and follow the discussion of emotional aspects so those correspondences may be readily noted. Those discussions are intentionally brief, since while they are of interest and relevance, they may be best explored in books devoted to Chinese spiritual philosophy.

Every organ has an associated external environmental factor by which it is most affected. Conversely, when an organ is out of balance, it often generates an internal analogue of its environmental factor. This can be a very useful observation when establishing a diagnosis. Those factors are introduced here and will be examined in more detail in Chapter 7, "Pathogenesis." Since each environmental factor is more prominent in a particular season, the seasonal associations with each organ are included. The interface between specific seasonal environmental energies and related organs is a unique feature of the holism of Chinese medicine.

Every organ has an ascendant time of day called its "open" time, when the Qi of the organ is at its peak within any twenty-four hour period. If a pathology obviously affects primarily one organ, it may be best to treat that organ at its ascendant time. For example, Lung time is 3 a.m. to 5 a.m. If a patient suffers from asthma, bronchitis, chronic cough, tuberculosis, or any other breathing disorder, their symptoms will usually be worst at that time. Historically, an acupuncturist who followed the principle of chronoacupuncture might sleep at their patient's house and wake at 3 a.m. to treat them. Alternatively, the patient might be prescribed a Qigong practice that strengthens the Lungs, told to practice between 3 a.m. and 5 a.m., and given an herbal formula to drink during those hours.

The organs' ascendant times may serve as an aid to diagnosis. Shortness of breath is usually thought of as a Lung problem, but if a person regularly suffers from breathing difficulties between 11 a.m. and 1 p.m., the Heart's ascendant time, it could indicate that the breathing difficulty stems from a Heart weakness. The organs' affinity for the cycle of diurnal energies is another unique feature of the holism of Chinese medicine.

Chapter 5

Zang: The Yin Organs

The Heart

Main Functions of the Heart

- Governs the Blood and dominates the Blood Vessels

Other Functions and Attributes

- Opens to the tongue and controls taste and speech
- Houses the mind (consciousness) and *Shen* ("spirit"). In a medical context, any of these four words may be used interchangeably. (See Appendix 2, Note 5.1.)
- Manifests on the facial complexion
- Controls sweat

Additional Correspondences

- Its associated emotion is joy. Joy slows and scatters Qi.
- Its healthy emotional expressions are compassion, empathy, and love.
- The Heart's virtue is *Li*, or "Order."
- In Five Element theory, its elemental representation is Fire. Accordingly, its seasonal correspondence is summer, and it is most affected by the environmental factor of Heat.
- Its influencing taste is Bitter. The significance of taste is discussed in Chapters 8 and 15.
- Its ascendant time of day is 11 a.m. to 1 p.m.

Analysis of Physical and Energetic Aspects of the Heart

The primary function of the Heart, governing the Blood and dominating the Vessels, is almost identical to the Western view of the heart, even if the language is different. This means that the Heart, specifically the Heart Qi, is the motive force driving blood circulation, and the Blood Vessels are the physical structures through which Blood is circulated. When the Heart Qi is strong and the Heart Blood is abundant, blood circulates well throughout the entire body, nourishing all body tissues. Another meaning is that the condition of the Heart is reflected in the quality of the pulse, as assessed through the Vessels. When the Heart Qi and Blood are strong and abundant, the pulse will be even, strong, and regular. If they are deficient, the pulse will feel weak and very thin (thready, in Chinese medical terminology) and may be irregular.

A distinctly non-Western aspect of Heart function is unique to Chinese medicine. The Heart is responsible for converting the Qi acquired from food, drink, and air into Blood. Other organs, the Lungs and Spleen, are involved in this process, but the actual transformation occurs in the Heart.

The Heart opens to the tongue. The tongue is considered "a sprout of the Heart," so, as with all organs and their related sense organs, there exists a close physiological, structural relationship between the two. The Heart meridian also connects with the tongue internally, and this connection is primarily responsible for the Heart's control of taste and speech. If the Heart is functioning normally, the tongue will appear moist and light red, it will move freely and easily, and the sense of taste will be normal.

Various pathologies alter the tongue's color, moisture, size, and shape. For example, Heart Blood Stagnation will cause the tongue color to become purplish, while Heat will turn it red. Heart Blood or Yin Deficiency may make it dry and thinner in shape. A fuller range of possible changes in the tongue is covered in Chapter 10, "Diagnosis."

A freely moveable tongue is required for the basic function of speech, but the quality and content of speech—coherence—relates more to the Heart housing the mind. This concept is both broad and complex, as it involves philosophy and spirituality, which are integral to classical Chinese medicine, as much as it does clinical medicine. For our purposes, we'll stick to the basics, which are more straightforward and easier to apply practically.

We've learned that the Heart governs Blood and Blood Vessels throughout the body. Because there are many blood vessels in the face and head, the quality of the Blood can be readily assessed there, so the Heart manifests on the complexion. This is in part due to the heart's physiological function of pumping blood. Whether standing or sitting, the heart has to pump blood upward, against gravity, to get to the face and head. This is an aspect of Heart Qi. If the Blood is healthy and abundant, and the Qi is strong, the facial complexion will have a light red glow and a luster. If there are Heart problems, the complexion can appear sallow, white or gray, and dull.

All body fluids are on the Yin side of the Yin-Yang continuum and share a common source. In Western as well as Chinese medicine, there are well-known correlations between blood, heart function, and body fluids. The Western biomedical condition of edema is caused by blood vessels becoming excessively permeable from various factors, allowing the fluid portion of the blood to leak into surrounding tissue and cause swelling. Two examples include an obstruction of blood flow by blood clots in the deep veins, causing leg edema, and congestive heart failure, which can cause leg edema and pulmonary edema (a fluid buildup in the lungs). In Chinese medical terms, clot obstruction is an example of a failure of the Heart to adequately govern the Blood, while Heart Qi Deficiency can cause the consequences of congestive heart failure. Both involve the failure of the Heart to adequately govern the Blood Vessels, allowing leakage.

Sweat is another body fluid that shares a common source with Blood, and because there can be an immediately observable correlation between sweat and Heart function, the Heart is said to control sweat. When the Heart is functioning normally, its control of sweat contributes to the healthy luster of the complexion. In the case of Heart pathologies, Heart Yin Deficiency causes night sweats, and more severe Heart problems can cause profuse, cool, and usually clammy sweat. Conversely, conditions that may cause profuse sweating, including excessive exercise and prolonged exposure to high heat or dryness, can deplete Heart Blood and cause such things as heat exhaustion or stroke. Some classic texts observe that "the Heart loathes Heat" for this reason. In these cases, it is notable that speech may also become incoherent.

Analysis of Emotional Aspects of the Heart

The Heart's associated emotion is joy. It may be difficult at first to understand how joy can be considered a pathological manifestation. In this case, the joy is excessive, approaching mania. A common example used to explain this is a person who may become so excitedly overjoyed at winning a fortune in the lottery that he has a heart attack. This may be an extreme example, but it does illustrate how excessive joy can be detrimental to heart health, scattering the Qi to the point where there is none to provide heart functionality. There are less obvious ways in which joy can be problematic, but remember that it's only when joy is excessive or prolonged that it will be destabilizing. Since the Heart houses the mind, prolonged and excited joy can lead to mania, delirium, or a loss of the ability to perceive or function in the world that everyone else experiences.

The Heart's healthy emotional expressions are compassion, empathy, and love. These emotions can engender a more balanced, healthy experience of joy.

Analysis of Psychospiritual Aspects of the Heart

The Heart houses the mind. The Chinese word *Shen* is translated as "mind," "consciousness," and "spirit." Here, "spirit" relates most to aspects of consciousness, and is similar to the idiomatic English usage in the phrases "having a spirited conversation," or "being in high (or low) spirits." It encompasses all mental activity, thinking, and emotional experience, involves memory, and is associated with sleep. So when the Shen is strong, supported by healthy Heart Qi and abundant Heart Blood, the mind is peaceful, clear, lively, and aware of and responsive to the environment, emotions are balanced, and sleep is sound and restful. Speech is orderly and coherent, as it will be directed by a healthy Shen. If the Shen is housed insecurely by an impaired Heart, a person may experience poor sleep, excessive and often disturbing dreams, depression, sluggish thinking, and poor memory. In extreme cases, the result can be delirium, mania, or loss of consciousness. In those instances, speech will be less organized, possibly incoherent, or absent.

Beyond the standard concerns of Chinese medicine, clear Heart consciousness influences a person's ability to make supportive, beneficial choices about various life issues over the long-term arc of one's life. When we consider the time component involved in those types of decisions, it becomes easier to understand how the Heart plays a role in the long-term aspects of memory. This becomes more important as a person advances to old age, since short-term memory may decline under the dominion of the

Kidneys, but long-term memory will remain intact for as long as the Heart is functioning reasonably well.

The Pericardium

The pericardium is the protective membrane that surrounds the heart. Its name is its description and is practically identical in English and Chinese. The English word is derived from Latin: "peri-" means around or surrounding, and "cardium" means heart. The Chinese word is *Xinbao*. *Xin* means "heart." *Bao* means "wrap" or "a wrapping." Both mean "surrounding the heart" or "the heart wrapping."

Its main function is to protect the Heart. Accordingly, almost anything external to the Heart that may harm it will first affect the Pericardium. Its secondary functions are largely identical to those of the Heart. This means that clinically, while the Pericardium has some unique qualities and functions, it is almost never treated as a separate organ but more as an appendage of the Heart. This is alluded to in its Five Element correspondence, where its element is designated as Supplemental Fire.

The Pericardium does have its own meridian, which is needled independently from the Heart. Some schools of acupuncture almost never needle the Heart meridian directly, preferring to treat it through the Pericardium whenever possible. In many styles of Qigong, the Pericardium meridian is of extreme importance. The eighth point of the Pericardium meridian, *Laogong*, is located at the center of the palm and is one of the most energetically sensitive points on the body. It is used to tactilely sense Qi for medical and other purposes as well as to emit and absorb Qi.

The Pericardium has an internal/external relationship with its paired intangible Yang organ, the Sanjiao (or Triple Burner), discussed later.

The Lungs

Main Functions of the Lungs

- Govern the Qi and respiration
- Control the channels and blood vessels
- Control dispersing and descending
- Regulate water passageways
- Dominate and manifest on the skin and body hair

Other Functions and Attributes

- Open to the nose, control smell, and control mucus
- House the corporeal soul (*Po*)

Additional Correspondences

- Its associated emotions are grief and sadness. Grief and sadness constrict Qi.
- Its healthy emotional expressions are exuberance, zest, and vitality.
- The Lung's virtue is *Yi*, or "Integrity."
- In Five Element theory, its elemental representation is Metal. Its seasonal correspondence is autumn, and it is most affected by the environmental factor of Dryness.
- Its influencing taste is Spicy.
- Its ascendant time of day is 3 a.m. to 5 a.m.

Analysis of Physical and Energetic Aspects of the Lungs

One of the primary functions of the Lungs, governing respiration, is almost identical to their Western function. That is, pure air is drawn into the lungs through inhalation, oxygen and other gasses are exchanged in the blood, and carbon dioxide and other wastes are expelled through exhalation. When we take into account that one translation of the word "Qi" is "air," that explains half of what is meant by the Lungs' function of governing Qi. (When used in the context of Chinese medicine and Qigong, the translation "air" is a limited, partial meaning of the word "Qi".) On the inhalation, clear Qi (*Qingqi*, atmospheric or celestial Qi) is drawn in, and on the exhalation, waste Qi is expelled. This is the main point of the Lungs' function of governing the Qi of respiration. But the Lungs also govern the Qi of the whole body, the second meaning in its governance of Qi, and this relates to many of their other functions.

As the Lungs draw in atmospheric Qi, that Qi combines with the Qi extracted from food by the Spleen, to form *Zongqi* (Zong Qi), most simply translatable as "chest Qi." (Other traditional translations include "gathering Qi" or "ancestral Qi," but the meanings of those translations are more complex and obscure—less suitable for practical use here.) That is a form of Qi more useable by the entire body. The Lungs' "control of descending and dispersing" function circulates this Qi throughout the body, nourishing all its tissues and promoting healthy physiological functioning. Because it's formed in the chest, it directly aids in strengthening Heart function, especially in regard to circulating Blood, and a portion of Zongqi is combined with Heart Qi to help form Blood.

The Lungs' function of controlling the channels and blood vessels can be partially understood by its role in aiding the Heart in its circulation of Blood. However, Zongqi forms nutritive Qi, which circulates internally both with the Blood in the blood vessels, and within the meridians. Since the Lungs control the Qi of the entire body and help form and power the circulation of nutritive Qi, it is said to control the channels and Blood vessels.

The Lungs are the uppermost of the Zangfu organs, known traditionally as "the canopy" of the organs, and because they interface directly with the atmosphere, they are also the most external of the Yin organs. These qualities play a role in the following Lung attributes.

As the uppermost Yin organ, its Qi must descend. We've seen how it descends Qi to nourish the body and improve functionality, providing nutritive Qi throughout the vessels and meridians. Another portion of Zongqi helps create Weiqi (defensive Qi) which circulates just under the surface of the skin and serves as the first line of defense against pathogenic invasion. This is nearly equivalent to the general immune system of Western medicine. This also relates to the Lungs being the most external of Yin organs, since it directs Qi to the most external parts of the body.

The Lungs descend and disperse body fluids as well as Qi. As it dominates and manifests on the skin and body hair, including the sweat glands, the Qi and fluids warm the skin and provide nourishment and moisture, keeping the skin supple and lustrous. Dominating the skin also means control of the opening and closing of the pores. When the Lung Qi is strong, the surface of the body is consolidated and strengthened against colds, flus, and other external pathogens, and sweat is normal. If the Lung Qi is weak, the pores of the skin may become more flaccid and open. This provides an entrance for disease, and sweat can be spontaneous, profuse, and often cool or clammy.

The Lungs descend body fluids to the Kidneys and Urinary Bladder. Some of that fluid is "steamed" by the Kidneys, which rises as a vapor to moisten the Lungs. The rest is converted into urine to be excreted by the Urinary Bladder. In this way, the Lungs' function of regulating water passageways plays a role in the elimination of waste fluids through sweat and urine. Lung Qi Deficiency affecting the water passageways can cause various urinary disturbances and edema.

The nose is the direct opening to the Lungs. Air and clear Qi enter the Lungs through the nose. When Lung Qi is normal and healthy, the nasal passages remain open, respiration is full and easy, and the sense of smell is normal. When the Lungs are invaded by pathogens that cause a cold or sinus infection, breathing becomes obstructed, excess mucus is produced and causes either a stuffy or runny nose, and a person may sneeze and have a reduced sense of smell. Excess Heat in the Lungs can cause the nose to bleed and also reduce the sense of smell.

Analysis of Emotional Aspects of the Lungs

Grief and sadness are the emotions associated with the Lungs. Any emotion can be situationally appropriate. It's only when an emotion becomes prolonged or habitual that it can cause health problems. So any period of protracted grief can depress Lung function and cause a person to breathe more shallowly, drawing in less clear Qi and thus lowering energy overall. Conversely, when the Lungs are out of balance with the rest of the body (possibly affected by Damp through phlegm accumulation from poor Spleen functioning, for example), or suffering a deficiency of Qi or Yin from other causes, a person may experience a lingering sadness or grief for no apparent reason. When grief constricts Qi, there is a sense of being shut down, withdrawn, and disengaged from life.

The emotional expression of healthy Lungs is exuberance and a zest for life. A natural antidote for sadness and grief, this is the outcome of strong Lungs effectively bringing in more Qingqi, which energizes the entire body and makes a person feel full of life. This is one reason why regulated breathing is an important part of all Qigong practices and makes a person healthier and more vital.

Analysis of Psychospiritual Aspects of the Lungs

The Lungs house the *Po*, the corporeal soul. While this has more to do with Chinese spiritual philosophy than with practical Chinese medicine, it does have some contemporary clinical relevance. The Po is the densest, most Yin part of the human soul. It has a particular sensitivity to the emotions associated with the Lungs, sadness and grief. Sometimes grief can be so profound that even in English it is referred to as being "soul sick." In that case, the quality and depth of breath is usually affected, becoming short, shallow, and restricted, an indication of its association with the Lungs. In those cases, treating the Lungs can strongly rectify emotional disturbances and restore balance. There is even a point on the Urinary Bladder meridian called Po Hu that tonifies the Lungs for just such conditions.

Being the densest, most Yin part of the soul, at death the Po descends and is absorbed back into the earth.

The Liver

Main Functions of the Liver

- Governs the smooth flow of Qi

- Stores Blood

- Dominates the Sinews (tendons and ligaments)

Other Functions and Attributes

- Opens to the eyes, controls sight, and controls tears

- Manifests on Nails

- Houses the ethereal soul (*Hun*)

Additional Correspondences

- Its associated emotions are anger and depression. Anger makes Qi rise.

- Its healthy emotional expressions are fortitude, the ability to get things done, a creative drive, and the ability to make life plans. This latter can be thought of as a quality of "having vision," a metaphorical association with the eyes.

- The Liver's virtue is *Ren*, or "Kindness."

- Its Five Element representation is Wood. Its seasonal correspondence is spring, and it is most affected by the environmental factor of Wind.

- Its influencing taste is Sour.

- Its ascendant time of day is 1 a.m. to 3 a.m.

Analysis of Physical and Energetic Aspects of the Liver

The Liver's nature is typified by the qualities associated with the first of its functions, governing the smooth flow of Qi. The Liver likes to grow in a healthy, lush, vigorous way, thriving in a favorable environment while similarly supporting such a favorable environment throughout the body. That is best accomplished through its governance of the smooth flow of Qi, which creates a sense of relaxation, a free looseness (contrasting tension and a feeling of being bound up), and a functional ease in every Organ System. The Liver dislikes depression. It will both be adversely affected by prolonged periods of depression and will generate feelings of depression when it is functionally compromised, primarily from various types of deficiency.

The smooth flow of Qi can be subdivided into three distinct yet interrelated aspects: its relationship to emotions, its role in digestion, and its relationship with Qi and Blood.

There is a traditional herbal formula designed to support and promote the smooth flow of Liver Qi. Its name, *Xiao Yao Tang*, means "Free and Easy Wanderer" formula, conjuring the image of an enlightened, peaceful, and carefree Daoist monk roaming the countryside unencumbered and untroubled by conflict yet able to help resolve conflicts between others and restore neighborly harmony. This is a useful image to keep in mind, since that is exactly the Liver's role in this context.

The Liver and Emotions

When a healthy Liver ensures the smooth flow of Qi, a person experiences emotional balance and is able to enjoy the full range of emotions while rarely being prone to emotional excess or fixation. While every organ has a particular emotional affinity, the Liver's larger role is in allowing all the emotions a harmonious expression. We've seen how the Heart houses consciousness and therefore encompasses all mental and emotional experience, yet the free, smooth flow of Qi is required for the free and strong flow of Blood, allowing Qi and Blood to be harmonized and the mind to be peaceful and at ease.

Any strong or prolonged emotional experience can disrupt the flow of Liver Qi, and any Liver imbalance can be responsible for a variety of emotional upsets. Some of those upsets can be directly associated with the emotional state of another organ, since Liver Qi is responsible for the free flow of Qi in every organ. For example, if Lung Qi is not flowing freely due to Liver Qi Stagnation, a person may experience grief or sadness, the emotions that are most closely linked with the Lungs.

More commonly, those upsets first affect the Liver's primary associated emotions. In the case of Liver excess or hyperfunction, Liver Qi Stagnation or Obstruction, those emotions include anger and the related emotions of frustration and irritability. In the case of a Liver deficiency or hypofunction, depression is most common. Depression can easily coexist with frustration, irritability, and anger, so those emotions cannot be used as the sole determinant of the exact type of Liver dysfunction.

The Liver and Digestion

The smooth flow of Liver Qi is very influential in the proper functioning of the Stomach and Spleen. The Stomach's main function is the breakdown of foods into useful nutrition. The Spleen is responsible for extracting food Qi, transforming the nutrition into a more bioavailable form, and transporting it throughout the body. The normal direction of Stomach Qi is downward, since the Stomach sends processed food material down to the Small Intestine, while the normal direction of Spleen Qi is upward, since the Spleen sends part of the food Qi up to the Lungs and Heart for conversion to Blood. The Liver supports those normal digestive activities of the Stomach and Spleen. If the Liver function is disturbed and its Qi does not move freely, there can be abdominal discomfort and distention, and the accompanying disruption can cause the normally descending Stomach Qi to reverse, causing belching, hiccups, nausea, and vomiting. A disruption of the normally ascending flow of Spleen Qi can lead to diarrhea. This type of digestive disturbance is from a local excess of Liver Qi, which, in an attempt to disperse, moves laterally to the Stomach and Spleen. This is called "Liver Invading the Stomach and Spleen."

The Liver also secretes bile, another aspect of its role in digestion. The free flow of Liver Qi is necessary for proper bile flow. Bile is necessary for the digestion of dietary fats. A disruption in bile flow can cause belching and jaundice, a yellowing of the skin and eyes.

The Liver's Relationship with Qi and Blood

"The Qi is the commander of the Blood," a saying in Chinese medicine, means that all blood flow relies on the functional energy of Qi. While the Heart and Lungs play the largest role in blood circulation, the Liver ensures that the Heart Qi and Lung Qi are smooth and unobstructed, so they can perform their role as efficiently as possible. Additionally, Qi flow throughout the body must be smooth and unobstructed if Blood is to freely circulate to all body tissues. A disruption in Liver Qi can cause Qi stagnation or Blood Stasis anywhere in the body. This can cause minor, dull aches to severe, sharp pain, abdominal distention, loss of appetite, a sense of pressure in the chest, various menstrual disorders, and even the formation of cysts, tumors, or other masses.

While these three aspects of governing the smooth flow of Qi have been presented separately, keep in mind that they are entirely interrelated, and each aspect is a part of the others.

The Liver stores Blood based on physiological need. When the body is active, the Liver releases more Blood so that it can moisten and nourish the muscles, as well as other tissues. This helps supply the body with needed energy. We learned that "the Qi is the commander of the Blood," and the corollary to that is "the Blood is the mother of the Qi." This means that Qi requires a material substrate out of which to grow, and the Blood is that substrate. Healthy, abundant Blood brings abundant Qi with it.

When a person is at rest, as during sleep at night, more of the Blood returns to the Liver, since the circulating Blood volume requirements are less. The Liver can then assist in restoring a person's energy during sleep. Following the principles of Chinese medicine, being soundly asleep by 11 p.m. each night is considered especially important. The Gall Bladder's ascendant time is from 11 p.m. to 1 a.m. The Gall Bladder is the Yang partner to the Liver. Both are Wood-element organs, and 11 p.m. begins Wood time and influences the functionality of the Gall Bladder and Liver.

If there are problems with Liver Blood, the body is not as well nourished, and a person may become easily fatigued. Since the Liver opens to the eyes, there can be blurred vision or other visual disturbances. Since it dominates the tendons and ligaments, the muscles and limbs can become tight, achy, or numb. Because of the Liver's strong relationship with Blood and Qi, most gynecological complaints are directly attributable to the Liver during a woman's menstrual years, including headaches, cramps, breast tenderness, irregular cycles, scanty menstrual blood, and clots in the menstrual blood, among other possibilities.

The tendons and ligaments, collectively referred to as "the Sinews" in most Chinese medical texts, are what connect muscle to bone (tendons), allowing for all body movement, and what connects bone to bone at the joints (ligaments). We've seen how Liver Blood nourishes and moistens all body tissues and how Liver Qi influences smooth movement and all functionality in the body. A healthy Liver provides for free, open, relaxed, and easy movement in the four limbs and the joints. If the Liver is compromised, the Sinews will not be nourished properly and can cause stiffness and tight, painful muscles and joints. In more severe cases, where there may be strong pathological Heat affecting the Liver, there can be tremors, spasms, and opisthotonos, a type of whole-body rigidity primarily affecting the muscles of the back.

The fingernails and toenails are considered to be extensions of the tendons. When the Liver Blood is healthy and abundant, the tendons and nails are strong, moist, and healthy. When the Blood is deficient, the nails will appear dry, brittle, and with indentations or cracks.

The eyes are the sense organs most closely associated with the Liver. Liver Blood nourishes the eyes, allowing for clarity of vision. The Liver meridian also connects internally with and brings Qi to the eyes. A healthy Liver produces bright, lively eyes that shine and move quickly and easily. If Liver Blood is deficient and fails to nourish the eyes, they may become dry, red, or itchy, and there can be visual disturbances like nearsightedness, floaters (spots in front of the eyes), or poor night vision. I've explained that some Liver diseases affecting bile flow can cause jaundice, a yellowing of the eyes and skin. There are even idiomatic English language references to the Liver's association with the eyes. If a person is angry (the emotion associated with the Liver), he is said to be "seeing red," a visual connection to that emotion. If the Liver has been compromised by too much alcohol consumption, a person is said to be "seeing double" or "blind drunk."

Analysis of Emotional Aspects of the Liver

Since the Liver has a relationship with all of the emotions as part of its governance of the smooth flow of Qi, we introduced some of the emotions that are specific to the Liver above. Let's examine the Liver's emotions more closely now.

The emotions commonly associated with the Liver are anger and depression. Anger is most often seen in excess conditions, such as Liver Qi Stagnation, in which there is an undesirable buildup of Liver Qi due to some type of obstruction. When anger causes Qi to rise, anger can become more intense, flaring up unpredictably like a blazing fire, out of control. Lesser manifestations of the same condition include frustration and irritability. These are unhealthy counterparts to emotions that are generated by a normal, healthy Liver. Those include fortitude and the abilities to get things done, to accomplish something, and to have vision in a conceptual way that allows for effective life plans. If someone does not have vision—does not feel they are able to accomplish life goals—they will become frustrated and irritable, may appear hyperactive and volatile, may use anger as a pathological substitute to get people around them to do the things they want, and may attempt to destroy anything they perceive as an obstacle in their path.

Depression is most often seen in some type of deficient condition, such as Liver Blood Deficiency, for example. In this person, the same feeling of not being able to accomplish positive life goals will generate feelings of hopelessness, like there is no point in even trying to make one's life better. This is a mild to moderate depression, as opposed to the bleak despair of clinical depression, which comes from the Kidneys.

Analysis of Psychospiritual Aspects of the Liver

The Liver houses the *Hun*, or the "ethereal soul," which is the counterpart to the Po, or the corporeal soul housed by the Lungs. While the Hun is not of great importance relative to the contemporary practice of Chinese medicine, there is a notable correspondence with an aspect of the Liver's emotional health. The Hun is influential in giving a person the ability to create a life plan and find a sense of direction, or life trajectory. This can be thought of as a type of practical physics, since the Hun must be aligned with and firmly rooted in space and time in order to fulfill this purpose. Without such a root, possible in Liver Blood or Liver Yin Deficiency, a person may suffer from mental confusion and a sense of aimlessly wandering through their own life.

The Hun is the more active, Yang aspect of the soul, relative to the Po. Without the stability of adequate Liver Blood or Liver Yin, the Hun is inclined to roam. This can cause spontaneous astral projection, the sense of floating above the body just before sleep or of entirely leaving the body during sleep. At death, while the Po descends into the earth, the Hun unites with the subtle energies of the nonmaterial world.

The Spleen

Main Functions of the Spleen

- Governs transformation and transportation
- Controls blood
- Dominates muscles and the four limbs

Other Functions and Attributes

- Opens to mouth, controls taste, and controls saliva
- Controls the raising of Qi
- Manifests on lips
- Houses thought

Additional Correspondences

- Its associated emotions are worry and pensiveness. Worry knots the Qi.
- Its healthy emotional expressions are centeredness, groundedness, calm focus, and presence.
- From a Confucian perspective, the Spleen's virtue is *Xin*, or "Trust."
- In Five Element theory, its elemental representation is Earth. Its seasonal correspondence is late summer, and it is most affected by the environmental factor of Damp.
- Its influencing taste is Sweet.
- Its ascendant time of day is 9 a.m. to 11 a.m.

Analysis of Physical and Energetic Aspects of the Spleen

The Spleen's main functions of transformation and transportation have to do with its role in the digestive process. Specifically, it separates and extracts pure, useable nutrients, the "clear" or "clean" portions of the *Guqi* (Gu Qi, "grain" Qi or food Qi) from food and drink held in the stomach (its paired Yang organ), transforms those nutrients into useable substances as part of their becoming Qi and Blood, and then transports those nutrients both for further processing and to disseminate them throughout the body for nourishment. The impure parts of food are left in the Stomach, which sends it down into the intestines either for further processing or for elimination.

The initial transportation of Guqi is upward, part of the Spleen's ability to control the raising of Qi, to the Lungs for transformation into Zongqi (chest Qi), and to the Heart to be transformed into Blood. These aspects of the Spleen's function have earned it the distinction of being considered the primary Yin organ for the generation of Qi and Blood and the foundational source of postnatal Qi. Postnatal Qi—that is, all the Qi acquired after birth until the time of death—is important to all of Chinese medicine, but perhaps most important to the practice of Qigong, whose sole purpose is the acquisition, preservation, and utilization of Qi for numerous specific objectives.

The Spleen also transforms and transports water and other body fluids. As with food, it first separates the useable portions (the "clear" or "clean" portions) from any liquid that has been consumed. The clean portions are transported to the Lungs, which distribute moisture to the skin, and are further used to moisten all the tissues of the body. The impure parts of the fluids are sent down into the intestines either for further processing or for elimination. The Spleen also transports excess fluids from meridians, tissues, and organs for elimination from the body. So the Spleen's role in water metabolism includes transportation of clean fluids to ensure proper moistening of all body tissues and the elimination of excess or unclean fluids to prevent the accumulation of Damp. Damp is a pathological manifestation of moisture and can be produced by Spleen Qi Deficiency.

Looking at just this part of Spleen function, a healthy Spleen is responsible for good appetite and nutrient absorption, normal digestion and elimination, the production of energy, and the generation of Blood and other body fluids. A poorly functioning Spleen can cause poor appetite, abdominal distention, low energy, loose stool, or diarrhea (from poor nutrient absorption with an accumulation of Damp), as well as swelling, edema, and phlegm (from an accumulation of Damp). (See Appendix 2, Note 5.2.)

The Spleen's control of Blood has two main parts. We've looked at one part already, the Spleen's role in generating Blood. The second part is that the Spleen is responsible for holding the Blood within the blood vessels. When the Spleen is healthy and working properly, there is no obvious indication of it performing this function, since the body is simply functioning normally. However, a deficiency of Spleen Qi can cause a variety of bleeding disorders if the Blood extravasates, or leaves the blood vessels inappropriately. This can include the tendency to bruise easily, having frequent nose bleeds or bleeding gums, bloody stool, excessive uterine bleeding or bleeding at various time throughout the menstrual cycle, and frank hemorrhaging with a poor ability of the blood to clot normally.

The Spleen's domination of the muscles and four limbs is related to functions already discussed. As the Spleen transforms nutrients into Qi, Blood, and body fluids and transports them to all the body's tissues, it nourishes the muscles, providing for good muscle development and strength, and it lubricates muscle tissue, providing for suppleness and proper functionality. While the Spleen dominates all muscles, it has a special affinity for the muscles of the arms and legs. If the Spleen Qi is weak, a person will tire easily, and the muscles will be weak, stiff, dry, and less flexible and may even atrophy.

The Spleen's opening to the mouth and controlling taste and saliva is the very first step in its bringing nutrients into the body for transformation and transportation. A healthy Spleen creates a healthy appetite, and the mouth is able to enjoy the full spectrum of tastes to support that appetite. (In any illness, one of the main indicators of a good prognosis is the maintenance or return of a good appetite.) Spleen deficiencies may cause a poor appetite and dull the sense of taste or may cause an unpleasant, abnormal sweet taste in the mouth.

The production of adequate saliva is necessary to break down starches and lubricate other food for better mastication, the beginning of good digestion. The Spleen's manifestation on the lips is a reflection of the quality of its transformation and transportation. A healthy Spleen produces ample Qi and Blood, and so the lips will appear pink, moist, and lustrous. Various Spleen pathologies will make the lips appear pale, dry, or cracked.

The Spleen controls the raising of the Qi. We've seen how the Spleen sends nutrients upward to the Lungs and Heart to produce Qi and Blood, one aspect associated with the raising of Qi. (This quality is counterbalanced by its paired Yang organ, the Stomach, which descends Qi.) Another raising function involves holding the internal organs in their proper place, to prevent organ prolapse. While many internal organs such as the stomach, kidneys, or urinary bladder are subject to prolapse, in prolonged Spleen weakness, the uterus or anus may abnormally lower to the point of protruding from the body. The final aspect of raising Qi is that the Spleen causes clear Yang Qi to rise to the head, aiding in the function of all the sense organs and in clear thinking. If the ascent of the Qi is blocked, as can be the case in an accumulation of Damp, there can be dizziness, blurry vision, a sense of heaviness in the head, and fuzzy thinking.

Analysis of Emotional Aspects of the Spleen

The Spleen's associated emotions are worry and pensiveness. Since it houses thought, some sources say thinking or meditation is an associated emotion. Keeping in mind that from a medical perspective the primary emotions of an organ are its pathological manifestations (an aid to diagnosis), for this association to hold, the quality of that thinking has to be interpreted as obsessive or at least excessive, bringing it into the realm of worry or pensiveness (brooding). Pensiveness in this case means overthinking or excessive mental work. All of these things can damage the Spleen functionally, in all of the ways discussed previously. When worry causes Qi to knot, a person will become stuck fretting over a troubling thought or stuck in a nonproductive, circular thought pattern. This is very similar to the obsessive portion of an obsessive-compulsive disorder.

If a person has a constitutional Spleen weakness, one common manifestation is being flighty or ungrounded, with an inability to stay focused or present—the stereotypical "space cadet." A person with a healthy Spleen will have exactly the opposite presentation and will be grounded, solid, focused, and present. Their thoughts are clear and organized, and they may be able to engage in prolonged mental work with relatively little detrimental effect.

Analysis of Psychospiritual Aspects of the Spleen

The Spleen houses thought, but this is a different function from the Heart housing the mind or consciousness. There is some relationship between the two, as illustrated by the function of the first acupuncture point on the Spleen meridian, which is said to clear the Heart and stabilize the spirit. The Kidneys play yet another role in thinking and memory as we will soon see.

Housing thought primarily has to do with clear thinking, having the ability to concentrate and memorize easily, absorbing information in the context of schoolwork, any type of extended study, or related mental tasks. This absorption can be seen as yet another aspect of the Spleen's governing of transformation and transportation. Just as the Spleen absorbs nutrition from the outside world and makes it useable within the body, it grasps or apprehends concepts and ideas, absorbing and transforming them through thought to make them useable and accessible for many purposes by the person who has assimilated them.

As in its emotional correspondence, overthinking and excessive studying can weaken the Spleen. This is a relatively common concern for high-achieving students. Strengthening the Spleen can minimize this, and there is even one point on the Spleen meridian that is used for students who think too much.

The Kidneys

Main Functions of the Kidneys

- Govern birth, growth, reproduction, and development and govern Water
- Store *Jing* (essence)
- Dominate bones, produce Marrow, and fill the Brain

Other Functions and Attributes

- Control the reception of Qi
- Open to ears and control hearing
- Control the two lower orifices and control urine
- Manifest on the head hair
- House willpower

Additional Correspondences

- Its associated emotions are fear and fright. Fear and fright make Qi drop.
- Its healthy emotional expressions are self-understanding and clear perception, leading to true wisdom.
- The Kidneys' virtue is *Zhi*, or "Wisdom."
- Its Five Element representation is Water. Its seasonal correspondence is winter, and it is most affected by the environmental factor of Cold.
- Its influencing taste is Salty.
- Its ascendant time of day is 5 p.m. to 7 p.m.

Introduction to the Kidneys

The Kidneys are perhaps the most complex organ in all of Chinese medicine. They have more functional interrelationships with every organ than any other individual organ. Being the origin of both Fire and Water in the body, the Kidneys have many unique and seemingly paradoxical attributes. Although there are two kidneys, some sources include a third, nonphysical (although functionally very apparent) structure called the *Mingmen* as an integral part of the Kidneys, while others consider it to be separate from but functionally related to the Kidneys.

The Kidneys occupy a unique place among all Yin organs in that they store "prenatal essence," or *Yuan Jing* (also translated as original, preheaven, or congenital essence), which is inherited from one's parents and is loosely equatable with being the repository of all our genetic information. While other types of Jing are found throughout the body, the Kidneys are the only place where Yuan Jing is stored. Combined with "acquired essence," it composes Kidney Jing. Kidney Yin, Yang, and Qi are separate things and are included as part of Kidney Jing. Since so many of the Kidneys' functions rely upon it storing Jing, some consideration is warranted.

General Characteristics of Jing

In simplest terms, Jing is a Yin fluid with a high-energy functional Yang Qi aspect. Present in many places throughout the body, Jing is most often thought of as exclusively residing in the Kidneys, since Kidney Jing is a one-of-a-kind essence that underlies the health of the entire body.

Most organs store or generate their own type of Jing essence. Every organ has a Yin substantive nurturing aspect, and a Yang energetic functional aspect. These are mutually supportive qualities that are typically separate, although some part of an organ's Yin fluid can be imbued with an energizing Yang quality, which makes it a Jing essence. This Jing is manufactured or otherwise acquired through various physiological processes after birth and throughout the course of one's life, so it is an acquired essence, a postnatal Jing.

For example, we've seen how saliva is a fluid controlled by and associated with the Spleen. Saliva is not commonly thought of as Spleen essence, but if we examine its role, we see how it fits the criteria. It is a Yin fluid substance that moistens the mouth and lips, which are associated with the Spleen. It moistens food for easier mastication, another part of its Yin attribute. But beyond moistening food, it also breaks down some components of food, beginning the process of digestion, under the Spleen's governance of transformation. This is a functional Yang attribute of saliva, due to saliva containing Yang Qi, energy blended with the Yin fluid. From Western medical science, we know that saliva contains salivary amylase, an enzyme that breaks down carbohydrates. The salivary amylase is the most Yang part of saliva—an example of the Yang within the Yin as illustrated by the Taiji symbol—and is what makes saliva a Jing and not just a moistening Yin fluid.

Using this example as a model, we can define Jing as any Yin fluid that contains a functionally Yang quality, an energy that initiates, mediates, or maintains any functional activity in the body. This analysis is supported by the definition of Jing from the Beijing Medical College *Dictionary of Traditional Chinese Medicine* found in the following section. With this understanding, we can draw correlations between Jing and Western medically defined substances such as enzymes (which catalyze all biological chemical reactions), hormones, and other secretions of most endocrine and exocrine glands.

Jing and Qi

Jing has a unique relationship with Qi, in part because Jing may be thought of as Qi in the form of a fluid substance. In his book *The Foundations of Chinese Medicine*, Giovanni Maciocia states, "[Original Qi] is closely related to Essence. Indeed, Original Qi is nothing but Essence in the form of Qi, rather than fluid. It can be described as Essence transformed into Qi."[8] While describing Jing (essence) *as* Qi, the clear implication is that original Qi is contained in and transformed from the fluid essence.

Some Chinese medical references inseparably link Jing with Qi, calling it *Jingqi*. In the Beijing Medical College *Dictionary of Traditional Chinese Medicine*, Jingqi is considered both a "vital substance, chiefly referring to that derived from food essence," and as "vital essence and vital energy as material basis for visceral functioning. The vital essence and energy stored in the kidney are closely related to sexual activity and

---

8. Giovanni Maciocia, *The Foundations of Chinese Medicine: A Comprehensive Text for Acupuncturists and Herbalists* (London: Churchill Livingstone, 1989), 41.

reproduction." [9] From these statements we begin to see how Qi and Jing have an interdependent relationship of mutual influence. We also see that when Jing or essence is referred to by itself, it is almost always Kidney Jing being discussed.

Jing is a highly refined substance, the quality and quantity of which influences every aspect of our health and life. In *The Web That Has No Weaver*, Ted Kaptchuk explains,

> Jing, best translated as Essence, is the Substance that underlies all organic life. ... [It is] the source of organic change. Generally thought of as fluid-like, Jing is supportive and nutritive, and is the basis of reproduction and development.
>
> Jing has two sources. ... Prenatal Jing ... is inherited from the parents. In fact, the fusion of this prenatal Jing is conception. ... The quantity and quality of prenatal Jing is fixed at birth and, together with Original Qi, determines a person's basic makeup and constitution.
>
> Postnatal Jing is the second source and aspect of Jing. It is derived from the purified parts of ingested food. The Postnatal Jing constantly adds vitality to the Prenatal Jing. Together, they comprise the overall Jing of the body. [10]

This passage provides a workable definition of Jing, primarily focusing on Kidney Jing, and introduces its two sources, prenatal Yuan Jing and postnatal acquired Jing.

Kidney Jing

There is a lot to be explored in the expanded understanding of Yuan Jing (prenatal Jing) and acquired Jing. Throughout the rest of this book, we'll focus primarily on Kidney Jing and its role in general and medical health.

Kidney Jing is what's most often meant in discussions of Jing. While every organ has its essence, the Kidneys are unique in that they also store the arguably finite Yuan Jing from one's parents and a significant quantity of acquired Jing, more readily avail-

---

9. Xie Zhufan, Huang Xiaokai, *Dictionary of Traditional Chinese Medicine* (Hong Kong: The Commercial Press, Ltd., 1984), 34.

10. Ted Kaptchuk, *The Web That Has No Weaver: Understanding Chinese Medicine* (Chicago: Congdon and Weed, 1983), 43.

able from food and other sources. This blend of Yuan and acquired Jing is typically identified simply as "Jing," most physically manifesting as sperm and ova. Kidney Jing contains both inherited Yuan Jing and acquired Jing, and by extension Kidney Yin, Yang, and Qi.

Kidney Jing has at its root the energy of sex, which in many people's experience embodies the strongest concentration of the energy of life. That sexual association is also responsible for much of the Kidneys' role in governing birth, growth, reproduction, and development, and, later in life, inevitable decline.

Sexual essence, specifically Kidney Jing, is not only the root of sexual vitality and reproduction but of *all* vitality, not just sexual activity. Many people take up the practice of Qigong or Taiji in their later years for the expressed purpose of conserving or restoring their sexual vitality and consequently their overall health and longevity.

Qigong and Jing

Qigong can be practiced as a part of Chinese medicine, as is taught in this book. When Qigong is cited as the only practice that can restore Jing, it is almost always taken to mean sexual Jing essence, Kidney Jing. Since Yuan Jing is stored in the Kidneys and makes up a part of Kidney Jing, some contend that Qigong may also restore Yuan Jing. Many practitioners consider Qigong to be the best way, possibly the only way, to replenish Yuan Jing. Some highly cultivated contemporary Qigong masters have stated that the practice of Qigong allows one to access and alter the genetic code itself. This clearly addresses Yuan Jing, and at an advanced level of practice, it may in fact be possible to replenish or otherwise positively alter Yuan Jing. More commonly, scholars, teachers, doctors, and other authorities agree that Kidney Jing, since it is largely composed of acquired Jing, can be replenished and nourished, and its Yuan Jing component can be conserved or spared.

Conservation is no small thing. As people age and experience the associated decline and degenerations that typically accompany aging, it is the depletion of Kidney Jing (the Kidney Yin and Yang Qi components separately as well as the totality of essence as their material foundation) that is the primary cause of that decline. While sensible, healthy lifestyle choices help slow that decline, the skillful practice of Qigong can stop or reverse many of those changes. When that occurs, it is evidence that the Kidney

Jing, including Yuan Jing, is being restored, and this is what is meant by most who state that Qigong can replenish Jing.

Mingmen

Some of the oldest Chinese medical texts (notably the *Classic of Difficulties*, Chapter 36, produced circa 100 CE) consider that the left Kidney is the "true" Kidney, the source of true Yin. This makes it the origin of Water. At that time, the right Kidney was not thought of as a true Kidney at all, but instead as the seat of the "Gate of Vitality," a common translation of *Mingmen*, which contains Kidney Yang. That makes the right Kidney, or Mingmen, the origin of Fire. When referred to in this context, its full name is *Mingmen Hou*, meaning "Life Gate Fire."

Two herbal formulas from that time, still in use today, are named to neatly capture that thought. *Zuo Gui Wan*, or "Restore the Left" pill, nourishes Kidney Yin. *You Gui Wan*, "Restore the Right" pill, tonifies Kidney Yang.

Physicians from later periods revised this thought and considered Mingmen a separate energy center located between the Kidneys. That perspective is prevalent today and is in keeping with what most cultivated Qigong practitioners assert from direct experience. While the Mingmen is still called the Gate of Vitality, or the Gate of Life, it is also colloquially referred to as "the rear Dantian," since it is located behind and slightly above the Dantian, can be perceived as a discrete energetic entity, and serves functions similar to the Dantian while maintaining its role as the origin of Fire.

For our purposes, we will consider the right and left Kidneys and the Mingmen as one functional unit unless otherwise stated for a specific purpose or clarification. In contemporary clinical settings, the right and left Kidneys are seldom treated separately (although Kidney Yin and Yang are frequently addressed separately), and except in advanced Qigong practices, the Mingmen is almost never directly addressed separately. (See Appendix 2, Note 5.3.)

Analysis of Physical and Energetic Aspects of the Kidneys

The Kidneys' function of governing growth, reproduction, birth, and development is related to its storing of Jing essence. The union of parental Kidney Jing creates a new life and is the clearest indication of Kidneys governing reproduction. Equally important, each parent must have enough sexual vitality to have the health and sexual desire to initiate conception, another aspect of reproduction.

Original essence along with its original Qi governs the growth and development of the fetus inside the womb. After birth, that essence is stored within the Kidneys of the newborn as part of its original essence, along with the Kidney Yin and Yang that makes the baby a unique individual. Original essence is responsible for the baby's constitution and vitality and governs its continued growth through all the stages of life, including puberty/reproduction, maturation, menopause/andropause, and the decline that precedes the finality of death.

Acquired essence, the refined essences extracted from food and transformed by the Stomach and Spleen, is added to Kidney Jing after birth. It replenishes and adds vitality to original essence, and together they form the totality of Kidney Jing.

Kidney Jing is the material base for Kidney Yin, Yang, and Qi, all of which can be transformed from Kidney Jing and exist simultaneously with it. Some medical texts say it is the essential Kidney Qi that governs the phases of birth, growth, development, and reproduction, which are all functional activities and so naturally rely on Qi, but since even in that case it's derived from Kidney Jing, essence is its ultimate source. Accordingly, Kidney Yin and Yang also have Jing as their foundation.

Kidney Yin is the foundation for all the Yin fluids of the body, which moisten and nourish all the organs and body tissues. Kidney Yang is the foundation for all the Yang Qi of the body, which warms and promotes the functional activities of all the organs and body tissues. This is how the Kidneys are the origin of Water (Yin) and Fire (Yang), an important aspect in their government of all the developmental stages of a person's life.

The Kidneys' relationship with Bones and Marrow is again dependent on their storage of Jing. Essence generates Marrow. This Marrow has two aspects, one that is similar to Western medicine, bone marrow, and one that is very different, Marrow as the substance that makes up the spinal cord and Brain.

Marrow is produced in the core matrix of bone cavities. The strength and density of bone is dependent upon its nourishment by Marrow. If the Kidneys are strong and Marrow is abundant, bones will be firm and hard, with a suppleness that makes them difficult to break. If the Kidneys are deficient and Marrow is insufficient or of poor quality, there can be bony malformation in children and weak, achy back, knees, and feet in adults. Bones will be brittle and prone to break more easily. (See Appendix 2, Note 5.4.) The teeth are an extension of bone and are therefore subject to the same considerations. Healthy, abundant Marrow creates teeth that are strong, dense, resistant to cavities, and rooted firmly in the gums and jaw. Weak Kidneys cause teeth to be softer, prone to chipping and cavities, and liable to become loose or to fall out.

Marrow generates the spinal cord and Brain, a perspective unique to Chinese medicine. Marrow is said to fill up the Brain, so the Brain is referred to as "the sea of Marrow." If the Kidney Jing is strong, it will nourish the Brain and produce clear thinking with good memory and concentration. If the Jing is weak, there will be forgetfulness, poor concentration, and fuzzy or dull thinking. The Kidneys' involvement with memory and concentration is primarily related to short-term memory. The loss of short-term memory can be distracting and disruptive to a person's ability to follow an immediate sequence of events, reducing concentration. This is most often seen in the elderly, who have a marked decline in Kidney Jing. Milder versions of this can happen at any age, whenever Jing is sufficiently depleted. We've seen that the Heart houses consciousness, and the Spleen houses thought. This function of the Kidneys completes the picture of the organs' roles in consciousness, thought, and other mental processes.

The Kidneys receive Qi from the Lungs. They are said to "grasp" the Qi, assisting the Lungs in their descending function. This is what is meant by controlling the reception of Qi. Working in concert with the Lungs, when Kidney Qi is strong, respiration is smooth, even, and full. If Kidney Qi is weak and fails to grasp the Qi, Lung Qi can stagnate in the chest, causing shortness of breath and difficult inhalation, especially after any type of exertion. This is a common cause of asthma.

We've seen that the left Kidney is the origin of Water, and the Kidneys' Five Element representation is Water. The Kidneys' governance of Water is yet another water correlation, and relates to its function of controlling the lower orifices. The Kidneys are very involved with every aspect of water metabolism and play an important role in the regulation and distribution of all body fluids.

Fluids are first received by the Stomach and then transported by the Spleen up to the Lungs. The Lungs' function of descending and dispersing sends fluids down to the Kidneys. Here, the Kidney Yin Qi and Yang Qi come into play and separate the clear, pure fluids from the waste fluids. The pure fluids are sent back up to the Lungs by the "steaming" function of Kidney Yang Qi, for distribution to all of the organs and tissues in the body. The waste fluids are sent to the Urinary Bladder to be converted to urine and excreted.

Kidney Qi is also responsible for the Kidneys' opening and closing function, in which it acts as a sort of sluice gate. This function is most commonly thought of in its connection to urination, but since the Kidneys regulate all aspects of water metabolism, it is equally important in their receiving fluids from the Lungs. When the Kidneys' Yin and Yang Qi are balanced and normal, the Kidneys will receive, separate, and transmit fluids normally. Urination will be normal, and the body will be hydrated and nourished by ample amounts of pure fluids. If Kidney Yang Qi is deficient, the sluice gate will be too open, there will be less efficient separation of the pure fluids from the waste fluids, and urination will be profuse and pale. If prolonged, dehydration may occur. If Yin Qi is deficient, the gate will be too closed, urination will be scanty and dark yellow, and there may be an abnormal accumulation of fluids, causing edema.

The lower orifices include the anterior orifice (urethra and sex organs), involved in urination and reproduction, and the posterior orifice (the anus), functioning to excrete feces. While it is the Urinary Bladder that discharges urine, Kidney Qi powers that function and similarly powers the anus in its excretory function. In addition to the urinary considerations addressed above, weak Kidney Qi can cause incontinence or enuresis (the inability to control urination). It can also cause diarrhea and anorectal prolapse. Semen is the external manifestation of Jing, so a deficiency in either Kidney Qi or essence can cause spermatorrhea (leakage of sperm), nocturnal emission, premature ejaculation, or impotence. It can cause infertility in both sexes. There can be other less common presentations, but primarily, healthy functioning lower orifices will prevent any type of leakage, while compromised functioning will allow leakage of sperm, urine, and feces.

The Kidneys open to the ears and control hearing. This is a less obvious connection than many organs have with their related sense organ, yet the *Huangdi Neijing* (*The Yellow Emperor's Inner Cannon*, a classic Chinese medical text produced circa 100 BCE) states, "The Kidney Qi goes through the ear. If the Kidney is harmonized, the ears can hear the five tones." [11] The ears rely on nourishment from Kidney Jing and

---

11. Giovanni Maciocia, *The Foundations of Chinese Medicine: A Comprehensive Text for Acupuncturists and Herbalists* (London: Churchill Livingstone, 1989), 97.

Qi for healthy functioning. With such nourishment, hearing is acute. If the Kidneys are weak, hearing can become reduced even to the point of deafness, or there can be other hearing abnormalities, such as tinnitus (a persistent ringing in the ears). This connection becomes more apparent in the presence of pathology, since many hearing problems are resolved by treating the Kidneys, and in the aging process.

The Kidneys manifest on the hair. The hair relies on Kidney Jing to grow. Jing supports the production of Blood, and hair is called a "surplus of Blood" in some texts. In any case, Blood is required to nourish hair and give it luster. When the Jing is abundant and able to promote healthy Blood, the Kidneys create hair that is full, thick, lustrous, and with good color. If the Kidneys are weak and Jing is deficient, the hair will be dull or brittle, will lose color and become gray or white, and will fall out easily. Hair is considered a secondary sex characteristic in most cultures and can be a subliminal cue in assessing a person's sexual (and overall) vitality, since both depend on Kidney health. Accordingly, during reproductive years hair appearance may be a factor in selecting a potential mate.

As people age, it's natural that Kidney Jing, Yin, Yang, and Qi will decline, causing all of the symptoms of aging. Taking into account what we've learned about the Kidneys, we can easily see that correspondence. In aging people, sexual vitality diminishes until in menopause women can no longer conceive and bear children, and at some point most men will have too low a sperm count or too weak an erection to be able to father children. Bones become brittle, become osteoporotic, and tend to fracture easily. They may change in other ways, causing various spinal curvatures or arthritic deformities. Teeth become loose and fall out, hair becomes dull, brittle, thin, and white; and hearing diminishes. Short-term memory becomes poor. Incontinence and breathing difficulties are common. Many elderly people become fearful and sensitive to cold. When the Kidneys become too weak to provide the ultimate support that other organs rely on, those organs become functionally impaired.

Analysis of Emotional Aspects of the Kidneys

The emotions associated with the Kidneys are fear and fright. These can arise from various Kidney deficiencies, although Qi deficiency is most usually involved. Fear is typically a more prolonged, pervasive state of being. Fright has the quality of an immediate shock, a sudden fear from a perceived real-life danger, or the feeling some might seek out in an amusement park fun house or at a horror movie. Since fright has a rapid onset, its effects manifest rapidly and obviously, so we'll discuss that first.

Fear and fright cause Qi to drop. When frightened, that drop can happen suddenly and strongly and can make a person lose control of the lower orifices, the anus and urethra. Most people have encountered instances, either in real life or in the movies, of someone getting so frightened that they wet themselves. This is also the origin of the descriptive if somewhat crude phrase of being "scared shitless." The sudden drop also causes a loss of Qi, so the Kidneys must convert and release some Jing to make up for that loss, which can be temporarily stimulating and energizing. That's why fright is used as entertainment in amusement parks, movies, public haunted houses, and other similar diversions. They are especially popular with young people and those with abundant Jing, who are less likely to notice the depleting effects in the short term. People who are addicted to extreme sports (also known as "adrenaline junkies"), transform fear into excitement and get their high from the same source, Kidney Jing. If prolonged, this expenditure of Jing will eventually lead to adrenal fatigue or adrenal burnout, one Western correlation with Kidney deficiency.

Fear produces many of the same consequences as fright. A person may be fearful because of a constitutional Kidney deficiency, but if it's situational, it may be more insidious because it can grow slowly, linger, and be interpreted as a person's nature. In children, lingering fear can be caused by insecurity about family matters, for example, which is often a significant factor in bed-wetting. In adults, fear is caused by a perception of danger, a feeling that their life is threatened. This can take the form of chronic anxiety from concerns about job security or other financial matters, an unsettling or hostile work or home environment, or the more immediate danger of occupations that put a person in emergency situations on a regular basis. The loss of Jing may happen more slowly, and includes a depletion of Kidney Yin, producing Dryness and Heat. In this case, symptoms of Kidney Yin Deficiency can include heart palpitations, night sweats, dry mouth, and insomnia.

If fear with its concomitant depletions is prolonged, it can lead to a bleak, hopeless depression, much more debilitating than the depression caused by Liver Blood Deficiency or Qi Stagnation.

The Kidneys' healthy emotional expressions of self-understanding and clear perception can thwart the manifestations of fear or can be the natural antidote to fear, especially if the fear is not well-grounded in reality. With some work, the bed-wetting child can be reassured that her family is stable, loving, and supportive. The adult who feels fearful about job security, finances, family, or other daily life situations can learn either how to change his circumstances or how to change his perception of those circumstances, whichever may be most appropriate. In these examples the clarity and understanding empowers the person and dispels the fear at the root of the problem.

Analysis of Psychospiritual Aspects of the Kidneys

The Kidneys house willpower. This is an aspect of the mind that allows a person to focus on a goal and pursue it to completion. It's related to the healthy emotional expressions of clarity and self-understanding, since those qualities provide a person with the ability to see which goals are in their ultimate best interest and with the motivation with which to direct the drive of will. With strong Kidneys, a person can work purposefully for extended periods of time with focus and concentration and can effectively store and retrieve information in short-term memory.

When the Kidneys are suffering an imbalance, the motivation to work can become excessive and cause the compulsive working habits of the workaholic. If the Kidneys are weak, then concentration is poor, the mind can be easily distracted from primary goals, determination wavers, and the person can become discouraged.

Chapter 6

Fu: The Yang Organs

The Yang organs are hollow. Their main shared physiological functions are the receiving and processing (digesting) of food and other nutrients and transmitting and excreting wastes. The Yang organs are considered the more superficial and external organs, both Yang attributes, because most of them open directly to the outer environment. The Stomach opens to the mouth, the Large Intestine opens to the anus, and the Urinary Bladder opens to the urethra. The small intestine communicates with the outside world through the large intestine. The Gall Bladder is the exception, although even it connects with the small intestine through the common bile duct. The Gall Bladder is further exceptional in that it does not receive food or excrete wastes, earning it the distinction of being the only Yang organ that is also an Extraordinary Organ, a separate organ classification. The Sanjiao is an insubstantial organ and therefore not able to physically connect with the outside world. Its very insubstantiality is a Yang attribute, contrasting with the heavy denseness of Yin.

The Five Element associations of Yang organs are almost identical to those of their Yin organ counterparts. So while the Heart corresponds to Yin Fire and the Small Intestine to Yang Fire, the Fire attributes are common to both organs. Similarly, they share the same associations with body tissues, sense organs, and emotional correspondences as their Yin counterparts, although the Yang organs typically play a smaller role in those functions. Any significant divergences are included in each organ's description.

Some of the Yang organs have a strong, obvious anatomical and physiological relationship with their paired Yin organ. Others are less obvious, but in all cases there are strong energetic relationships because their meridians are directly linked at or near their endpoints, within each paired organ, and at linking points (*Luo* connecting points) along the meridian pathway.

As the Yang organs do not produce or store essences and are mainly involved with nutrient absorption and waste elimination, their list of functions and attributes is smaller than those of the Yin organs. They are presented to you here in more or less the order in which they fulfill those functions.

The Stomach

The Stomach has an internal/external relationship with the Spleen, its paired Yin organ. Having a primary role in nutrient assimilation, the Stomach is considered to hold a place of special importance among the Yang organs. In fact, in the clinic it is often noted that one of the best indicators of a favorable prognosis is the return of a healthy appetite, a sign of good stomach functioning—that is, healthy Stomach Qi—while a worsening appetite usually indicates a decline in health.

Main Functions and Attributes of the Stomach

- Governs the rotting and ripening of food
- Controls the transportation of food essence
- Rules descending Qi
- Its ascendant time is 7 a.m. to 9 a.m.

Analysis

While "rotting and ripening" might be an unappealing image, it serves as a metaphor for the initial stages of digestion, where received food begins its decomposition, being mechanically broken down by the churning action of the stomach and chemically broken down by the stomach acid's effects on proteins. After this transformative process, the pure portions are transported to the Spleen for Qi and other nutrient extraction, while the impure (still undigested) parts are sent down to the Small Intestine for further processing. This is how the Stomach controls the transportation of food essence.

The pure food essence is further transformed by the Spleen and then transported throughout the entire body. This cooperative partnership between the Stomach and Spleen's functions of transformation and transportation is the origin of Qi for the whole body, so together they are considered to be the acquired foundation, or the root of acquired Qi.

The Stomach normally sends Qi downward. This is apparent through its function of sending the impure food down into the Small Intestine. This is balanced by the Spleen's function of raising Qi, in its sending Qi up to the Heart for the production of Blood and in its holding all the internal organs in their proper place, preventing organ prolapse. If the Stomach's descending function becomes impaired, it causes a syndrome called Rebellious Stomach Qi, and a variety of ailments will occur. In mild cases, the syndrome can be simple hiccups or belching. If it worsens, it can cause lack of appetite, feelings of abdominal heaviness, fullness, and distension or acid regurgitation, nausea, and vomiting.

The Small Intestine

The Small Intestine has an internal/external relationship with the Heart, its paired Yin organ. Its upper end connects to the stomach, and its lower end connects to the large intestine. It continues the stomach's role in nutrient assimilation, primarily digesting fats and carbohydrates.

Main Functions and Attributes of the Small Intestine

- Controls receiving and transforming of food, aiding in digestion
- Separates fluids, separating the clear from the turbid
- Its ascendant time is 1 p.m. to 3 p.m. (See Appendix 2, Note 6.1.)

Analysis

The Small Intestine receives the impure (incompletely digested) portion of food sent to it by the Stomach. It continues the digestive process, transforming the food by further separating the pure from the impure parts, and absorbs essential nutrients and fluids from the food. As part of the Spleen's job is to transport all nutrients throughout the body, the pure nutrients separated by the Small Intestine are sent to the Spleen. The Small Intestine sends the impure portion of remaining food to the Large Intestine for final processing and excretion. The pure portion of fluids, primarily water, is also sent to the Large Intestine for reabsorption, while the impure fluids are sent to the Urinary Bladder for elimination.

If the Small Intestine's function is impaired, symptoms can range from simple intestinal rumblings and gas to poor digestion, abdominal pain, and abnormal bowel movements (either constipation or diarrhea). Since the Small Intestine's function of separating the pure from the impure fluids is controlled by Kidney Yang Qi and the impure fluids are sent to the Urinary Bladder, other symptoms of Small Intestine dysfunction can include either excessive or scanty urination. Additional urinary symptoms may also be present.

The relationship between the Heart and Small Intestine may be illustrated most easily on the psychological/emotional level. We've seen that the Heart houses the mind and so governs all mental activities. The Small Intestine's role here is in supplying clear discernment, providing the guidance necessary to assist in making the best life choices. While still under the province of the mind, this distinction is unique to the Small Intestine.

The Gall Bladder

The Gall Bladder has an internal/external relationship with the Liver, its paired Yin organ. It sits nestled against and connected to the liver, just to the right of the solar plexus. Its main physiological role is to store bile secreted by the liver and then expel relatively large quantities of it into the small intestine through the common bile duct whenever fats enter the small intestine. The bile emulsifies the fats and aids the small intestine in that aspect of digestion.

Main Functions and Attributes of the Gall Bladder

• Secretes bile
• Controls Sinews (tendons and ligaments)
• Controls judgment and decisions
• Its ascendant time is 11 p.m. to 1 a.m.

Analysis

The Gall Bladder is a unique Yang organ in that it is the only one that does not receive nutrients nor excrete wastes, and it is the only Yang organ that does not connect with the external environment.

Its function of secreting bile is identical with the Western understanding of the organ's function, with these additions. The functional energy of the Liver, Liver Qi, is responsible for the production of bile. The Gall Bladder's secretion of bile is dependent on the Liver's function of regulating the smooth, free flow of Qi. Any disruption of Liver Qi will have an adverse effect on the Gall Bladder's ability to properly secrete bile, and any Gall Bladder dysfunction will likewise adversely affect Liver function. They are dependent on each other. In this way, the physiological and energetic connection between Liver and Gall Bladder is as close as that between the Stomach and the Spleen. In fact, the Liver and Gall Bladder together are said to govern the free flow of Qi.

The Gall Bladder controls the Sinews, or tendons and ligaments, in a way similar to the Liver, which shares that function. Being a Yin organ, the Liver's control is mediated more by the nourishing, moistening, softening effect of Blood than by Qi, providing suppleness. Being a Yang organ, the Gall Bladder's control is mediated more by the functional energy of Qi than by Blood, providing smooth agility of movement.

The Gall Bladder normally sends Qi downward. This downward flow directs bile properly, assists in some of the digestive functions of the Stomach and Spleen, and supports normal Liver functions. If there is Gall Bladder impairment, bile, which is bitter and yellow, may rise and cause a bitter taste in the mouth or vomiting of bitter, yellow fluid. The Stomach and Spleen may be adversely affected, causing nausea, belching, abdominal distension, and diarrhea. Liver functions may become impaired, causing Liver Qi Stagnation and possibly jaundice.

Along with these functional relationships, the Gall Bladder shares in most of the Liver's emotional characteristics. It has an additional related role controlling judgment, the ability to make decisions. This supports the Liver's ability to plan a life trajectory. The Gall Bladder facilitates the decision-making process, providing the courage, decisiveness, and strength of will to implement the most desirable life plan. If the Gall Bladder is weak or impaired, a person may be too timid to realize their life's path.

Idiomatically, the Chinese will refer to a courageous person as having (or being) a "big gall bladder," while a timid or weak-willed person is said to have a "little gall bladder."

The Large Intestine

The Large Intestine has an internal/external relationship with the Lung, its paired Yin organ. It begins at the lower right quadrant of the abdomen, connects to the small intestine through the ileocecal sphincter, and ends opening to the outer environment at the anus. Once the small intestine completes the digestive process, the large intestine receives waste from the small intestine, absorbs whatever useable fluids remain, and transports and excretes the resultant feces.

Main Functions and Attributes of the Large Intestine

- Receives food/waste from the Small Intestine
- Reabsorbs fluids
- Excretes wastes
- Its ascendant time is 5 a.m. to 7 a.m.

Analysis

The physiological functions of the large intestine are the same in Chinese and Western medicine, as described above. If the large intestine is not functioning properly, there can be intestinal rumblings and gas, constipation or diarrhea. Of note, in Chinese medicine the Spleen has the ultimate control over every aspect of digestion throughout the entire digestive system. Accordingly, these same symptoms are often attributed to a Spleen dysfunction. Other diagnostic information, including pulse and tongue diagnosis, may be required to make a differential diagnosis, revealing the exact source of such symptoms.

Energetically, there are some unique connections between the Lungs and Large Intestine. We've seen that the Lungs have a function of descending Qi. That Lung Qi can assist the Large Intestines in the elimination of feces. When Lung Qi is weak, a person may become constipated. If constipation arises from another source and becomes chronic, that can obstruct the descent of Lung Qi and cause shortness of breath.

While not a definitive indication of an energetic connection between the Lungs and Large Intestine, it is nonetheless noteworthy that one of the most common sites of colon (large intestine) cancer metastasis is the lungs. It is much less common for it to move the other way; that is, it's rare that a primary lung cancer metastasizes to the large intestine. This may be explained by the Large Intestine's energetics being Yang, having the qualities of being more superficial and protective. Our environment is loaded with carcinogens, and any external carcinogenic pathogen or chemical attempting to affect the body will first be intercepted by protective Yang Qi. In the case of a carcinogen that might affect either the lungs or large intestine, the Large Intestine will be the first line of defense. If it fails, then colon cancer will occur. As the cancer moves deeper, it will then affect the deeper, more sensitive paired Yin organ, the Lungs. If the Lungs are affected first, from smoking, airborne chemical exposure, or constitution/genetics, the cancer has bypassed the defensive Yang Qi, is already a deeper problem, and is therefore much less likely to move exteriorly to its paired Yang organ.

The Urinary Bladder

The Urinary Bladder has an internal/external relationship with the Kidneys, its paired Yin organ. It is located in the central part of the lower abdomen. Physiologically, it receives urine, temporarily storing it until enough has accumulated, when the urge to urinate will then cause it to be excreted.

Main Functions and Attributes of the Urinary Bladder

- Stores and excretes urine
- Excretes fluids by Qi transformation
- Its ascendant time is 3 p.m. to 5 p.m.

Analysis

The Chinese and Western understanding of the functions of the urinary bladder are nearly identical, although Chinese medicine has a different view of how and why those functions occur and adds some information related to the role of Qi.

The Urinary Bladder receives the impure portion of fluids separated out by the Small Intestine and to a lesser extent by the Large Intestine and Lungs. Some sources state that urine is made in the Kidneys and then sent to the Urinary Bladder, which is consistent with the Western medical view. Most sources state that the Kidneys receive fluids from the Small and Large Intestines and Lungs, further separate pure from impure fluids, and send the impure fluids to the Urinary Bladder to be converted into urine.

The transformation of impure fluids into urine requires Qi, which is supplied by Kidney Yang Qi. All Yang Qi is warm or hot, so this transformation requires heat as well. It is the heat that contributes to urine's yellow color. (See Appendix 2, Note 6.2.) This is the process of the creation of urine and what is meant by the Urinary Bladder's function of transforming fluids with Qi. The Urinary Bladder performs that function, but it is assisted by the Kidneys. Qi is required for the functional act of urination, and that Qi is also supplied by the Kidneys. This is why the Kidneys are said to control urine and the two lower orifices. In this way, it's easy to understand the close relationship between the Urinary Bladder and the Kidneys.

If the Urinary Bladder is not functioning properly, a variety of urinary problems can arise, including frequent or urgent urination, difficulty in or lack of urination, burning or otherwise painful urination, excessive and clear urination, incontinence, and bed-wetting.

The Sanjiao

Sanjiao is translated as "Three Burners," "Triple Burner," or "Triple Heater." (*San* means "three," and *Jiao* means "burner.") It has an internal/external relationship with the Pericardium, its paired Yin organ, and has the distinction of being an insubstantial organ, meaning it has no physical form. In fact, in the classic Chinese medical text the *Nanjing* (*The Classic of Difficulties*), the Sanjiao is said to have "a name but no shape." Lacking such physiology, it has no discrete Western medical counterpart with which to compare physiological functions. It is often thought of more as a collection of interrelated functions, but that does not mean it isn't "real." It does possess distinct qualities and can be treated through its meridian like any other organ, with the same type of expected outcomes.

Still, the exact nature of the Sanjiao is the most ambiguous of all Yang organs. Over the centuries, it has been the subject of much debate among Chinese physicians and medical scholars. Here we'll examine only the aspects that are most agreed upon and which may most easily be put to practical use.

Main Functions and Attributes of the Sanjiao

- Governs various forms of Qi
- Provides a pathway for *Yuanqi* (Yuan Qi, "original Qi" or "source Qi") and body fluids
- Delineates and divides the body into three primary regions, the Upper, Middle, and Lower Jiao
- Its ascendant time is 9 p.m. to 11 p.m.

Analysis

The Sanjiao's functions are interdependent and best explained in a less sequential way than was used with the other organs. It assists and combines with the receiving, transforming, transporting, and excreting functions of the Zangfu organs in each body region.

Clinically, the Sanjiao is most often thought of as a water or fluid passageway. Some classical sources include the transportation of food within that function. That passageway is what links the functional activities of each of the Three Burners. Its role of governing various forms of Qi and the division of the Three Burners is largely associated with its effects on fluid metabolism. Classically, it has been referred to as an "irrigation official who builds waterways." The Fire quality of a Burner is required to control and balance Water processes.

The Upper Burner is the body region above the respiratory diaphragm and contains the Heart, Lungs, Pericardium, and everything within the head. Here, despite being paired with the Pericardium, the Lungs and Heart are the main organs influenced by the Sanjiao. (See Appendix 2, Note 6.3.) The Sanjiao meridian additionally influences the sense organs, primarily the ears, hinting at its close relationship with the Kidneys through its role in fluid metabolism.

The Upper Burner governs dispersing and distribution in conjunction with those functions of the Heart and Lungs. It assists the Heart in distributing essential Qi extracted from food and water to nourish the entire body, and it plays a stronger role in assisting the Lungs both in dispersing fluids to moisten the body and in regulating the skin and pores. These fluids are in a clear, fine state, vaporized and pervasively disseminated throughout the body, so the Upper Burner is classically described as being like a "mist" or "fog." Assisting another Lung function, it governs the movement of Weiqi (defensive Qi), releasing it and providing unobstructed passage to the skin, where Weiqi does its primary work of protecting against external pathogenic invasion. The acupuncture point Sanjiao 5 (*Waiguan*, or "Outer Pass") is used to stimulate this function.

The Middle Burner is the body region between the diaphragm and the umbilicus and contains the Stomach, Spleen, and Gall Bladder. It governs the digestive processes, promoting those functions of the Stomach and Spleen. The Middle Burner governs transformation and transportation where food Qi is extracted, and other nutrients are absorbed and transformed into useable forms of Qi, beginning the generation of healthy new Blood.

Aided by the Sanjiao's releasing function and by the Sanjiao providing clear passage for Qi and fluids, the Spleen transports this extracted and transformed nutritive Qi throughout the body. The Sanjiao is instrumental in guiding the portion of it to the Heart that will be used to create Blood and guiding the Weiqi portion to the Lungs. This demonstrates one connection between the Upper and Middle Burners and the Sanjiao's governance of various forms of Qi.

The Stomach is considered to be central to the Middle Burner. Accordingly, the Middle Burner is alternatively described as being like a "foam" or "froth," referring to the state of digested food, or like a "bubbling cauldron," describing the churning action of the stomach during digestion.

The Lower Burner is the body region below the umbilicus and contains the Liver, Large and Small Intestines, Kidneys, and Urinary Bladder. (In purely anatomical terms, the largest portion of the liver is not below the umbilicus, and in younger people, the kidneys are not either—they tend to descend somewhat with age. Functionally, they are contained within the Lower Burner.) It governs the separation of the pure from the impure, directing those functions of the Kidneys, Intestines, and Urinary Bladder, assisting in urination and defecation. Because the Lower Burner continuously directs the impure fluid and solid wastes downward for excretion, it is commonly described as "a drainage ditch."

Regardless of whether they are located in the Upper, Middle, or Lower Burner, all of the Yin organs and most of the Yang organs have numerous functions. The Sanjiao primarily influences only those functions having to do with water metabolism, made clear by the classical imagery of mist or fog, froth or bubbling cauldron, and drainage ditch.

The last Sanjiao function is also dependent upon it being a passageway. *Yuanqi*, "original Qi," is located within the Kidneys. Yuanqi needs the Sanjiao passageway in order to be distributed to all the internal organs and their related twelve meridians. Yuanqi supports, stimulates, and promotes all physiological functions throughout the body, perhaps the most important being providing the heat necessary for digestion, which is the source of all of our acquired Qi and nutrition.

Chapter 7

Pathogenesis: The Origins of Disease

Like most other aspects of Chinese medicine, pathogenesis (the things that cause illness, pain, debility, and degeneration) is viewed differently in Western medicine. In the West, a diagnosis is made, increasingly by technological means, and then the disease is named based on that information. Treatment is given for that named disease, and in most cases, people with the same disease are given exactly the same treatment.

Chinese medicine recognizes the same diseases that Western medicine does, although some may be called by different names. A Western disease diagnosis represents one collection of symptoms that figures into a pattern of disharmony that the Chinese physician seeks to identify in order to treat the patient in the best way possible. The disease isn't treated; it's just a clue to the entire pattern. The whole person is treated to restore a healthy balance. That is one of the hallmarks of all holistic practices. Once balance is restored, the symptoms of the disease disappear.

For example, if someone's pancreas is not able to produce the hormone insulin or produces it in insufficient quantities, they are said to have Type 1 diabetes (insulin dependent, formerly called juvenile onset). If they can produce insulin but their cells are not able to utilize it properly, they have insulin resistance and are said to have Type 2 diabetes (formerly called adult onset). Type 1 or Type 2 diabetes becomes the person's diagnosis and the name of their disease. For the most part, everyone with Type 1 diabetes is treated exactly the same (taught to give themselves insulin injections, monitor blood sugar levels, and possibly make lifestyle modifications), while everyone with Type 2 diabetes is prescribed glucophage (metformin), thiazolidinediones, or related drugs to promote insulin uptake and may be instructed on leading a healthier lifestyle. For Type 1 diabetes, the Western approach is a true life saver and is the best first choice. This example serves to illustrate that different paradigms are used in each medical system, as we'll see throughout the rest of this chapter. The Chinese view of diabetes is discussed in Chapter 8.

The Causes of Disharmony

What causes things to go wrong with our health, disturbing the harmonious balance among our organs and other aspects of our body, mind, and emotions and creating these patterns of disharmony?

Primary Causes of Pathology

1. **External pathogenic factors** (EPFs): These are the predominant climatic factors of the external, natural environment, along with the more subtle associated energies that are present even in parts of the world where observable seasonal changes are not very pronounced. As a category, they are characterized by their sudden onset.

2. **Internal pathogenic factors** (IPFs): These are commonly emotional in origin. Additionally, imbalances within and among the internal organs can create internal "climates" similar to those of the external environment, mimicking EPFs. Typically these produce a slower onset of symptoms than EPFs.

3. **Epidemic diseases (pestilence)**: These are almost always from a combination of Wind and Fire EPFs.

4. **Trauma:** Any type of injury.

5. **Miscellaneous factors** such as insect and animal bites.

6. **Diet and lifestyle** considerations.

Note that while trauma and diet and lifestyle are presented here separately for greatest clarity, they are often considered to be categories of miscellaneous factors.

Individual constitution is also a factor, affecting a person's susceptibility to EPFs and some IPFs. In comprehensive contemporary clinical practices, additional environmental factors are considered, due to so many toxic industrial pollutants in our air, food, and water, numerous side effects to most common over-the-counter and prescription drugs, and exposure to many types of destabilizing electromagnetic fields and other man-made radiant energies through various electronic devices and pervasive wireless technologies. Those are outside of the scope of this discussion.

Overview of External Pathogenic Factors

Most EPFs are seasonal aspects of nature, sometimes translated from the Chinese as "climates." These are the six climates:

- Wind
- Summer Heat
- Fire
- Damp
- Dryness
- Cold

Under normal circumstances, healthy people will usually not be adversely affected by these seasonal changes, which are the "Six Qi" of the natural world. It's only when they are observed causes of disharmony that they are considered pathogenic and are then traditionally called the Six Pernicious Influences or the Six Excesses.

Seasonal energies can cause disease if they are prolonged or intense, if they are perverse (a period of unusual Cold during the summertime or Heat during the wintertime, for example), if a person has a constitutional imbalance predisposing a sensitivity toward a particular environmental factor, or if a person is already suffering an imbalance from another cause that makes them susceptible to an environmental energy. Additionally, some people are very sensitive to energetic shifts and can feel unsettled, feel out of sorts, or become prone to illness during seasonal transitions.

Most EPFs have a typical seasonal association (Cold during the winter and Heat during the summer, for example), but almost all can occur during any season. In fact, multiple EPFs can and often do occur simultaneously. Being external, they only become pathogenic once they invade the body through the nose, mouth, or pores of the skin. All EPFs can affect every internal organ, but each organ is most sensitive to disruption or injury from a single specific EPF.

Of note, contemporary indoor environments often create human-made EPFs. For example, fans create Wind, air conditioners create Wind and Cold, and heating systems create Heat and Damp (radiators) or Heat and Dryness (central/electric heating).

Overview of Internal Pathogenic Factors

The main IPFs are emotional in origin. The range of human emotional experience is normal and healthy, but as with the climatic energies, they can become problematic and pathogenic when very intense or prolonged. These are the Seven Emotions:

- Joy
- Anger
- Sadness/Melancholy
- Grief
- Pensiveness/Worry
- Fear
- Fright

Each emotion has an affinity for a particular organ, although other organs may be affected secondarily. While emotions can injure specific organs, an organ compromised from another source can produce inappropriate emotional responses. For example, if a person harbors long-standing anger or resentment toward another, that will eventually create a pattern of disharmony within the Liver.

Conversely, if a person damages their Liver function from excessive alcohol consumption, anger is often inappropriately evoked, leading to the infamous barroom brawl or to the surly, grumpy, acerbic personality as a common manifestation of the chronic alcoholic.

Taken as one part of diagnostic criteria, the emotions can play a significant role in determining the correct diagnosis, which is the pattern of disharmony affecting the individual. This is an aspect of the holistic nature of Chinese medicine. All parts of the person's life must be considered integral to the whole.

Examining that holism further, the individual person can be viewed as a microcosm of the larger macrocosmic environment, inseparably linked. IPFs can be generated by patterns of disharmony arising from organ imbalances when the organ's function is compromised by an EPF, another IPF, or other causes of pathology. Many of these organ-generated IPFs reflect the same environmental factors found in the outside environment. There can be internally generated Wind, Damp, Heat, Dryness, and Cold, and the primary organ associations are the same as those found with EPFs. As all of the organs share a holistic interconnection, these IPFs can and often do affect more than the primary organ.

An EPF can work its way deeper into the body and become an IPF of the same type or transform into a different IPF altogether. In this case, the EPF is defined as external when it primarily affects the more external parts of the body: the skin, muscles, and sense organs. As it penetrates deeper into the body and directly affects the internal organs, it will be identified as internal. For example, external Wind on the surface of the body can cause fever or chills, sweating, nasal congestion, itchy eyes, and body aches. If it is allowed to penetrate deeper, it can easily affect the Liver. This can cause internal Liver Wind, or it may congest the Liver Qi sufficiently to generate internal Heat and cause a Flare-Up of Liver Fire, transforming into a Heat IPF.

The Six External Pathogenic Factors

It bears repeating that all environmental factors discussed here are only pathogenic when they produce a discernable adverse effect in relation to the body, which is the result of the body's reaction to the environmental factor. Except in the most extreme circumstances, there is nothing intrinsically pathogenic about the seasonal energies as they exist in nature.

The symptoms given are typical presentations associated with each EPF. Not every person afflicted by an EPF will have all of the associated symptoms, and other symptoms besides those included here may be present.

Wind

- Prominent season: Spring
- Organ most affected: Liver
- Nature: Yang

Main Attributes and Associated Symptoms

Wind is the most ubiquitous and pervasive of the EPFs. While spring is its predominant season, it is present throughout the year. Because each season has its own energetic quality, capable of affecting people in numerous subtle ways, even robust people can be more vulnerable to Wind during spring.

Wind readily carries other EPFs along with it. This is why it's referred to as "the agent of 1,000 diseases," noted in the *Suwen* (*The Book of Plain Questions*), a Chinese medical classic originally dating as far back as 400 BCE. Wind can facilitate and combine with Damp, Heat, Dryness, and Cold when invading the body, making it the primary EPF in all infectious and epidemic diseases.

Wind Qi is characterized by upward and outward movement. It therefore readily affects the head and upper body and is a component of all types of colds and flus, along with many other ailments of the head. Wind alone can cause headaches, eye twitches, an aversion to wind, and itchy eyes, skin, and throat. Combined with Cold, it can cause a cold characterized by nasal congestion and sneezing with white or clear mucus, chills more than fever, and body aches. Combined with Heat, the cold is characterized by nasal congestion with yellowish mucus, fever more than chills, thirst, and a sore throat. In either case there may be a puffy face and absent or profuse sweating.

Wind can freely blow anywhere and is associated with movement and rapid change. Wind disorders are characterized by their sudden onset, with symptoms that can appear then disappear or appear in one part of the body, disappear, and then emerge at another part of the body. Hives, itchy skin bumps that appear suddenly and randomly change location, are caused by Wind. The Western biomedical name for this condition is urticaria, but even in the West it is colloquially called "wind rash." Another example is joint pain that intermittently appears and disappears, moving among various joints throughout the body. This can be a presentation of some types of arthritis. It is called "Wandering Bi" or "Wind Bi" in Chinese medicine. (*Bi* Syndrome means "Painful Obstruction Syndrome" and is caused by pathogenic factors blocking the meridians.)

Internal disharmonies can generate Internal Wind, an IPF with many of the same presentations as External Wind. This is usually, although not exclusively, caused by some sort of Liver disharmony. Some common Liver patterns that produce Wind include Liver Wind, Liver Yang Rising, and Flare-Up of Liver Fire, in order of increasing severity. Each has its own distinguishing signs and symptoms, but the related Wind IPF symptoms are dizziness and vertigo (both are subjective sensations of internal movement), tremors, convulsions (physical movements, associated with the Liver's governance of tendons and ligaments), headache, painful or red eyes (affecting the head from Wind's upward movement), and both the biomedical and figurative versions of apoplexy. Medically, that means unconsciousness, usually from a stroke, again affecting the head. Used figuratively, it means "rendered speechless by extreme anger." Anger is the emotion most associated with the Liver.

Summer Heat

- Prominent season: Summer
- Organ most affected: Heart. Clinically, all organs may be affected.
- Nature: Predominantly Yang, but as Summer Heat frequently combines with Damp (summer humidity), a Yin pathogen, it can have a mixed nature.

Main Attributes and Associated Symptoms

Unlike all other EPFs, Summer Heat, being defined as such, only occurs during the summer. While there is no exact IPF match for Summer Heat, Damp Heat has some presentations that are a close analogue that can be generated internally and is also an EPF that can occur in any season.

Summer Heat is a strong Heat that both scatters and consumes Yin fluids. Being a Yang pathogen, it has an upward directionality. Its ability to scatter will leave the pores open and induce profuse sweat. At the same time the nature of Heat is very drying. This combination can lead to dehydration, dry lips, mouth, and tongue, and a strong thirst. It will also cause urination to be scanty and dark yellow. Parts of the body, or the entire body, may look or feel hot, the complexion is usually red, and the person will avoid heat and prefer cold foods, beverages, and environments.

Heat's upward surge can cause a high fever, dizziness, and mental restlessness. If it becomes more severe, it will cause heatstroke/sunstroke, where the exposure to high heat causes the body to lose the ability to cool itself down. This serious condition induces fainting and possible coma. Since the Heart both generates sweat and houses the mind, these demonstrate primary ways in which Summer Heat affects the Heart.

When mingled with Damp from summer humidity, symptoms of Spleen involvement occur, as the Spleen is most sensitive to Damp. These include low energy, poor appetite, loose stool or diarrhea, and a heavy sensation in the head or throughout the body, combined with the previous Heat symptoms.

Fire

- Prominent season: Summer
- Organ most affected: Heart. Clinically, all organs may be affected.
- Nature: Yang

Main Attributes and Associated Symptoms

Fire exists on a continuum of Mild Heat, Heat, and Fire. While summer is its predominant season, Fire can occur at any time of the year. It shares some of the same presentations as Summer Heat, excluding the Damp symptoms.

Its excess Yang nature consumes Yin fluids and induces an upward directionality. The image of fire in nature makes those traits easy to see, as fire consumes all it burns and prefers to rise whenever that is possible. The consumption of Yin causes dry lips, mouth, and throat, scanty, dark urine, and a drying of the intestines, causing constipation, with a desire for cold foods, beverages, and environments.

The upward burning quality of Fire can cause high fever, dizziness, mental restlessness, insomnia, profuse sweating, and red, painful swelling or ulceration of the lips, mouth, tongue, and gums.

Fire is an EPF that readily penetrates the body, disrupting organ functions and creating IPFs. Fire attacks the Liver both directly and by drying the tendons and ligaments, the Liver's associated tissues. This generates Liver Wind, an IPF, with Wind symptoms such as dizziness, vertigo, headache, eye disorders, tremors, convulsions, and loss of consciousness.

When Mild Heat penetrates deeper and affects the Blood, it will initially quicken the pulse. Penetrating Fire can cause a syndrome called Reckless Marauding of Blood, a potentially serious bleeding disorder that forces blood out of the vessels. Symptoms may include nosebleeds, bleeding gums, coughing or spitting blood, blood in the urine and stool, and heavy uterine bleeding or hemorrhage.

Damp

- Prominent season: Late summer
- Organ most affected: Spleen
- Nature: Yin

Main Attributes and Associated Symptoms

Traditionally, Damp is the pathogen most prominent in late summer—what we might call "Indian summer"—mainly because in China that's a particularly rainy season and Damp is found everywhere. While there is a seasonal Qi, an energetic quality, that makes people more predisposed to an invasion of Damp during late summer, in practice Damp is present year-round. Extended rainy weather, foggy environments on mountaintops or by the ocean, moist forests, and indoor environments like a damp basement apartment are all capable of generating pathogenic Damp. In most cases it takes prolonged exposure for Damp to create a health problem. There can, however, be an acute sudden onset of Damp. For example, if a person gets caught in a downpour, falls into a body of water, or sweats profusely and by choice or necessity keeps their wet clothes on, Damp can readily invade the body.

Damp is thick, heavy, sticky, cloying, and turbid. These qualities make it perhaps the most stubborn, intractable pathogen to eliminate. When it affects the head, it can cause dizziness, heaviness in the head, and a persistent dull headache around the entire head. This can cloud thinking and dull emotional expression, as its turbid quality creates an opaque muddiness and lack of clarity. When it enters the meridians, Damp can cause a heavy sensation throughout the body or in the arms, legs, and head and can cause stiff, achy, or sore joints. Combined with Wind, it generates Wind Damp Bi, a painful joint obstruction common to many types of arthritis.

Damp can manifest on the surface of the body, always with an unwholesome fluid aspect such as festering sores, weeping eczema, or profuse vaginal discharge. When combined with Heat, the fluids appear yellowish and often produce a bad odor. When combined with Cold, they will appear whitish or clear and have no odor.

As a Yin pathogen, the heaviness of Damp has a downward, sinking movement and often affects the lower body first. It readily obstructs the flow of Qi and can literally dampen the expression of Yang. This can cause a heaviness and fullness in the chest, abdominal distension, scant and difficult urination (often with dribbling), and incomplete bowel movements.

The Spleen is most affected by Damp, and if compromised by other factors, it will generate Damp as an IPF. The EPF and IPF manifestations of Damp are identical in relation to the Spleen. The heaviness of Damp suppresses the Spleen's role of causing Qi to rise. As the Spleen struggles against the onslaught of Damp, Spleen Qi Deficiency is a common result. The combination of Damp and Deficiency causes abdominal fullness, loss of appetite, nausea, low energy, and loose stool or diarrhea. The Spleen's transformation and transportation functions are also impaired. This further allows the already cloying Damp pathogen to linger. The downward trajectory can involve the Kidneys and impair aspects of their fluid metabolism, leading to edema.

As the pathogenic fluids linger, they produce mucus and Phlegm. Mucus is normally secreted by mucous membranes, primarily in the head and in the lining of the lungs and alimentary tract. Mucus in the nasal passages causes either a runny or stuffy nose and is most often no more than a temporary inconvenience from a cold or allergy. In the case of chronic sinusitis, a long-term nasal obstruction that does not respond to antibiotics or decongestants, or a chronic post-nasal drip, Damp is most often responsible and must be treated to resolve the condition.

In Western medical terms, phlegm is formed in the lungs and is always relatively thick and sticky when compared to mucus, which may appear watery. The Chinese perception is not exactly the same. It observes both "substantial" and "insubstantial" phlegm. Substantial phlegm is identical to the Western understanding: the thick, gelatinous substance you may cough up from your lungs from a cold or allergy or as a complication from smoking or other diseases. Insubstantial Phlegm is less dense, is less purely physical, and may obstruct channels as well as body tissue.

Insubstantial Phlegm can appear anywhere and is stagnant and obstructive. When lodged in the channels, its stagnant quality can cause surrounding tissue to aggregate. In the body, anything stagnant blocks the flow of Qi, Blood, or other body fluids. In doing so, it causes a type of friction that generates Heat. The Heat "cooks" the obstructing Phlegm, forming nodules, cysts, or tumors. Insubstantial Phlegm is also responsible for a pattern of disharmony called Phlegm Misting the Heart. Here there are no overt physical tissue changes, but there is an impairment of the Heart function of housing the mind. Symptoms may be as mild as confused or fuzzy thinking or as serious as wildly erratic behavior, mania, complete dissociation, and insanity. A stereotypical example is an unfortunate homeless person who may be seen having an animated conversation with or directing a shouting tirade at no one visible to others.

Dryness

- Prominent season: Fall
- Organ most affected: Lungs
- Nature: Yang

Main Attributes and Associated Symptoms

Dryness is the environmental energy of autumn, when the air becomes much drier in many parts of the world. Dryness is an EPF in its own right, but a person invaded by Heat or Fire during the summertime can have a resultant internal Dryness as an IPF. In such cases dry symptoms can be obscured, muted, or delayed by the Damp of late summer, but they readily manifest in autumn, exacerbated by external Dryness. In all cases Dryness consumes body fluids, resulting in dehydration. If Heat was the initial cause and still lingers, there will be additional Heat signs, such as redness and feverish sensations.

Dryness typically invades the body through the nose and mouth. As it is a Yang pathogen causing upward and outward movement, many of its external signs appear in the upper and outer parts of the body, such as dry mouth and lips and dry nasal passages and throat, accompanied by thirst. When Dryness moves more interiorly, it can cause constipation and reduced urination.

The Lungs are most affected by Dryness. They have the function of descending, dispersing, and moistening, as well as dominating the skin, all challenged by the effects of Dryness. Other signs include dry or chapped skin, dry body hair, possible shortness of breath, and a dry cough with little phlegm. If Heat is present, the phlegm may be bloody.

Cold

- Prominent season: Winter
- Organ most affected: Kidneys
- Nature: Yin

Main Attributes and Associated Symptoms

Cold is the predominant environmental energy of winter but can affect a person in any season when it may be unusually cold, when exposed to environments that are by nature cold, like hiking up mountaintops and swimming in cold rivers, or due to human-made environments, as when entering air-conditioned buildings after being out in the high heat of summer, which leaves the pores open and especially vulnerable to invasion by Cold.

As with every EPF, some people are more prone to Cold disorders than others, due to their constitution or a preexisting Cold disharmony. A common example occurs when two people walk into the ocean together. One may immediately dive in and feel invigorated, while the other may only be able to slowly wade in to their thighs or waist before needing to retreat to the shore. The latter person has an aversion to cold, one symptom factored in to the diagnosis of a possible Cold disorder.

The primary characteristics of a Cold disharmony are often the most obvious ones. The afflicted person will avoid cold environments and seek warm ones, exhibit a preference for warm or hot beverages, will feel cold subjectively and often be cold to the touch, and will wear more or heavier clothing than other people. The person's complexion is pale or white. Other symptoms can include various clear or white bodily secretions, such as clear or white nasal mucus or phlegm, clear or watery vomit, and profuse clear urination. Cold can impair the digestive functions of the Stomach and Small Intestine, causing diarrhea with undigested food.

Cold is a Yin pathogen causing things to both slow and to constrict or condense, in the same way that flowing water will freeze into an unmoving block of ice. Such constriction obstructs the flow of Qi and by extension reduces Blood flow, causing painful contraction of the muscles and tendons, and closes the pores, causing a lack of sweat.

As Cold moves more interiorly, it can diminish or damage the body's warming Yang Qi, notably of the Kidneys and Mingmen. In addition to the above symptoms, this causes inactivity, an excessive desire for sleep, reduced sexual energy and interest, and an overall loss of vitality.

Epidemic Diseases

Epidemic diseases are sometimes thought of as a separate class of EPFs, in that they affect a large segment of the population at the same time. From a Western perspective, these are usually caused by a virus, whether the latest strain of influenza or the polio epidemics of the twentieth century. Because they are most often airborne contagions, they are a type of Wind EPF, generating expected Wind symptoms, and because they typically cause feverish symptoms, they are also a Heat EPF, often a particularly virulent Wind Heat pathogen. Other EPFs and IPFs may be part of the clinical picture depending upon the exact presentation, but Wind Heat is almost always primary.

The Seven Emotions as Internal Pathogenic Factors

The six EPFs are considered external, although they can penetrate the body to create internal changes that generate IPFs. The Seven Emotions are exclusively IPFs. All emotions are normal and usually healthy expressions of human experience. Like the environments, they can become pathogenic if extreme or prolonged, and they may be the result of an internal disharmony within any Organ System. Also as with EFPs, while there is a primary organ associated with each emotion, the emotions can and do often influence more than one organ, since all the organs have various unique interrelationships. Some examples are provided below. Generally, the organs most susceptible to emotion-based disharmonies are the Heart, Liver, and Spleen.

The Seven Emotions and their healthier, more balanced counterparts were discussed in detail with their associated organs in Chapter 5. The following is a brief review with additional information about them as IPFs.

Joy

Joy is the emotion primarily associated with the Heart. Moderate joy is healthy and beneficial, not pathogenic. Its main pathogenic qualities arise from its ability to induce overexcitement or overstimulation, which scatters the Qi and may cause heart palpitations, arrhythmia, headaches, or fainting; when very excessive, it has a manic quality that disturbs the mind (the Heart houses the mind) and Shen/spirit. Milder manifestations include insomnia, vivid and unsettling dreams, and confusion. In more extreme cases, there can be wild mood swings, true mania, and other psychological disturbances.

One stereotypical example of joy injuring the Heart is that upon receiving very good news, such as winning the lottery, a person may become so excited that they have a heart attack.

Anger

Anger is the emotion primarily associated with the Liver. It can be an appropriately healthy response to life circumstances, and if expressed and resolved in a reasonable amount of time, it is not pathogenic. It can become pathogenic when it is a prolonged response to unchanging external events or when it is a person's choice or nature to hold on to their anger.

Associated emotional variations include frustration and irritability, which can persist due to unsatisfying work or personal relationships, for example. Resentments held for a long time will injure the Liver, with passive-aggressive behavior being one result of a Liver disharmony. Depression is a related emotion that arises more from a deficient Liver condition, often a result of a long-standing frustration or from repressed anger.

Anger makes Qi rise and can cause headaches (especially migraine headaches) and dizziness, as anger may cause any of a few Liver patterns that generate Wind as an IPF. Liver Qi Stagnation is one common pattern that generates internal Heat due to its obstructive quality. Heat also rises and will add symptoms such as a red face. An idiomatic expression denoting anger is "hot under the collar," referring to this phenomenon.

Anger causes Qi to rise and Heat rises, which can easily disturb the Heart, causing many Heart symptoms like restlessness and insomnia. Liver Qi Stagnation can cause abdominal distension and discomfort and can invade the Spleen and Stomach, with the accompanying symptoms of belching or nausea, loss of appetite, and diarrhea. These are examples of ways in which anger can affect both the Heart and Spleen secondarily to affecting the Liver.

Anger and any of its related emotions (frustration, irritability, resentment, or depression) will result if the Liver is damaged by an EPF, another IPF, or through the toxic effects of alcohol, recreational drugs, or prescription drugs. Since the Liver is responsible for the smooth, free flow of Qi, the instability and unpredictability inherent in these emotions adversely affects the flow of Qi and Blood, causing a generalized physical and psychological tension.

Sadness and Grief

Sadness and grief, two similar emotions related by degree of intensity, are primarily associated with the Lungs. Sadness consumes Qi. Since the Lungs govern Qi, they are the organs initially most affected by sadness. Grief, a more intense and often lingering form of sadness, consumes Qi more seriously.

All emotions affect breathing in their own ways, causing different, distinctive breathing patterns. Since the Lungs are intrinsically involved with the mechanics of breathing, it's easiest to see how sadness and grief affect them. In grief-stricken people, the sound of their voice is described as "crying" in a Five Element context, even when they are not actually crying. Their inhalation is shallow, often sharp and brief, while their exhalation is more prolonged, and they usually take fewer breaths per minute. This is nearly identical to the breathing pattern of a person who is actively crying or sobbing. So while sadness is consuming their Qi, they are simultaneously taking in less atmospheric Qi on their inhalation and expending or dispelling more Qi with each exhalation, increasing the rate of Qi depletion.

While sadness may make someone feel tired and listless, unable to feel excited by or engaged in life, grief is much more debilitating and can seriously impact health when prolonged. This can happen to varying degrees at any age, but it's most pernicious in the elderly, who may be facing age-related health problems. For example, when one spouse dies, it's not uncommon for the other to die soon after, often within a few weeks or months. This can be directly attributed to grief consuming Qi, which is life force.

Sadness may also affect the Lungs secondarily, through the Heart. Joy primarily affects the Heart, but sadness is its polar opposite and so may also first affect the Heart. In that case, while joy scatters Qi, sadness makes it constrict and creates obstruction in the Upper Jiao, causing the feeling of "heavy-heartedness." If persisting over time, this obstruction spreads and interferes with Lung function.

Lung 9, "The Great Abyss," is the Influence Point of the vessels and can be used to strengthen a weak pulse from weakened Heart Qi. This demonstrates another relationship between the Heart and Lungs.

Because sadness depletes Lung Qi, most of its symptoms are related to the Lungs, including shortness of breath, heaviness in the chest, low energy, and possibly lowered immunity, especially in relation to the respiratory tract. Due to the Lungs' pairing with the Large Intestine, constipation is often present. Depression and emotional fragility are also common. Afflicted this way, a person may become distant, avoiding further emotional attachment rather than face the potential pain of loss.

Pensiveness/Worry

Pensiveness, sometimes translated as contemplation or rumination, includes worry and overthinking. It is the emotion primarily associated with the Spleen.

Overthinking most obviously affects those involved in rigorous mental activities, such as students, and those who are engaged in mental work, whether academics, scientists, lawyers, or accountants. Worry usually involves an element of overthinking as well, as when a mother may obsessively worry about her children when they are out of her sight or when a person may worry about their job or financial security in uncertain economic times. Worry may create a pattern of circular thought, a compulsive way of viewing things from which there may seem to be no escape. This can have a stronger impact on emotional and physical health than overthinking alone.

Worry and overthinking both cause Qi to stagnate or "knot," disturbing the Spleen's functions of transportation and transformation and weakening Spleen Qi overall. This manifests as low energy, loss of appetite, poor digestion, abdominal distension (often with a tendency to accumulate body fat), and loose stool or diarrhea.

Fear and Fright

Fear and fright are two related emotions primarily associated with the Kidneys. They are sometimes considered different intensities of the same emotion, but there are some differences. Fear is a more generalized, pervasive, and often lingering sense of dread—a state of being. Fright is more situational, involving an element of immediate surprise or shock. A horror movie fan may experience numerous frights throughout the course of the movie, reflexively covering their eyes or grabbing the person next to them while gasping from fright. Once the movie is over, the frights are gone, but there may be a disturbing sense of fearful unease that lasts a while longer.

Both fear and fright deplete the Kidneys and make Qi descend. This affects Kidney function in numerous ways. With fright alone, the abrupt sinking of Qi may make a person lose control of their bladder and involuntarily urinate. Since the Kidneys control the two lower orifices, when fear and fright are both strongly present, as when a person may suddenly realize they are facing imminent death, they may lose control of their bladder and bowels. Since the Kidneys dominate growth and development, children are very susceptible to fear and fright and may feel insecure and powerless. Such children may be prone to bed-wetting or have other developmental problems. A fearful adult may have similar insecurities and lead an isolated life as a pathological form of self-protection. That emotional hardening may translate physically into arthritis, as the Kidneys dominate the bones, and to deafness, as the Kidneys open to the ears.

Fear and fright secondarily damage the Heart, causing palpitations or insomnia. Since the Heart houses the mind, anxiety and mental confusion can result and, if persistent, can set the stage for Alzheimer's or similar mental deterioration.

Miscellaneous Factors

Most remaining causes of disease that follow are designated as miscellaneous, traditionally categorized as "not external, not internal," since they are not caused by EPFs or IPFs. Diet and lifestyle are under the control of any sufficiently motivated individual and are often given the separate designation of lifestyle factors, especially in contemporary times.

Trauma

Trauma includes any type of injury involving bodily harm. The effects of emotional trauma are contained within the context of the Seven Emotions.

Trauma may be caused by a slip and fall, a workplace accident, a sports injury, a car accident, burns, a knife or gunshot wound, or any number of similar events. Its immediate effects range from minor cuts, scrapes, bruises, sprains, strains and contusions, and blistered or raw skin to broken bones, severe blood loss, and organ damage.

The pain, swelling, and discoloration of bruising comes from Qi stagnation, as the meridians and freely circulating Qi may both be damaged by injury, and from Blood Stasis, often accompanied by extravasation, which is blood leaving damaged blood vessels and pooling under the skin or within the body as well as causing visible external bleeding.

In trauma, Qi stagnation rarely exists by itself. The pain from Qi stagnation is characterized by a diffuse, dull ache most often seen in chronic pain conditions. However, Qi stagnation does occur to varying degrees in almost all traumatic injuries and is an additional factor in Blood Stasis, since Qi moves Blood. If the Qi is not moving, Blood will not move. Blood Stasis pain is sharp and focal, existing in a readily identifiable location except in some cases of deep internal bleeding. The stronger pain of Blood Stasis is able to mask the milder pain of Qi stagnation.

There are secondary issues around trauma that can be both long lasting and less apparent. If the Qi stagnation or Blood Stasis is not completely resolved within a short while after the initial injury, it can lodge within the body, causing lingering ache and intermittent pain, while laying the foundation for further degeneration. This can occur even when the initial injury seems to be healing normally.

Chinese traumatology is well able to deal with injuries, although it is not often used for emergency care in the Western world. Acupuncture may be useful in both acute and chronic pain management, to allay Qi stagnation, and to encourage tissue repair, but herbs are the main modality of choice. They can strongly break up Qi stagnation and Blood Stasis while at the same time stop bleeding and reduce inflammation. They also add things to the body that are necessary to rebuild it after tissue damage.

Many Chinese healers are martial artists and may be deeply disciplined in spiritual practices. Whether sparring with friends to improve one's skill or fighting in earnest, traumatic injuries frequently occur. Not surprisingly, in communities where that is common, many herbal remedies for trauma have been formulated and refined for hundreds, and in some cases thousands, of years. The Shaolin monks, known since around 500 CE for their extraordinary martial skills, have hundreds of extremely effective "strike formulas" to treat everything from simple bruising to broken bones, severe bleeding, concussions, loss of consciousness, paralysis, and organ damage. Some Chinese physicians specialize in bone-setting and can reset dislocated joints as well as treat other joint dysfunctions in similar ways to chiropractors. (Bone-setting services are not legally available in the United States under Chinese medical licensure.)

Qigong, Taiji, and other movement practices are very beneficial in remedying chronic pain from Qi stagnation and Blood Stasis. While improving health in general, specific Qigongs exist to address specific conditions, and many standard Qigong practices can be modified to address those same concerns. Practitioners who are sufficiently adept can easily sense exactly where they may have pockets of obstruction or deficiency of any sort and consciously direct their Qi there to heal themselves.

This can also be very useful in acute conditions. As an example from my own life, in 2009 I suffered a serious bike accident and fractured my pelvis in four places. Since I wasn't able to put any weight on my left leg for fear of displacing the fractured bones, potentially causing life-threatening organ damage, I was basically housebound for six weeks. While I did give myself acupuncture treatments and took the appropriate herbs,

I spent a couple of hours each day running Qi through my pelvis while either sitting or laying on my back to accelerate my healing. After six weeks, the doctors told me my X-rays showed no signs that I'd ever fractured my pelvis.

Animal and Insect Bites

Animal bites cause many of the same complications as other types of trauma, including pain, swelling, broken skin, torn muscle, inflammation, and bleeding, all with accompanying Qi and Blood obstructions. Most common insect bites produce relatively mild Wind Heat symptoms, including redness, swelling, itch, and possibly pain.

Some insect and animal bites are more venomous and may induce numbness, convulsions, and paralysis, sometimes causing death. While recognized as being caused by a venomous bite, these symptoms indicate a severe Liver Wind disorder, possibly with Heat or other factors included. Some animal and insect bites contain infectious agents, bacteria, and viruses. They may cause high fevers with possible delirium, muscle aches, skin lesions, and bleeding disorders, indicative of a severe Blood Heat condition. They may also introduce parasites into the body, which can either cause skin nodules or cause poor appetite, low energy, abdominal distension, and bloody stool, indicative of Spleen Qi Deficiency.

Depending on the type of bite and the nature of the infection, many other symptoms are possible. While the obvious initial cause of the disease must be addressed and the toxic or parasitic agents expelled, the pattern of disharmony (Liver Wind, Blood Heat, and Spleen Qi Deficiency in these examples) must also be recognized and treated in order to alleviate the symptoms and return the patient to full health as soon as possible, just as in all other causes of pathology.

Imbalances in Diet and Lifestyle

When diet and lifestyle are out of balance, disrupting the natural harmony between Yin and Yang, they become causative factors of poor, declining health. They deplete Qi and make it more difficult to replenish what is lost, progressively weakening the body and reducing functionality at every level. This increases susceptibility to most other external and internal pathogenic influences, setting the stage for numerous patterns of disharmony.

Many of these factors will be familiar, as they are the type of common sense advice you might get from your family, friends, and media "health gurus" on TV or the Internet as much as you'd hear them from your healthcare provider. You may find some surprises and new slants on old ideas. Here are the basics of Chinese medical thought on dietary and lifestyle factors:

- Poor diet
- Too much or too little exercise
- Overexertion and stress with inadequate rest
- Excessive sexual activity

Diet

The first aspect of diet that can become imbalanced is the quantity of food consumed. Too much food eaten on a regular basis will cause a person to become overweight. This is the most prominent concern in the minds of most Westerners, where the weight loss industry is big business. From a Western point of view, excess weight directly causes or contributes to high blood pressure, heart disease, diabetes, metabolic syndrome, sleep apnea, fatty liver disease, kidney diseases (secondary to high blood pressure and diabetes), and even some types of cancer. Before those diseases manifest, the Chinese recognize imbalances in the Spleen and Stomach due to overeating, early warnings presenting symptoms such as bad breath, belching, acid reflux, vomiting, diarrhea, and a swollen or painful abdomen. Some common associated patterns of disharmony include Food Stagnation, Spleen Qi Deficiency, and Rebellious Stomach Qi. When these patterns are identified and remedied, the progression to the above Western diseases can be prevented.

Undereating is the counterpart to overeating and is a dietary imbalance leading to malnutrition. Whether by choice (following a strict weight-loss regimen) or life circumstance (poverty, for example), undereating reduces the amount of sustenance a person takes in. Inadequate nourishment weakens the Spleen, causing deficiencies of Qi and Blood. This sets up a downward spiral, since a weakened Spleen is less able to absorb nutrition, one of its primary functions. Any food eaten is not well absorbed and is consequently less nourishing, further weakening the Spleen.

Because the Spleen is responsible for transporting Qi throughout the body and is involved in generating Blood, the entire body is compromised. The weight that's lost is largely muscle weight, so a person will feel weak and have low energy. Weiqi (defensive Qi) is also diminished, causing increased susceptibility to all types of EPFs. Paradoxically, a weakened Spleen will cause a loss of appetite, so a sufficiently under-nourished person may not want to eat. Common associated patterns of disharmony include Spleen Qi Deficiency, and Qi or Blood Deficiencies of any organ are possible.

The next dietary concern involves eating one type of food excessively or to the exclusion of other foods. This can be due to geographical constraints and most often causes disease from specific nutritional deficiencies. For example, in some remote parts of the world polished white rice may be a common staple food, and even with the additions of some vegetables, a severe vitamin B1 deficiency may develop, causing beriberi. In other regions, the dietary staples may lack iodine, and an abnormal en-largement of the thyroid gland (a simple goiter) may result. These conditions are less common in the contemporary Western world, but diabetes, which is caused in large part by overeating sweet foods and carbohydrates that readily convert to sugars when digested, is nearly an epidemic. The related conditions of metabolic syndrome and nonalcoholic fatty liver disease, along with widespread obesity, are also caused by ex-cessive consumption of sugary foods.

Another type of overconsumption of a food type relates to the Five Tastes and their organ correspondences. They can be causative factors of disharmony when one flavor is favored over all others.

Sweet is the flavor associated with the Spleen. While a small amount of sweet food can tonify the Spleen, a large quantity will damage Spleen Qi and adversely affect all its related functions. In the Chinese way of thinking, carrots and beets are considered sweet foods, while most fruits are very sweet. I know one Qigong master who is careful to eat no more than two or three fruits per week to avoid overtaxing his Spleen.

The Spleen is disrupted by eating predominantly cold and raw foods. Cold means both the common temperature of foods, such as ice cream or iced beverages, and foods whose energetics are cold. Mint is an easy flavor to identify as energetically cold, since it is used to create a sensation of coolness when added to food or drink. However, most vegetables and fruits are energetically cool or cold. Another example is watermelon, a favorite cooling, summertime treat. Raw foods, including salads, are also cooling.

Since balance is key in every aspect of Chinese medicine, eating a moderate amount of cool foods during the hot summer months is usually not harmful, unless a person already has a compromised Spleen. When eaten predominantly or in cold weather, they may easily damage Spleen Yang, strongly impairing digestive, transformation, and transportation functions and may cause Internal Cold and Damp syndromes. This can elicit abdominal distension and pain, low energy, diarrhea, and a tendency to feel chilled easily. Damp additionally causes Phlegm, with accompanying symptoms such as sinus congestion, heaviness in the chest with a phlegmy cough and other upper respiratory problems, dizziness, a dull, pervasive headache, fuzzy thinking, mucus in the stool, and a clear or whitish vaginal discharge.

Greasy foods also engender Damp, which the Spleen dislikes. Some examples include dairy products (cheese, milk, ice cream) and deep fried or fatty foods. Alcohol, drying in some contexts, engenders Damp when consumed. Damp causes obstruction that often creates Heat, so Damp Heat syndromes can occur. In addition to the above digestive problems and Damp symptoms, Damp Heat can cause bleeding hemorrhoids, bloody mucus, and severe abscesses or clusters of boils anywhere on the skin.

Spicy flavors influence the Lungs. Small amounts of spicy foods can benefit the Lungs, stimulate its functions, and be energizing. Too much, especially if spicy and hot, can dry the Lungs and disturb its functions of opening and closing the pores, which causes profuse sweating, and a reduced ability to descend and disperse, which causes dryness throughout the body, including dry skin and hair, with increased thirst and possibly a dry cough. Since spicy foods scatter Qi and any functional activity such as sweating expends Qi, there is an accompanying loss of energy, and Weiqi diminishes, making the body more vulnerable to external pathogens.

The Stomach receives all foods consumed and is vulnerable to excessive consumption of spicy hot foods. Stomach Yin is most easily injured in this case, both from the spicy heat and from the Lung's reduced ability to moisten. This can cause heartburn, acid regurgitation, excessive hunger, bad breath, bleeding gums, and thirst for cold liquids.

Salty flavors influence the Kidneys. As with all flavors, used appropriately and in small quantities, salt can be beneficial to the Kidneys. Domesticated animals are given a little extra salt through salt licks so they will retain fluids and be encouraged to drink more water to stay well hydrated, especially in hot weather or when required to perform strenuous activities. Some wild animals seek it out for the same purposes. Salt was given to soldiers during World War II to prevent dehydration in hot jungle or desert environments, and it's still an old-school supplement used by many athletes, particularly in football training camps during the preseason hot months of July and August.[12] Specific to Chinese medicine, salty tastes can help break up cysts and nodules and are used to direct the healing effects of herbs to the Kidneys.

Since the Kidneys play a primary role in fluid metabolism, if salt is consumed excessively or for extended periods, it injures the Kidneys in ways that first manifest through their functions related to fluid metabolism: their governance of water, controlling the lower orifices, and grasping the Qi from the Lungs. Diarrhea is common, due to salt's disruptive influence on the Stomach as well as its disruption of the functioning of the lower orifices. Other early symptoms may include scanty urination and fluid retention with swelling, a simple edema. Over time this may progress to the Western diseases of high blood pressure, pulmonary edema (fluid buildup in the lungs, causing breathing difficulties and heart problems), and a few types of kidney disease. It is a factor in adrenal insufficiency and some types of sexual dysfunction.

Sour is the flavor associated with the Liver, and bitter is associated with the Heart. In the United States, these present almost no problems since they are not popular flavors and are rarely overeaten the way sweet, spicy, and salty foods are. The main exception is coffee, a very popular bitter beverage, but most chain coffee shops hide its bitterness with multiple types of sugary flavorings and milk or cream, which are also sweet flavors. The bitter quality is there even if not fully tasted, and it affects the Heart.

Coffee scatters Heart Qi in a similar way to the IPF of joy. Both can be very exciting and make the heart beat faster. Caffeine itself is a very bitter alkaloid, largely responsible for coffee's bitterness. Its effects on the Heart are very noticeable to anyone who drinks a cup more than once in a while. In many people the stimulation rapidly transforms into jitteriness and a big drop in energy—the "crash." The energy drop comes both from the scattering of Heart Qi, and the depletion of Kidney Yang Qi. (Caffeine causes you to tap into your Kidney Yang reserves.) Both are initially stimulating, but the apparent energy boost one feels from coffee is not due to any energy

---

12. "Salt Tablets," Internet FAQ Archives, The Gale Group, accessed May 10, 2016, http://www.faqs.org /sports-science/Pl-Sa/Salt-Tablets.html.

contained within the coffee. If that were true, coffee, or caffeine, could be used to power many other things. What it does is deplete your own body of its stored reserves. It's a little like spending time with a thief who takes you out and spends all kinds of money with you doing fun things. Only it's not free money; it's money that the thief is stealing from your own savings without your knowledge. What do you think happens when all your funds are gone? If you feel jittery from coffee or need to sleep soon after the stimulation wears off, those are indications that you are significantly depleting your reserves.

The final dietary cause of pathology is eating unclean food—that is, food that has spoiled, is moldy, or is contaminated with parasites. This is fairly straightforward, since it is a common cause of disease no matter what medical system is employed to diagnose it. The Chinese perspective includes impairment of the functions of the Stomach and Spleen, with symptoms such as stomach and abdominal swelling and pain, nausea, vomiting, and diarrhea. Fever may or may not be present. These symptoms are consistent with various types of food poisoning. The symptoms associated with parasites vary according to the type of parasite involved.

Other Lifestyle Factors

Balance is a key element in Chinese medical thinking when considering lifestyle. Activity is balanced by rest, wakefulness by sleep, work by play. When any component becomes excessive, the body becomes out of balance and prone to injury and illness.

Activity often becomes imbalanced due to the demands of work. That can mean excess mental work, physical work, or both. Mental overwork does not necessarily mean high-level intellectual endeavors. While people who work in the fields of high finance, medicine, academia, legislature, and science might seem to be most prone to mental overwork, those who do accounting, office work, computer programming, or any number of other jobs can expend just as much mental energy and are just as vulnerable to resultant job-related stresses.

Whether you put in long hours because you're ambitious, find your work exciting, or want to get ahead or because it's a necessity just to make ends meet, overwork causes the same imbalances. Overwork and mental expenditure depletes your Qi overall but in particular the Qi of your Heart, Spleen, and Kidneys. We've seen in Chapter 5 that the Heart houses the mind (consciousness), the Spleen houses thought (related to concentration, memorization, absorbing information, and other mental tasks), and the Kidneys house the willpower (primarily associated with goal-related activities, purposeful work, focus, and short-term memory).

Job-related stress is known to cause many heart conditions, such as hypertension, cardiovascular disease, and mental health problems, which are included in the Chinese understanding of the Heart. While usually not life-threatening, digestive disorders (related to Spleen and Stomach) and various sexual dysfunctions (related to the Kidneys) are widespread due to overwork.

Mental overwork is commonly accompanied by harmful secondary factors: eating low-quality "fast food" at irregular times and foregoing adequate sleep. These are particularly detrimental as they compound the exhaustion caused by mental overwork alone. The dietary irregularities further injure Spleen and Stomach Qi and possibly Stomach Yin. The Stomach and Spleen are responsible for restoring Qi and Blood on a daily basis. If they are not functioning normally, Qi and Blood are not adequately replenished. Sleep provides the deep rest necessary to restore and regenerate Qi, recharging your vitality. With inadequate sleep, that won't happen.

Excessive physical work can cause many of the same types of Qi depletions as excessive mental work and can create a few other problems. Physical strain can cause Qi stagnation, with or without Heat (as inflammation), and additional Spleen and Kidney harm.

The Spleen dominates the muscles, so any overuse of muscle can weaken Spleen function. Overuse of any particular muscle group causes local Qi stagnation in the overused muscles and their related joints. That's the root cause of the pain of repetitive stress injury, carpal tunnel syndrome, and other similar afflictions found in relatively sedentary people who type, mouse, or play video games excessively.

Injuries are compounded when combined with carrying or repeatedly lifting heavy objects. Postal delivery workers carry heavy mailbags, usually over one shoulder, and commonly get neck, shoulder, and low back tension and pain. Trash collectors lift trash barrels and toss their contents into trucks, using the same muscles in the same way repeatedly throughout the day.

The heavy lifting done by most construction workers can injure their low backs and knees, two parts of the body that reflect and influence Kidney health. The rapid, heavy vibrations endured by jackhammer operators damage muscle, bone, and nerves, causing numbness and pain. In addition to Spleen and Kidney injury, the Liver may be adversely affected in this case.

A variation of excess physical work is excessive exercise. Sensible exercise should be part of a healthy lifestyle, but when done improperly or excessively it causes overstrain and unhealthy physical stress, often leading to injury. If you typically sit at a desk all week, it's not a good idea to push yourself to extreme limits during the weekend. This is exactly the cause of the "weekend warrior" syndrome that lands many people in the hospital emergency room with exercise-induced injuries. Similarly, some people seem to wake up one morning and realize they've gotten out of shape and immediately begin exercising at or beyond their physical limits in order to lose weight and feel stronger and healthier. Many do lose weight but often have poor muscle tone, appear gaunt, have digestive problems, and have lower energy caused by Spleen Qi depletion from overexercise.

Even when done properly, some exercises are more likely to cause the same types of Qi stagnation caused by overwork. Anyone involved in weight training (whether with free weights, with resistance machines, or by using their body weight for resistance) should incorporate cross-training, including cardio and flexibility exercises. Both promote the flow of Qi and blood, reducing the likelihood of Qi stagnation induced by weight lifting. In China, the wisest among people engaged in the most rigorous and demanding of physical martial practices balance those practices with others specifically designed to move Qi and blood, such as Taiji and Qigong, to reverse harmful stagnations and to increase the amount of Qi available, replenishing what was exhausted. Among those who don't incorporate softer harmonizing practices, some may become very powerful in the short term but often die young from the accumulated effects of repeated injury (unresolved Qi stagnation and Blood Stasis), and from the declining health of the internal organs due to unreplenished Qi exhaustion.

In the short term, none of these excesses may cause a significant problem. If you need to occasionally make a big push to complete a work project or prepare for a final exam at school, it can cause some immediate Qi depletion. If you then revert back to a more balanced lifestyle, giving yourself the time and rest you need to replenish, you'll be able to restore your healthy balance in a matter of days. It's only when overexertion becomes your lifestyle that serious depletion can occur, causing long-term health issues.

Lack of exercise can be just as harmful as overexertion. Recently, even Western medicine has come to realize that excessive sitting, for example, poses many significant health risks, including a higher risk of death in general and from heart disease and cancer in particular. It causes high blood pressure, obesity, and high cholesterol (each of which produces a host of other diseases) as well as milder but still harmful problems such as back pain, muscle degeneration, and foggy thinking. Since the harmful effects of excessive sitting are not fully reversed by exercises, even among those who exercise regularly, a most recent slogan among media pundits and health-conscious Americans is, "sitting is the new smoking." [13]

Chinese medicine understood this approximately 2,200 years ago, as recorded in *The Yellow Emperor's Inner Classic* (*Huangdi Neijing*), a book in two parts. The first part, *Simple Questions*, lists the Five Exhaustions: Excessive use of the eyes injures the Blood (Heart), excessive lying down injures Qi (Lungs), excessive sitting injures the muscles (Spleen), excessive standing injures the bones (Kidneys), and excessive exercise injures the tendons and ligaments (Liver).

The first four Exhaustions are due to physical inactivity (arguably, most people are physically inactive when overusing their eyes), while the fifth addresses the previously discussed dangers of overwork.

Excessive Sexual Activity

Aside from concerns about sexually transmitted diseases, the idea of sexual activity as a possible cause of pathology is a foreign one in the minds of most Westerners. Chinese medicine contends that excessive sex damages Kidney Jing, the importance of which is discussed in Chapter 5. The depletion of Kidney Jing from any cause creates many health complications and accelerates aging.

Sex can be a charged topic involving significant emotional issues, intimacy and esteem considerations, personal and religious morality, and still a fair amount of titillation—all of which are fodder for the ubiquitous manipulations of advertising, entertainment, and politics—and it shapes our perceptions independent of health considerations. In a memorable exchange between characters on the classic TV show

---

13. Marc T. Hamilton, et al., "Too Little Exercise and Too Much Sitting: Inactivity Physiology and the Need for New Recommendations on Sedentary Behavior," *Current Cardiovascular Risk Reports* 2, no. 4 (July 2008): 292–98, doi:10.1007/s12170-008-0054-8 PMCID: PMC3419586 NIHMSID: NIHMS182380.

M*A*S*H, Major Charles Winchester, asking about Captain Hawkeye Pierce, says "Why this constant preoccupation with sex?" Captain B.J. Hunnicutt quips, "A lack of occupation with sex." [14]

As much as it is one of the greatest sources of love and joy capable of being shared between two people, sex can also be a source of frustration and misery. In previous times the onus of sexual dissatisfaction was largely borne by women, who were labeled as frigid if they were unwilling or unable to experience sexual pleasure. Now with erectile dysfunction (ED) being the more prominent media focus, that onus has shifted to men. ED has become more of a health problem over the last few decades. This is in large part due to the inescapable plethora of man-made hormone-disrupting pollutants in our food, water, and air from various industrial contaminants and from the inclusion of similar hormone-disrupting chemicals found in plastics (including those in which our food is packaged), the can linings of canned foods, the ink in cash register checkout receipts, and in various cosmetic and personal hygiene products, to name just a few. Since these things appeal to consumer convenience as well as commercial profitability, they are not likely to change any time soon. While these factors were not part of the original landscape of Chinese medicine, they do play a role in contemporary sexual health.

For Men

Men are more at risk of depleting themselves through excessive sex than are women, and this potentially causes many health problems. Every ejaculation expends Kidney Jing and contains between 200 and 400 million sperm, along with hormones and other nutrients. Theoretically, each sperm is capable of creating a new life. This explains in part the stereotype of a man needing to sleep immediately after having sex. Much more energy has been expended than what can be accounted for from the physical activity of sex, even when rigorous. Chinese medical thinking contends that if a man has frequent ejaculatory sex, he expends a great deal of life energy and will consequently age faster, while experiencing the various declines of health that accompany typical aging.

Determining what constitutes excessive sex varies in part according to the criteria of the purpose of the sexual activity. For example, when using sex for spiritual cultivation,

---

14. *M*A*S*H*, season 6, episode 5, "The Winchester Tapes," first broadcast 18 October 1977 by CBS, directed by Burt Metcalfe and written by Everett Greenbaum and James Fritzell.

as in higher-level tantric yoga and Daoist sexual practices, men are taught to control their ejaculations and have injaculations, rarely actually emitting semen—the famous Tang Dynasty physician and Daoist adept Sun Simiao recommended one ejaculation out of every hundred instances of intercourse—so that energy can be channeled internally for physical rejuvenation and spiritual development. When having such nonejaculatory sex, there are no limits on sexual activity. The practice of ejaculation control is outside the scope of this book, but it is referred to in order to stress the importance the Chinese and other non-Western cultures place on semen retention and its role in preserving health and increasing longevity.

The Qi cultivation practice of Qigong has different criteria that can vary among different systems. Many advanced Qigongs require sexual abstinence for one hundred days while a person begins the practice in order to conserve Jing and Qi, helping to strengthen and consolidate the Qi body so that it may better hold the energetic charge of the practice and speed cultivation. In most Qigong systems, it is at least recommended that men avoid sex for up to two hours before and after their practice times. This ties in with the above understanding that ejaculation depletes a man's Jing and by extension his Qi, Yang, and Yin. Having sex too soon after a practice will discharge too much energy and undo much of the benefit of the practice. After sex, the body continues to lose Qi for a period of time, until the man is rested and the Qi body is again consolidated. Practicing too soon after sex isn't harmful, but it's a waste of time, as it won't store the Qi from the practice; it's like pouring water through a sieve.

For men who are not involved in any such practices and are engaging in sex primarily for intimacy, procreation, or recreation, the criteria are purely for preserving health by avoiding undue depletion, which means aligning with the rhythms of nature. Even here there can be some variability, as not every person is physically and energetically the same. What's excessive for one man may not be for another, based on relative strength, health, and age. It's important to honestly gauge your personal circumstances to determine what that is for yourself. In his book *The Tao of Health, Sex, and Longevity*, Daniel Reid cites from "The Plain Girl" (the second book of the *Huangdi Neijing*, written around 100 BCE) these general guidelines recommended for ejaculatory frequency: At twenty, a man in good health may ejaculate twice per day. For a man of average health or less, no more than once per day. At thirty, a man in good health may ejaculate once per day. For a man of average health or less, no more than once every other day. At forty, a man in good health may ejaculate once every three days. For a man of average health or less, no more than once every four days. At fifty, a man in good health may ejaculate once every five days. For a man of average health or less, no more than once every ten days. At sixty, a man in good health may ejaculate once every ten days. For a man of average health or less, no more than once every twenty days. At seventy, a man in good health may ejaculate once every thirty days. A man of average health or less should abstain from ejaculation entirely.[15]

In his book *The Tao of Sexology*, Dr. Stephen Chang reports that some ancient Daoist texts recommend a stricter system, whereby ejaculation frequency in days should be limited to the man's age × 0.2. That would mean a twenty-year-old should limit ejaculations to once every four days (20 × 0.2 = 4), a thirty-year-old to once every six days (30 × 0.2 = 6), and so on.[16] While this too is a recommendation for health purposes and not spiritual cultivation, it is intended for those wanting superior rather than average health.

Since the seasons cycle each year, there is another consideration when aligning with rhythms of nature. Sexual activity should be at its peak during the springtime, when everything in nature is germinating and Yang is growing. During the wintertime, everything in nature is still and dormant, the peak of Yin. Sexual activity should be minimal during this time of conservation of Yang. Daniel Reid quotes the Han Dynasty master Liu Ching, recorded as having lived over 300 years: "In spring, a man may permit himself to ejaculate once every three days, but in summer and autumn he should limit his ejaculations to twice a month. During the cold of winter, a man should preserve his semen and avoid ejaculation altogether. … One ejaculation in winter is 100 times more harmful than an ejaculation in the spring."[17]

Except when working with spiritual, Qi, or longevity cultivation practices, these guidelines do not need to be strictly adhered to in most circumstances. They should serve as reminders, used to preserve or restore health in any instance where excessive

---

15. Daniel P. Reid, *The Tao of Health, Sex, and Longevity: A Modern Practical Guide to the Ancient Way* (New York: Fireside Publishing, 1989), 295.

16. Chang, Stephen T. *The Tao of Sexology: The Book of Infinite Wisdom* (San Francisco: Tao Publishing, 1986), 84–85.

17. Reid, *The Tao of Health, Sex, and Longevity*, 295.

sex, however that may be defined for you, may be causing health problems. Here are some indications to look for:

If you find yourself with lower energy for a day or two after having sex—one of my patients referred to it as having a "brownout"—your body is too weak to have sex at whatever frequency is causing that low energy. Other signs may include feeling cold after sex, chronic fatigue, irritability, catching colds easily or other signs of a weakened immune system, frequent day or night urination, dribbling after urination, and low back or knee pain. Loss of interest in sex, lowered libido, and ED are often the result of previously excessive sex. With serious imbalances, it might be necessary to eliminate sex until you have restored your health. Taking medication that treats ED only allows you to further deplete your body when it is already harmfully depleted. The hormone-disrupting pollutants and additives discussed at the beginning of this section accelerate and exacerbate these and other pathological changes related to sex.

For Women

While women are much more hormonally complex than men, they lose comparatively little Jing during sex and orgasm. Consequently, there are no recommended restrictions on frequency of intercourse for women. Women can lose Jing, Yin, Yang, Qi, and Blood during pregnancy and childbirth. Care should be taken to minimize those depletions and restore them to healthy levels as soon as possible postpartum.

One of the Six Extraordinary Yang Organs, the Uterus is both contained within the region of the Dantian and strongly related to the Kidneys. Anything that affects the Uterus can influence all of a woman's physical energy through the Dantian, including the functional energy of all the organs, as well as influence Kidney Jing, Yin, and Yang. So while pregnancy is a healthy, natural process, it can stress the uterus and other parts of the body, and women may feel changes in their energy levels and overall health while some of their vitality is directed toward growing a healthy baby.

In a normal pregnancy, there are often signs of Liver Qi Stagnation (swollen, tender breasts, dizziness, and emotional changes), Spleen Qi Deficiency (fatigue, food cravings or aversions, hemorrhoids, and bleeding gums), Rebellious Stomach Qi (nausea, with or without vomiting, and heartburn, which may also come from Stomach Yin Deficiency), and various Kidney deficiencies (frequent and increased urination, backache, and vaginal discharge, which may also come from Spleen Qi Deficiency).

Headaches are common and may come from various patterns of disharmony, most often involving the Liver or Spleen.

Barring complications, the energy lost during pregnancy and labor should cause no lasting depletion or imbalance for the mother, assuming adequate time is allotted for rest, good nutrition is maintained, and moderate exercise and other restorative practices are followed. However, if a woman becomes pregnant again too soon, before she has had time to recover fully from the previous pregnancy, that can cause a Jing depletion as significant as excessive sex will cause in a man, and it presents many of the same symptoms. Additional symptoms may include menstrual irregularities and chronic vaginal discharge. If that pattern is frequently repeated so that the woman bears many children in a short period of time, it can seriously compromise her health and accelerate aging.

Chapter 8

Introducing Patterns of Disharmony

Patterns of disharmony are the ways in which the body responds to the pathogenic influences introduced in Chapter 7; they are the various types of imbalances possible as a result of those influences. When correctly diagnosed and treated, harmony can be restored long before a Western biomedical disease emerges. This is how Chinese medicine is used preventatively.

Once a Western-defined disease is present, Chinese medicine can still be employed to restore balance by reducing or eliminating all the symptoms of disease, but it can take longer if the pathogens causing the disease were present longer and created deeper, more disruptive imbalances. Even in this case, it is the pattern of disharmony that must be rectified, as that reflects the condition of the whole person and not just the disease and its symptoms. A Western diagnosis may be helpful as a shortcut to identifying a number of symptoms, but it cannot take the place of identifying the pattern of disharmony.

Many Patterns for One Disease; One Pattern for Many Diseases

In Chinese medicine the Western disease diagnosis is not so important. The same signs and symptoms present in those diseases are observed along with other symptoms that are only relevant to a Chinese physician. That collection of symptoms is a set of indicators guiding the physician to determine the imbalance within a particular organ or among various organs that constitutes a Chinese diagnosis.

Using the example of diabetes from Chapter 7, a Chinese correlation for one common constellation of diabetes symptoms is called *San Da*, or "The Three Bigs": big thirst, big hunger, and big urination. A person may have one, two, or all three of those symptoms. Big thirst is an indicator of an Upper Jiao disharmony, big hunger indicates a Middle Jiao disharmony, and big urination is a Lower Jiao disharmony. With just that understanding, there are already seven possible diagnoses based only on the involved Jiao. The organs in the related Jiao would be further examined for the full nature of the disorder, including variables in Qi, Blood, Yin, Yang, deficiency, excess, and so on. Additionally, a person's constitution is considered, along with contributing lifestyle and environmental factors. Only then would a diagnosis and treatment plan be made. It's entirely possible that ten patients with a Western diagnosis of Type 2 diabetes might be treated in ten different ways by a Chinese physician, based on the exact presentation of each patient. A Chinese physician cannot effectively treat a patient for Type 2 diabetes without a Chinese diagnosis.

Another category of disharmony, Wasting and Thirsting Syndrome, is seen in numerous types of Western-defined diseases, including tuberculosis, cancer, and AIDS. Depending on their presentations, which in almost every case includes the severe weight loss and dehydration that gives the syndrome its name, it's possible that a tuberculosis patient, a cancer patient, and an AIDS patient might be given exactly the same treatment by a Chinese physician. A Western diagnosis may be a helpful adjunct toward making a Chinese diagnosis, but it will never have a one-to-one correspondence and is of limited value in this context.

The Chinese diagnosis names the nature of the imbalance. In the example of diabetes, that might be Lung Yin Deficiency for an Upper Jiao disorder, Spleen Qi or Yin Deficiency for a Middle Jiao disorder, and Kidney Yin or Yang Deficiency for a Lower Jiao disorder. For Wasting and Thirsting conditions, the root disharmony often includes Kidney Yin and/or Jing Deficiency.

Examples of other pattern names involving more than one organ include Kidneys Failing to Grasp the (Lung) Qi, which often presents as asthma; Heart and Kidney Failing to Communicate, common in types of insomnia; or Liver Invading the Spleen, which is seen when appetite and digestion are disturbed by stress or emotional upsets.

These patterns of disharmony are not the cause of the distress but the result of the pathology that created the imbalance.

Any pattern of disharmony can have many possible causes as the root pathology. Sometimes the pathology is named in the pattern, as in Wind Heat Invading the Lungs, a diagnosis made in some types of common cold. In any case, the root pathology must be identified and addressed in order to completely resolve the condition, thereby restoring balance.

From a Western medical perspective, this is similar to restoring and maintaining homeostasis. The Chinese perspective is best encapsulated by the image of the Taiji (Yin Yang) symbol, a representation of the state of dynamic equilibrium introduced in Chapter 3. This includes restoring and maintaining balance within each individual organ, balance among all the internal organs, emotional balance; balanced dietary and lifestyle choices, balance between the individual and the environment, and (ideally and ultimately) balance and alignment among body, mind, and spirit. This is complete holistic balance, the highest realization of Chinese medicine.

The Lenses of Diagnosis

Chinese medicine has existed for thousands of years. During its long history, numerous medical philosophies emerged, each with its preferred diagnostic and treatment methods. Many still exist and are practiced today. Those most practiced in the West are Traditional Chinese Medicine (TCM) and Five Element. Despite its name, TCM is the newest system, developed in the 1950s as a way to incorporate and standardize most other Chinese medical systems in use today.

Those systems include Eight Principle and Zangfu (Internal Organs), which are among the oldest and most interrelated and are found to some degree in most other systems. Along with Pathogenic Factors, they are the systems most used in TCM. Channel and Collateral, Six Stage, Four Level (introduced in Chapter 3), and Sanjiao diagnoses are all discrete systems used primarily when a disorder clearly indicates one of those systems as the best model to choose, in specialized circumstances. In the diabetes example from the previous section, a Sanjiao model might be the most useful choice. A Four Level diagnosis of Heat in the Blood might be made in some types of bleeding disorders. There are further diagnostic systems focusing on Qi, Blood, and body fluid patterns. All these systems are contained under the TCM umbrella, often subsumed in an Eight Principle or Zangfu diagnosis, and weighted according to the needs of the patient.

When any one system is selected, it must be adhered to throughout pathology identification, diagnosis, and treatment principle. "Mix and match" is not applicable here, meaning you can't make a Six Stage diagnosis and then employ a Five Element treatment principle. For the purposes of this book, the particulars of those specialized systems are not important to include in your self-care practice, as they are most relevant to medical professionals. Mention is made only to acquaint readers with the possibilities included in the broad scope of Chinese medicine. Here, we'll primarily focus on the Eight Principle, Zangfu, and pathogenic factor aspects of TCM.

As the Five Element system is still widely practiced apart from TCM, a few additional comments are warranted before moving on. Five Element philosophy as included in other parts of this book presents the aspects that are most used in a TCM context. Such things as the Five Seasons with their corresponding Five Environmental Energies, the Five Tastes, the Five Emotions (with two having subdivisions, creating Seven Emotions), and the Five Elemental correspondences themselves (Wood, Fire, Earth, Metal, and Water) all originate within the Five Element/Five Phase system, and all are features commonly used by TCM practitioners. Remember that TCM is intended as a way to include and standardize all of the various traditional systems of Chinese medicine.

Strict classical Five Element practitioners have a somewhat different view of Chinese medicine, rooted in Daoist philosophies, with their own diagnostic criteria and treatment principles. Within that Five Element context, their methods are broader and deeper than the Five Elements as they are typically employed in TCM. Accordingly, the Five Element system has different patterns of disharmony, yet many of those patterns have close analogues in TCM, with slight variations. For example, the Zangfu diagnosis of Liver Invading the Spleen is nearly identical to the Five Element diagnosis of Wood Overacting on Earth. Including those variations here would be more confusing than helpful, especially for readers relatively new to Chinese medicine. Still, it's important to understand that there are many possibilities open to you, especially when considering professional Chinese medical help.

Criteria of TCM Pattern Identification

Everything presented in this book up to this point (Qi, meridians, Yin and Yang, internal organs, pathogenesis, and all systems of Chinese medicine) is considered in TCM pattern identification. The following are three of the main criteria and among the most commonly used.

The first criterion is the Eight Principles. This is covered in detail in Chapter 3. The Eight Principles are defined by the core polarities of Yin and Yang, fundamental to every Chinese medical system, along with three subsidiary pairs of versatile, diagnostically significant polarities.

The Eight Principles	
Yin	**Yang**
Interior	Exterior
Cold	Hot
Deficiency	Excess

The second criterion requires understanding the functions of the Zangfu, the internal organs. Knowing these functions allows for identifying what organs are affected by pathogenic influences—present symptoms point the way to the involved organs—and in what ways they are affected. Those ways can be determined through Eight Principle analysis and through identification of the pathogenic influences. The functions of the organs are covered in detail in Chapters 4, 5, and 6.

The third and final criterion we'll include is identifying the pathogenic influence(s) affecting the involved organ(s). Those are covered in detail in Chapter 7.

Before introducing the specific patterns, let's review and expand on the factors used in the Eight Principles. They inform all pattern identification and are the most simple, direct, and applicable diagnostics in all of Chinese medicine. A careful understanding of them is very helpful when selecting the most beneficial self-care practices taught in this book.

Eight Principle Considerations

Yin and Yang

Apart from representing every polar opposite, within the body Yin and Yang exist on a continuum between substance and functional energy. Yin substance includes blood and other body fluids, along with all body tissues, such as muscles, bones, organs, and so on. Yang functional energy includes Qi and its most active Yang aspect. It powers all cellular metabolism, the functions of every organ, every movement, and every thought.

Within Eight Principle diagnostics, Yin and Yang both summarize the other six principles—Interior, Cold, and Deficiency are Yin qualities; Exterior, Hot, and Excess are Yang qualities—and are related attributes used in differentiating and honing a diagnosis. For example, heat is a Yang quality, but the appearance of Heat in the body is not enough on its own to determine if it's caused by a Yang pathogen or syndrome. In the case of Excess Heat, there is in fact too much Yang, as you might expect. Cool or Cold is a Yin quality, which normally balances the warming Yang. In the case of a Deficiency Heat pattern, there is insufficient Yin to balance the Yang, and even if Yang is completely normal, there will be the appearance of Heat. There are numerous signs and symptoms used to make this distinction, discussed under "Cold and Hot."

The insufficiency of Yin illustrates a type of simple Yin deficiency, Deficiency Heat. There are comparable Yang deficiencies causing Deficiency Cold.

Interior and Exterior

Interior and Exterior, or Deep and Superficial, are used to determine the *location* of a disharmony.

The most interior parts of the body include nerves, organs, blood, and bones. Any pattern affecting these parts of the body is considered internal. IPFs (emotions and internally generated climates) and other Yin-Yang imbalances are internal and are the most typical causative factors.

The most exterior parts of the body include skin, muscles, and meridians. Any pattern affecting these parts of the body is considered external. The EPFs are external and are the most typical cause of external patterns.

There can be confusing presentations, as when an EPF may cause an internal disharmony. EPFs typically cause external patterns unless they invade deeper and transform into IPFs. External Wind Cold is an EPF, and if it causes a pattern that remains on the surface of the body, such as a simple cold with possible headaches, muscle aches, and sinus congestion, then it is an external pattern. But if the Wind Cold invades deeper, disrupts normal Lung functions, and causes the difficult breathing and wheezing characteristic of asthma, then the pattern is an internal one, regardless of its origins as an EPF.

Similarly, an internal pattern can cause external symptoms. Blood Heat, or Fire Toxins in the Blood, is frequently seen in biomedically defined conditions like viral infections or food poisoning and can cause rashes to appear on the skin. Despite the external symptom, further analysis will reveal it to be due to an internal pattern. As another example, Internal Heat from any cause will frequently cause the blood to dry and inadequately nourish muscles, presenting stiff, tight, achy muscles. By itself, superficial muscle tension may be taken as evidence of an external pattern, but here it is a symptom of an internal pattern, which may require further differentiation to ascertain.

Cold and Hot

Cold is Yin, and Hot is Yang. They help identify the basic *nature* of a pathology and are most advantageously viewed in combination with Deficiency and Excess to determine their most accurate nature.

Cold may be present from either a deficiency or an excess. There are distinguishing symptoms for each type. Excess Cold is a true Yin cold presentation. Yang energies may be completely normal, but Yin is present in excess, overwhelming Yang and causing Excess Cold symptoms. (In practice, excess Yin will consume some Yang, so it's likely there will be some Yang deficiency.) This is a Yin pathology. Deficiency Cold occurs when Yin energies may be normal, but Yang is deficient, unable to balance the cooling quality of Yin. This is a Yang pathology.

In just the same way, Heat may be present from either a deficiency or an excess. Excess Heat is a true Yang heat presentation. Yin energies may be completely normal, but Yang is present in excess, overwhelming Yin and causing Excess Hot symptoms. (In practice, excess Yang will consume some Yin, so it's likely there will be some Yin deficiency.) This is a Yang pathology. Deficiency Heat occurs when Yang energies may be normal, but Yin is deficient, unable to balance the warming quality of Yang. This is a Yin pathology.

Deficiency and Excess

Deficiency and Excess are used to describe the *strength* of the pathogenic influence relative to the body's defensive (Wei) and normal (Zheng) Qi. A strong EPF or IPF confronting strong defensive and normal Qi will produce symptoms consistent with an Excess condition. This is most common in acute conditions. Whether a pathogen is present or not, if the body's energy is low, the symptoms will almost always indicate a Deficiency condition. This is most common in chronic conditions.

The attributes considered in Deficient and Excess conditions are Yin, blood, Cold, Heat, Qi, and Yang. All can be deficient throughout the body. Yin, Cold, Heat, and Yang can be excessive throughout the body, but Qi and blood are almost always only excessive in relatively small, localized regions. Liver Qi Stagnation is a common pattern of disharmony indicating an excess of Qi localized within the Liver. Qi can become obstructed—excessive—in the channels, which can cause localized joint pain. Common to everyone's experience, the black and blue mark from a bruise is visible Blood Stasis, a local excess of unmoving blood under the skin.

Chapter 9

Selected Patterns of Disharmony

In TCM alone, there are scores of possible patterns of disharmony. The previous chapter introduced the three main criteria used in pattern identification. There may be only one or more than one organ involved in a pattern, and there can be complex presentations, in which Heat and Cold or Dry and Damp appear together, for example.

The Five Element system relies on some of the same criteria but has its own approach to pattern identification. There are patterns based on Qi and body fluids, along the spectrum of Yang, Qi, blood, and Yin. Other systems briefly introduced, Four Level and Six Stage, have their own patterns, as do other less common systems.

There can be some overlap among patterns, as Phlegm Misting the Heart is both a Zangfu and a body fluid pattern, and Spleen Qi Deficiency is both a Zangfu and a Qi pattern. This common pattern feature allows for great refinement and discrimination in pattern identification.

Some contemporary approaches may use Western disease names as an entry point to pattern identification, in part as an appeasement to the prevalence of Western medicine, in part because most Western-oriented patients are more comfortable with familiar terminology, and in part because the Western diagnosis offers one set of symptoms that can be included in a Chinese diagnosis. A pattern of disharmony will ultimately be used to differentiate among the many possible causes of the Western disease.

All of these patterns are important to the health professional. For our purposes, I'll share a few patterns here to give you a better idea of what they are and how they work. Pattern diagnosis is extensive and fairly complex to try to include in your self-care assessment. Still, it's useful to have some understanding of it both to further your knowledge of Chinese medicine and to have a frame of reference should you consult a Chinese physician for any health challenge. Readers wanting more detailed information about patterns are directed to Ted Kaptchuk's *The Web That Has No Weaver* for an accessible succinct account or to Giovanni Maciocia's *The Foundations of Chinese Medicine* for a comprehensive and professional yet still very approachable textbook presentation. (See Bibliography.)

These selected patterns are among the most common, and there is one for each Yin organ. The relevance of the included tongue and pulse diagnosis is discussed in Chapter 10.

1. Wind Cold Invading the Lungs

Main Symptoms

Cough, itchy throat, possible fever, aversion to cold, sneezing, nasal congestion or a runny nose with clear or white mucus, headache, most commonly at the back of the head, body aches, a reduced or absent ability to sweat, a thin, white tongue coating, and a floating (superficial) pulse, especially in the front (Lung and Heart) position.

Explanation

This is a common cold caused by the EPFs Wind and Cold attacking the Lungs.

The Lungs are the most external of the internal Yin organs. They are the canopy of the organs, protecting the other five Yin organs. They govern Qi (with a special connection to Weiqi, defensive Qi, which primarily circulates just under the skin) and respiration, open to the nose, and dominate the skin. Anatomically, they connect more or less directly with the throat via the trachea.

Being relatively external and protective, they are usually the first Organ System attacked by EPFs. As Wind and Cold obstruct the Lungs, their descending function is impaired, causing cough due to Qi rising inappropriately. That also obstructs the nose, causing nasal congestion or runny nose with sneezing. Wind is irritating, which contributes to the sneezing and causes the itchy throat.

If the EPF is strong and the Weiqi is strong, Weiqi will rise to fight off the EPF, causing the floating pulse, and the struggle between Qi and the EPF causes fever. If the

EPF is not very strong or the Weiqi is weak or unresponsive, there will be no fever, as this EPF is primarily Cold. Aversion to cold will be stronger than fever if fever is present. The combination of Cold and obstruction of the Lung channel closes the pores of the skin, leading to reduced sweat. The channel obstruction further causes headaches and body aches. (Any obstruction of Qi or Blood causes pain.) The warming aspect of the Weiqi is impaired, causing aversion to cold. While a thin, white tongue coating is generally considered normal, here white indicates Cold, and the thin quality only means that the EPF has not yet penetrated deeply to become Excessive.

A related pattern for comparison is a Wind Heat cold, which will be similar but with the following differences. The cough may be productive, and the phlegm, along with the nasal mucus, will be yellow instead of white. (Yellow indicates Heat, due to a "burning" of the mucus.) The throat will be sore instead of just itchy. There will be fever, possibly with aversion to cold, but the fever will be stronger. There will be some sweat and an aversion to Wind. The tongue may appear slightly red (indicating Heat) with a thin yellow coating. The pulse is still floating but rapid. All these changes are due to Heat replacing Cold as the EPF.

With the proper presentation, some Western diagnoses that may fit this pattern include bronchitis and emphysema.

Some common Lung patterns include Lung Qi Deficiency and Lung Yin Deficiency.

2. Heart Blood Deficiency

Main Symptoms

Heart palpitations, forgetfulness, anxiety, insomnia, excessive or very vivid dreaming, causing disturbed sleep, dizziness, a pale complexion, pale and possibly dry tongue, and a thready and weak pulse.

Explanation

This pattern can be caused by poor nutrition, either due to inadequate quantity or quality of food consumed, to a poorly functioning Spleen and Stomach that are unable to properly digest and absorb nutrition from any food that is eaten, or to extended periods of anxiety or stress that disturb the mind, eventually impairing Heart functions. It can also be caused by severe blood loss from any cause.

We've seen that Blood is the primary material foundation for Qi within the body, according to the Chinese phrase, "Blood is the mother of the Qi." Whenever Blood is deficient, there will inevitably be some Qi deficiency, and this is what causes palpitations—a tangible disturbance in the heart's functional energy.

As the Heart houses the mind, any weakening of the Heart will disturb the mind, as it is less securely housed. This causes the restlessness of insomnia, dream-disturbed sleep, and anxiety or generalized feelings of unease. The insufficiency of Heart Blood fails to nourish the brain, causing poor memory and dizziness.

The pale complexion and tongue—the Heart opens to the tongue—indicate Heart Blood Deficiency. Similarly, the thready pulse indicates insufficient blood, and the weakness indicates Deficiency.

A related pattern for comparison is Heart Yin Deficiency, which shows many of the same symptoms—remember that Blood is a Yin substance—with some differences. There will be some Deficiency Heat symptoms, since the Yin deficiency will allow for the warming aspect of Yang to go unchecked. This causes feelings of warmth in the palms of the hands, soles of the feet, and the center of the chest and feelings of agitation, all worse in the afternoon and evening. There may be night sweats. The tongue will appear light red and dry, and the pulse will be rapid.

With the proper presentation, some Western diagnoses that may fit this pattern include arrhythmia, tachycardia, high blood pressure, anemia, and some psychological disorders.

Some common Heart patterns include Heart Qi Deficiency, Heart Yang Deficiency, Phlegm Misting the Heart, and Heart Blood Stagnation.

3. Liver Qi Stagnation

Main Symptoms

Emotional: Irritability, frustration, inappropriate anger, and depression, possibly accompanied by sighing and a feeling of "a lump in the throat."

Gastrointestinal: Poor appetite, hiccups, belching, acid reflux, nausea, vomiting, abdominal distension and discomfort or pain often extending to just below the ribs, and diarrhea.

Menstrual irregularities: Long, short, or variable cycles, cramps, pain, premenstrual breast distension and tenderness, mood swings, and irritability.

The tongue may be normal or have a dusky, slightly purplish appearance, and the pulse is bowstring (strong, pounding, with a slight hardness).

Explanation

Due largely to its emotional correspondences and the menstrual problems that affect so many women, this Excess pattern is one of the most pervasive in the modern world.

Since the emotions associated with the Liver are anger and depression along with related emotions, Stagnant Liver Qi alters Liver function in ways that cause these emotions to become prevalent. In a Five Element context, sighing is the sound associated with the Spleen, which is easily affected by Liver Qi Stagnation. Sighing is also one of the body's ways to release or disperse Qi stagnation. When people get emotional, they often feel a sense of having a lump in their throat. When the emotions linger as they do in Qi stagnation, the sense of that lump will also linger, resulting in the Chinese designation "plum-pit Qi," the feeling of having a plum pit stuck in the throat. An internal branch of the Liver meridian runs through the throat, contributing to this sensation.

Most of the gastrointestinal symptoms in this pattern come from the stagnant, excessive Liver Qi moving horizontally to affect the Spleen and Stomach. This is a secondary pattern called Liver Invading the Spleen, commonly but not always found in cases of Liver Qi Stagnation. The hiccups, belching, acid reflux, nausea, and vomiting are due to the pattern of Rebellious Stomach Qi, an abnormal rising of Stomach Qi due to its being compromised by the invasion of Liver Qi. Poor appetite and diarrhea are due to a weakening of Spleen Qi, again caused by the invading Liver Qi.

The abdominal distension, discomfort, and pain extending to the sides and just below the ribs is due to the Qi stagnation in the Liver meridian, which runs through the abdomen and below the eleventh rib along the flanks. The organ may feel swollen or congested due to the primary stagnation occurring there.

Most of the menstrual concerns are caused by the Liver's function of storing Blood, which becomes impaired from Liver Qi Stagnation. This deranges (interrupts) Blood movement in the Chong and Ren meridians (see Chapter 2), directly affecting the uterus and causing menstrual irregularities and pain. Breast distension and tenderness are caused by the Qi stagnation in the Liver and Chong meridians, which have internal branches that run through and influence the breasts.

The tongue may appear dusky due to Stagnant Liver Qi poorly moving the Blood —"the Qi is the commander of the Blood"—causing the dark, purplish appearance common to Blood Stasis. The pulse is bowstring due to obstruction by Liver Qi. More force is required to move through, or against, the obstruction. Likewise pain, also caused by obstruction, produces a bowstring pulse.

With the proper presentation, some Western diagnoses that may fit this pattern include cervical lymphadenitis, mastitis, and various gastrointestinal, gynecological, and emotional disorders.

Some common Liver patterns include Internal Liver Wind, Flare-Up of Liver Fire, Liver Yang Rising, and Liver Blood Stasis.

4. Spleen Qi Deficiency

Main Symptoms

Poor appetite, low energy, fatigue, weak arms and legs, loose stool or diarrhea, heaviness after meals, abdominal distension, nausea, bruising easily, speaking in a very soft voice, a pale tongue with tooth marks on the sides, possibly enlarged (if Spleen Qi Deficiency engenders Damp), and a weak, forceless, and thin or thready pulse.

Explanation

As with Liver Qi Stagnation, Spleen Qi Deficiency is a very common pattern, caused by overwork, overthinking and worry, poor dietary choices, and irregular daily schedules.

The Spleen governs transformation and transportation, converting food and drink into useable substances and transporting nutrition and Qi throughout the body. When those functions are compromised by Qi deficiency, this causes the digestive symptoms of poor appetite, abdominal distension, heaviness after meals, nausea, and loose stool or diarrhea. A weak Spleen is not well able to transform fluids and causes internally generated Damp, contributing to the heavy sensations and nausea due to its obstructive qualities. In that case, this becomes a complex pattern, as it exhibits signs of both Deficiency from the primary pattern and Excess from the localized or systemic presence of Damp.

Qi is the body's functional energy, and when it is deficient, there are various signs of weakness, such as low energy, fatigue, speaking very softly and generally avoiding talking, and weak arms and legs. The Spleen dominates the muscles and the four limbs, so weakness appears there most obviously. If Damp is present, it causes the limbs to feel heavy.

The Spleen controls Blood. Part of that function means it is responsible for holding blood within the vessels. With Spleen Qi Deficiency, that function is impaired and a person will bruise easily.

A pale tongue with tooth marks along the sides indicates Qi Deficiency. Spleen Qi generates Blood, which is reduced in deficiency, so the tongue appears pale. The presence of Damp causes the tongue to enlarge. While it's easy to see how an enlarged tongue can have tooth marks, in Spleen Qi Deficiency without Damp, a normal-sized tongue can have tooth marks. With Damp from other causes and no Spleen Qi Deficiency, the tongue may be enlarged with no tooth marks.

The forceless pulse quality comes from Qi deficiency, and the threadiness is due to the Spleen's inability to generate adequate Blood.

A related pattern for comparison is Spleen Yang Deficiency, which includes all the signs of Spleen Qi Deficiency, but, as it is more severe and as Yang is a warming energy, there are additional signs. Fatigue and listlessness are worse. The person becomes easily chilled and feels cool or cold to the touch. Stool is watery and contains bits of undigested food as the Spleen's transformation and transportation functions are further impaired. This may cause edema, as fluids can accumulate under the skin, and the tongue can appear wet from excess fluid. The pulse is weak, slow from the Cold, and deep from the pathology moving deeper into the interior.

With the proper presentation, some Western diagnoses that may fit this pattern include ulcers, gastritis, enteritis, hepatitis, and dysentery.

Some common Spleen patterns include Sinking Spleen Qi, Damp Cold Invading the Spleen, Damp Heat Invading the Spleen, and Spleen Not Controlling Blood.

5. Kidney Yang Deficiency

Main Symptoms

Cold and sore low back, cold and weak knees, premature ejaculation, impotence, frequent profuse or scant clear urination, loose stool, a bright white complexion, aversion to cold, cold and weak arms and legs, low energy, fatigue, edema, a quiet voice, being withdrawn, listlessness, and apathy. If chronic, loose teeth and hearing loss are possible. The tongue is moist, swollen, and pale with tooth marks on the sides, and the pulse is thready, weak, deep, and slow.

Explanation

This Deficient pattern of Interior Cold is also called Deficiency of Mingmen (Gate of Vitality) Fire. It reflects numerous depletions most frequently caused by prolonged illness, excess sexual activity, or old age. As deficient Kidney Yang fails to warm the body, Cold signs are a prominent feature, including cold low back, knees, and limbs and an aversion to cold with a preference for warm environments, foods, and beverages. A bright white complexion indicates Cold. When prolonged, this condition may alternatively present pallor, which is a sickly, colorless, ashen complexion.

Kidney Yang Deficiency includes Kidney Qi Deficiency. With inadequate Qi, the Kidneys are unable to support the bones, low back, and knees—the kidneys are located in the low back and have a special relationship with the knees—so there is soreness there and weakness in the limbs. Since the Kidneys dominate the bones and open to the ears, teeth (an extension of bone) may become loose, and hearing diminishes. Deficient Qi and Yang cause low energy, fatigue, and a weak or quiet voice and make a person listless, apathetic, and withdrawn.

The Kidneys govern reproduction. The decline of Kidney Yang and Mingmen Fire fails to warm Jing (essence), and so sexual energy diminishes, causing premature ejaculation and impotence in men and infertility in women.

The Kidneys control the two lower orifices (urethra and anus) and urination, are the Origin of Water, and are involved with every aspect of fluid metabolism. When Kidney Yang is deficient, it loses its ability to effectively transform fluids and control the urethra, resulting in frequent profuse clear urination from the accumulation of fluids. Sometimes the Yang may be so deficient that it is unable to supply the power necessary to urinate, and in that case there will be scanty clear urination. The clear quality indicates Cold. Fluid buildup under the skin causes edema, which here will be more pronounced in the legs.

The Kidneys provide warmth, energy, and functionality to every organ—they have more patterns of disharmony involving other organs than any other individual organ—but here their inability to warm and nourish the Spleen is most prominent. That contributes to the weakness in the limbs and loose stool, as seen in Spleen Qi Deficiency symptoms.

The tongue is moist and swollen due to a buildup of fluids and pale due to insufficient Blood from weakened Spleen functions. Tooth marks indicate Qi deficiency. The pulse is thready and weak due to Qi and Blood deficiency and slow due to Cold. Deep indicates an interior condition.

With the proper presentation, some Western diagnoses that may fit this pattern include lumbago, arthritis, benign prostatic hypertrophy, adrenal fatigue, hypothyroidism, nephritis, and various sexual and urinary tract conditions.

Some common Kidney patterns include Kidney Yin Deficiency, Kidneys Failing to Grasp the Qi, and Kidneys and Heart Failing to Communicate.

PART 2

Holistic Self-Care with Chinese Medicine

In Part 2, you'll learn how to practice Chinese holistic self-care in a variety of ways, including acupressure, herbal remedies, Qigong, and food therapies. You can use any of those separately with many beneficial results. All are synergistically integrated for you in the prescriptions found in Chapter 18. That integration will optimize your health and wellness, providing the most comprehensive self-care and yielding the very best results. It will give you more control over every aspect of your health and greatly reduce the need for visits to the doctor.

There may be times when seeking professional medical help is the wisest course, as when a mild to moderate health challenge lingers for a long time despite your best self-care efforts or when facing a more serious medical condition. In those cases, remember the words of Canadian physician Sir William Osler, who famously stated in the 1800s, "A physician who treats himself has a fool for a patient." [18]

You may still opt for an integrated holistic approach, as a Chinese physician will often be of as much or greater help than a doctor of Western medicine. Most will advise you to seek Western

---

18. William Osler, *Sir William Osler: Aphorisms from His Bedside Teachings and Writings* (New York: Henry Schuman, Inc., 1950).

medical intervention if they believe that would be of greatest benefit for your individual circumstances.

For readers less familiar with practical Chinese medicine, Chapters 10 and 11 provide insight to what you can expect, so you'll be a better informed patient and can interact effectively with your physician. A Chinese physician will be able to guide you in most advantageously incorporating practices from this book to speed your recovery or improve your baseline of good health. You can still use everything here when seeing a Western physician, as long as you let them know what you are doing for self-care. Acupressure and Qigong are always safe, but herbs and some foods may interact with certain prescription medications.

Chapter 10

Diagnosis: Finding the Root of the Problem

If you've never been to a Chinese medical practitioner, this chapter and the next provide some insight into what you may expect. They outline various common procedures and go into some detail about exactly what they are and how they work. This will help you have an informed dialogue with your physician, and it offers a few tips you can use for assessment in your self-care.

Diagnostic Methods

The first and most crucial step in achieving the best therapeutic outcome from a Chinese medical course of treatment is a complete and accurate diagnosis. For reasons previously stated, a Western medical diagnosis is of limited help toward that end. It should be common sense that if you are seeking acupuncture or a more fully integrated Chinese treatment, you'll get the best results by using the diagnostics intrinsic to that medical paradigm.

Chinese diagnosis does not rely on technology. Even here, its methods are holistic, utilizing all of the physician's senses. Visual examination of the tongue (many physicians also examine their patients' eyes, complexion, and Shen/spirit) and tactile examination of the pulse points (some systems also palpate the abdomen, primarily in Japanese-style *hara* diagnosis) are standard. Sometimes acupoints are palpated for tenderness, and body parts may be palpated to determine *Ah Shi* points, painful regions of nonstandard points. Classically, the physician's senses of smell and taste were employed, with the patient's scent and the taste of some body fluids, chiefly urine, being diagnostically significant. While scent may still be surreptitiously included by some—few if any contemporary physicians in the Western world actively smell their patient, primarily out of social convention and prevailing sense of propriety—taste is no longer used due to hygienic concerns. Hearing is used for additional corroboration, as the sound quality and strength of a patient's voice and breathing are significant. Inquiry gathers specific information relevant to the patient's medical history, lifestyle, and constitution.

Inquiry

Inquiry is usually the first part of a medical intake. It allows the patient to talk about concerns and is useful in building a rapport. On a first visit, the questions may be very extensive, inquiring about occupation, diet, level and type of activity, aspects of familial and personal medical history, former surgeries, illnesses and injuries, problems with any sense organs, possible problems in every Organ System, number of pregnancies and possible complications, and other factors that fill in the patient's background and current life circumstances. This is where the physician learns of the patient's main medical concerns—the reasons they decided to come for treatment. That focuses most of the rest of the intake so that the patient's distress may be alleviated most quickly and effectively. The physician asks questions in order to expand on the patient's main concern, helping to arrive at the most accurate diagnosis.

The next aspect of inquiry is most detailed on a first visit but is included on all subsequent visits as a way to monitor the patient's progress and alert the physician to any possible new health challenges. These standard questions help evaluate the state of balance in a person's daily life and provide clues about which Organ Systems are most involved. These include the quality and amount of sleep, perceived energy throughout the day, appetite, regularity of bowel and urine functions, emotional states or changes, the regularity of menstrual cycles, length and quality of menses, any premenstrual discomforts, and any discomforts arising from perimenopause or menopause. If pain is present, questions are asked about the nature, location, and duration of the pain. If suffering from a cold, flu, or something similar, a patient is asked about fever, chills, perspiration, body aches, and other symptoms. Other relevant questions are asked about any new immediate concern that may arise.

Pulse Diagnosis

After the verbal intake, a pulse diagnosis usually follows. Chinese pulse diagnosis is more extensive than its Western counterpart of checking blood pressure and pulse rate.

Physician and patient sit facing each other across the interview table. (Some physicians prefer to have their patient laying on the treatment table; their fingers will still be placed on the pulse points exactly as described below, and they will make the same evaluations.) The patient's arms extend across the table, usually resting palm-up on a small cushion both for comfort and to open their wrists for unobstructed blood flow. The physician places their index fingers on both of the patient's wrists, just below the thumb, and then place their middle and ring fingers down just beyond their index finger. Each fingertip is now on one of six discrete pulse positions.

The first thing a physician may do is to take the pulse rate, exactly as a Western physician would do. Next, an assessment of the overall state of the patient's pulses may be made. The right wrist indicates the state of Qi throughout the body, and the left wrist indicates the Blood. The qualities of the overall pulses are determined, revealing the general state of the whole body. These two steps, rate and overall quality, may be taken in any order.

Next, the functionality of each organ is examined. Each of the six pulse positions has two depths (one close to the surface, the other deeper), yielding twelve positions in all (**Figure 10.1** on next page). The superficial pulses indicate the Yang organs, since they are more superficial, and the deeper pulses indicate the paired deeper Yin organ. On the right wrist, moving from wrist toward elbow, the first position indicates the condition of the Large Intestine superficially, and the Lungs, deeper; the second position includes the Stomach and Spleen; and the third position, the Urinary Bladder and the right Kidney. On the left wrist, the first position is the Small Intestine and Heart, the second position is the Gall Bladder and Liver, and the third position is the Urinary Bladder (again) and the left Kidney. The positions are frequently colloquially called by their Yin organ association, since those are most closely examined except in cases of suspected Yang organ pathology.

At each position, the physician feels for (sometimes called "listens to") specific qualities of diagnostic significance. A normal pulse feels smooth and even, has moderate force, with sixty to seventy beats per minute. There are volumes written on pulse diagnosis alone, so an exhaustive catalogue of those qualities is impractical, but here are some common qualities, their descriptions, and what they indicate.

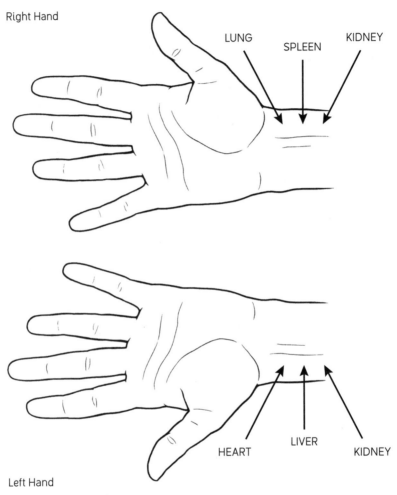

Figure 10.1 (Pulse Positions)

Pulse Qualities

• **Floating (Superficial):** This pulse is felt most distinctly at the superficial level, is discernible with a very light touch, and may be weaker or absent at deep levels. This most often indicates a superficial pathology, such as Invasion of Wind Cold.

In this case, the Qi rises to the surface of the body to fight off the EPF, causing the floating quality.

- **Sinking (Deep):** This pulse is felt most distinctly at the deep level, often requires a heavier touch to feel, and may be weaker or absent superficially. This indicates a deeper pathology, such as Kidney Yin Deficiency.

- **Slippery (Rolling):** This pulse has a smooth and bumpy quality that feels "like pearls rolling under the fingers," indicating "something extra" in the body. Most often, that something extra is Damp, either from an EPF or from an internal cause generating Damp, common in Spleen Qi Deficiency. This pulse is normal during pregnancy, as the fetus is seen as something extra in the mother's body.

- **Deficient:** A generally forceless pulse in all pulse positions, indicating Qi and blood deficiencies.

- **Excess:** A generally forceful pulse in all positions, indicating excess syndromes. Often seen when the body's normal or defensive Qi is strongly fighting a pathogenic Qi.

- **Bowstring (Wiry):** This pulse feels strong and hard, like the thump of a bowstring against the fingertips. This indicates excess, as in Liver Qi Stagnation, where the buildup of Liver Qi causes the obstruction that typically creates this pulse. This is also common in pain syndromes, as almost all pain is caused by obstruction of Qi, Blood, body fluids, or combinations of those.

- **Thready:** This pulse feels very fine, like a thread, yet distinct. It indicates deficiency, most often of Blood or Yin, but can indicate Qi deficiency especially when accompanied by Blood deficiency. Commonly found in Heart Blood Deficiency, with or without Spleen Qi Deficiency.

- **Slow:** A slow pulse is less than sixty beats per minute and usually indicates Cold syndromes. The Cold can be due to either deficiency or excess.

- **Rapid:** A rapid pulse is more than ninety beats per minute and usually indicates Hot syndromes. The Heat can be due to either deficiency or excess.

- **Leisurely:** A normal pulse of between approximately sixty and seventy beats per minute.

These pulses can be found in combination, giving a broader set of diagnostic indications. It's common for a pulse to be thready, bowstring, and rapid or floating and slippery, for example.

These qualities, and the many others that exist, can be subtle and difficult to distinguish. Most physicians spend years, even decades, refining their pulse-taking abilities while examining hundreds of patients. As an aid to your self-assessment, you can begin with the easiest pulse qualities of rate and general deficiency and excess. If you'd like to try, check your pulses in the following way.

Assessing Your Pulse

Place the back of your left wrist on the palm of your right hand at a right angle. Curl your right fingers so that the tips touch your left pulse points, with your right index finger closest to your thumb in the first position and your ring finger farthest from your thumb in the third position. Let your middle finger fall comfortably between. Check your rate by counting beats for fifteen seconds and multiplying the number of beats by four. Then get some sense of the strength of your pulse. If it feels strong and forceful, it may be an Excess pulse. If it feels weak or difficult to distinguish, it may be a Deficient pulse. Repeat on your right hand. Check these qualities at the same time every day for a week or so, preferably while you are feeling well, to establish a baseline of what is normal for you.

You can use this simple method to make some crucial distinctions if you become sick. For example, if you catch a cold, in the early stages you can note if your pulse feels stronger, indicating your Qi is strong and fighting off a strong EPF. If it feels weaker, that may mean the EPF is too strong for your Qi to effectively combat. In that case you will need to rest, nourish yourself, and work to build stronger Qi once the cold has passed. If your pulse feels faster than normal, that will tell you the EPF is Hot. If slower than normal, the EPF is Cold. That can help you determine which acupressure points and herbs will best address your condition.

With practice over time you will begin to distinguish some of the other qualities introduced above. You may begin to notice differences in pulse position qualities. For example, the Liver pulse (the middle position on your left wrist) commonly feels thin or thready and bowstring, especially in times of stress or pain, while the Heart and Kidney pulses may not.

Tongue Diagnosis

The tongue provides a wealth of visible information outside the scope of Western medical thought. The Heart, Spleen, and Kidney meridians have branches that directly end in the tongue, and most of the other organs connect with the tongue through collateral branches. Many aspects of the functional energy of the organs are thereby reflected on the tongue. Other factors that contribute to evaluating the tongue include the tongue body (size, shape, color, moisture, regions of organ correspondence), the coating, also referred to as "moss" or "fur" (its thickness, color, possible absence), and its mobility. A normal tongue fits comfortably in the mouth, is neither enlarged nor small, moves freely, is light red in color, is slightly moist, and has a thin, white coating.

As with pulses, there are volumes written on tongue diagnosis, but here are some common attributes and what they indicate.

The tongue body can be most simply divided into four regions: the tip, middle third, rear third (or "root"), and the sides (**Figure 10.2** on the next page). The tip of the tongue reflects the state of the Heart and Lungs, the middle third reflects the state of the Stomach and Spleen, the rear third reflects the state of the Kidneys, and the sides reflect the state of the Liver and Gall Bladder. It's possible for each of those regions to manifest entirely different changes, indicating different pathologies in the respective organs. Some possible changes include the following.

Tongue color can change. A pale color indicates Cold syndromes or Blood deficiency; red indicates Heat, from either Deficiency or Excess (a deeper red indicates stronger Heat); a light purplish color ("dusky") indicates Qi stagnation, where the obstructed Qi is less able to move Blood, causing mild Blood Stasis; and a purple or blue color indicates more significant Blood Stasis. A purple or reddish purple color indicates Stasis due to Heat, while a blue color indicates Stasis due to Cold. Different colors may appear on different portions of the tongue, giving clues about the state of the related organs.

The tongue body may be thin, indicating a deficiency of body substance, either Blood or Yin. It may be swollen or enlarged, indicating Damp. If swollen and pale, the Damp comes from Spleen or Kidney Yang Deficiency or both. If swollen and red, Damp Heat is present.

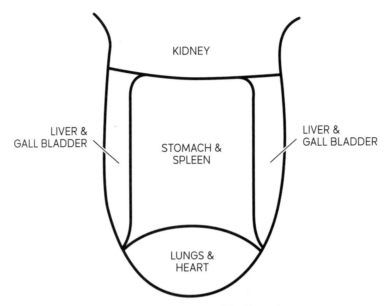

Figure 10.2 (Regions of the Tongue)

The tongue may have cracks or lines in it. This is caused by Dryness, which may come from Heat consuming fluids or from Yin Deficiency.

There may be uncontrollable tongue movement. A trembling tongue occurs in Qi Deficiency. A rigid, inflexible tongue may be caused by Heat attacking the Pericardium. Both a rigid and a deviated tongue (moved to one side or the other) indicate Internal Wind and may precede a stroke.

The tongue coating is equally important diagnostically, indicating the presence, absence, nature, and intensity of various pathological factors. It is produced by Stomach Qi, although the Qi of the other Yang organs also influence it. A normal tongue coating is thin and white, so the tongue body is clearly visible beneath.

A white coating can be from either exterior or interior Cold. A yellow coating indicates Heat, usually from interior syndromes.

A thick coating always indicates an excess condition, whether Hot, Cold, or Damp. So a thick, yellow coat indicates Excess Heat, while a thick, white coat indicates Excess Cold. A thickening of the coat indicates a worsening condition, while a thinning coat indicates improvement. If it is thick and greasy or sticky, the Stomach's digestive functions are weak, possibly indicating food retention and causing the dirty-appearing Damp residue.

A dry, coarse-looking coating lacks moisture, due to excess Heat (especially if yellow) or Yin deficiency. An absence of coating, a "peeled" tongue, indicates Yin deficiency, primarily of the Stomach or Kidneys or both. If only parts of the tongue are peeled, this is called a geographic tongue, indicating a Stomach Qi and Yin deficiency.

While there are many more possible presentations of the tongue body and coating, these provide numerous diagnostic clues to pattern identification.

Simple Self-Diagnosis

If you'd like to use basic tongue diagnosis to help assess your health, begin by examining your tongue at the same time each day, preferably first thing in the morning before you've had anything to eat or drink and before brushing your teeth. Eating changes the appearance of the tongue, bringing more blood to it and making it appear redder, and the coating often absorbs some of the color of the food you eat. Coffee always turns the tongue coating yellow for a time. If you can't examine your tongue in the morning, wait at least two hours after a meal, so it returns to normal.

Look for all the tongue qualities in its body, coating, and movement. For now don't be too concerned with organ correspondences to tongue regions, but you may notice that the tip of your tongue is redder than the rest of the body. While not "normal" (it indicates Heat in your Heart and Lungs), it is fairly common and an easy observation to make if it's there. Examine those qualities for a week or so to note possible changes and to establish a baseline frame of reference.

Follow the instructions from the section "Assessing Your Pulse."

If you do become sick, see how your pulse and tongue change. Ideally, as you incorporate the self-care practices found in this book, you'll see the positive changes reflected there.

For example, you know that if your tongue is consistently red with a thick, yellow coating, and your pulse is rapid and forceful, you likely have some syndrome of Excess Internal Heat. You can use the information in Part 1 to help refine that assessment.

In this case, you may select acupoints from Chapter 13 that sedate (to clear the Excess) and clear Heat. You might select herbs from Chapter 15 that nourish Yin and are cooling and moistening. However, if you have other troublesome symptoms, look through the index of conditions in Chapter 18 and see if there are any that are a good match for an Internal Excess Heat presentation. (Under "Digestive System Disorders," Constipation from Excess is one likely choice.) If so, select those acupoints and herbs, as they'll be the best choice for you. Include the recommended Qigong exercises(s) and foods. After a few weeks or a month, note the changes in your pulse, tongue, and overall health.

Remember, pulse and tongue diagnosis is challenging for health professionals too. Even with this simplified approach, take plenty of time, give yourself permission to make mistakes—you'll make a lot of them in the beginning—and eventually it will become clearer, easier, and immensely rewarding.

Chapter 11

Tools and Practice of Chinese Medicine: Holism and Integration

Each individual Chinese medical practice is holistic, treating the patient and not the disease. Each is very versatile yet has a main focus and strength. For that reason, most acupuncturists, Qigong doctors, and Tuina practitioners include herbs in their practice. Many Qigong and Taiji instructors teach their students and patients about lifestyle and dietary factors, and some offer acupressure or Tuina treatments. Not every physician integrates or even practices all modalities, but to get the fastest, most comprehensive resolution to a health problem or to live the healthiest possible life into a vital old age, all should be included and conscientiously integrated to best support each individual regularly, as is most often done in China. That will become more apparent as you proceed through the following chapters.

Acupuncture

Acupuncture is the art and science of encouraging the body to improve function and promote natural healing by inserting very fine surgical-grade stainless steel needles (see Appendix 2, Note 11.1) into select acupoints found along discrete, well-defined energy pathways called meridians. The diagnostic methods discussed in Chapter 10 are used to identify patterns of disharmony, and points are selected accordingly to restore the body to healthy balance by influencing the flow of Qi within the meridians and their related organs.

Each point has specific functions. The primary point functions usually relate to the function of the organ associated with the selected meridian or to the condition of the meridian itself, which can have its own related set of indications. No organ is ever needled directly. Examples of point functions for nearly one hundred points are found in Chapter 13.

Acupuncture's main strength is in moving Qi. The ways in which it moves Qi and for what purposes are discussed in the next two sections. Acupuncture on its own does not add Qi to the body. (By using the adjunctive therapy of moxibustion, Yang Qi can be added.) It builds Qi by strengthening the functions of the organs that are responsible for acquiring and producing Qi, primarily the Lungs and Spleen, so a treatment may feel immediately energizing, while building sustainable energy over time. More commonly, patients feel calm and relaxed. Acupuncture moves Blood by moving Qi, which is the commander of Blood. Acupuncture builds Blood by strengthening the functions of the organs that generate Blood, primarily the Spleen and Heart.

Needling Sensations: Deqi

It is a common misunderstanding that there is no sensation associated with acupuncture treatments. In fact, some sensation is required in order for the treatment to be most successful. The needling sensation is called *Deqi* (De Qi), or the "arrival of the Qi," and indicates that the Qi has been accessed.

For the physician, Deqi feels like a grabbing around the needle at the site of its insertion. Then the needle can be most effectively manipulated, guiding the Qi to produce a variety of effects and providing the best therapeutic outcomes.

For the patient, typical Deqi sensations include feelings of distension, heaviness, tingling, electricity, temperature change, internal motion, and tightness, among many other possibilities. Sometimes these sensations can be quite strong, and a new or very sensitive patient may interpret them as pain. Once a patient knows to look for a variety of needling sensations, they rarely perceive them as pain. It is possible to feel true pain when a needle is inserted, because there is a fine network of cutaneous nerves that spread across and just below the surface of the skin, and occasionally one of those nerves may be punctured. While that is not dangerous, it will provoke the type of pain usually associated with a pinprick, and it is usually much less painful than a hypodermic needle injection. Just as no organ is ever directly needled, no nerve is ever intentionally needled.

Needling Techniques

Acupuncture needles are manipulated using a variety of techniques to move Qi in specific ways, initiating or amplifying specific healing responses. One of the most dramatic techniques is used in acupuncture anesthesia. In that case, an acupuncturist selects the appropriate points and then twirls two needles very rapidly, 120 to 180 times per minute, for five, ten, or even twenty minutes. An acupuncturist must have a fair amount of personal Qi cultivation in order to be able to maintain such manipulation. While that was done historically, these days most acupuncturists opt for electroacupuncture, an electrical stimulation of the needles, to approximate the same effect.

In everyday use, less demanding manipulations are performed primarily to tonify (gathering Qi to the acupoint or encouraging Qi flow in the normal direction of the meridian pathway) or to sedate (dispersing Qi away from a point or encouraging Qi flow against the normal direction of the meridian pathway).

Tonification is performed to strengthen the functions of an acupoint and its related organ, to build Qi, Yang, blood, or Yin in a weak or deficient patient, or in other patterns indicating deficiency. Sedation is performed to dispel an external pathogen, to open a channel obstruction and reduce pain, or to reduce the presence of any internal excess (such as Damp accumulation) in any pattern indicating excess.

When a needle is not stimulated at all, it is a harmonizing treatment, providing a general balancing without overtly tonifying or sedating a point.

Points are combined in specific ways to create therapeutic effects. There are many classic two-point, four-needle combinations that have powerful effects, due to the unique attributes of the selected points. Usually, many more than two points are used in any acupuncture treatment. Dozens of point combinations used to treat common ailments are found in Chapter 18.

Treatment Frequency

Treatment frequency can vary some based on the severity of the condition being treated and whether an integrated approach, adding herbs and Qigong therapies, is being followed. With acupuncture alone, once a week is a standard minimum, though twice a week is better, and in China it's common to be treated every day or every other day for ten treatments as one course of treatment. This is because the effects of acupuncture peak in two to three days and then begin to decline. Boosting the effects of treatment every day or two maintains a steady increase of improvement. This is most important when treating any serious condition.

In minor to moderate conditions, one to two treatments a week are usually sufficient. If herbs are taken daily, they provide another benefit and enhance the effects of acupuncture. If the patient practices Chinese healing exercises, Qigong, Taiji, or the acupressure that's taught in this book, another layer of healing is added daily, and one acupuncture treatment each week is enough. For general health maintenance, a "tune-up" type of treatment, or a periodic energetic assessment and rebalancing, one or two treatments per month works well.

While this is a common protocol, acupuncturists can have differing strategies. If you are in treatment, follow the recommendations of your acupuncturist.

Three Case Histories

The following three cases will give you some context through which to understand how and why number and frequency of treatments can vary, and why your expected number of treatments may be ultimately unpredictable. Patient names and other minor details have been changed to protect their identities, but these are otherwise accurate synopses from my records.

Allergies and Eczema

John, a man in his midthirties, came to see me with two long-standing problems: a cat allergy and eczema that covered parts of his arms, legs, ears, and torso. At that point in his life, he was particularly motivated to get relief from his allergy. His fiancée had cats and told him in no uncertain terms that she was not getting rid of them, so he had to find a way to deal with it.

Since airborne allergens primarily affect the lungs, and since the Lungs dominate the skin, it was easy to see how these problems were related. It's fairly common for people with childhood asthma to develop eczema, psoriasis, or other skin conditions later in life as the pathology moves deeper and transforms. This was a variation of that pattern, now presenting with allergies instead of asthma, which had in fact afflicted John in his youth.

There were two difficulties in resolving these conditions: the length of time he'd suffered them (the longer a pathology is in place, the deeper it will penetrate the body), and the nature of the pathology itself, Damp.

Described as being thick, sticky, and cloying, Damp can be very intractable. It manifested as Phlegm swelling the mucous membranes in his sinuses, airways, and lungs, which compromised his breathing. It secondarily manifested through the eczema on his skin.

The other pathogenic factor was Heat, which manifested most as the redness, heat, and itch of the eczema. It caused symptoms in other parts of his body as well. Hot, damp environments exacerbated his eczema.

Examination revealed that Lung Qi Deficiency was the main pattern—this was likely constitutional—and the Spleen and Stomach were also involved. I explained these things to him and told him that it wouldn't be a fast and easy recovery. I recommended twice-weekly acupuncture treatments and daily herbs. As an additional therapy, I recommended some dietary modifications and a high-quality bovine colostrum supplement, which supplies immunoglobulins and balances immune response, to address the allergy from a nutritional/orthomolecular standpoint. Part of the Lungs' function of dominating the skin is roughly analogous to the role of the general immune system, so this approach made sense to me.

As he'd exhausted all other medical options, John agreed to this treatment plan. He was one of my most compliant patients, rarely missed an appointment, and was diligent in taking the herbs and colostrum daily. While we saw slow, steady improvement over time with some expected brief setbacks, it took six months to resolve the cat allergies. At that time, he was able to play with the cats and remain asymptomatic.

His eczema symptoms showed less improvement, but he was so encouraged that he continued treatment to fully resolve it. After a few months we reduced the frequency of his treatments to once a week, although he continued to take herbs daily. It took nearly an additional year and a half to resolve the eczema, but through all of that time, the cat allergy never returned. After two years of treatment, the eczema cleared, and he only experienced brief minor flare-ups in his elbow creases when he had to visit hot, humid environments for work. He reported that it was otherwise no longer a problem.

Everything about this case proceeded as expected. The constitutional component, the number of years the condition existed, and the Damp nature of the primary pathogen all indicated a long course of treatment, even with twice-weekly acupuncture and the daily use of herbs and supplements. As the eczema was a later, hence deeper, manifestation of the primary Lung weakness, it naturally took longer to resolve.

Sudden Onset Deafness

Ethan was a man in his early thirties who came to me through a referral about a week after he awoke one morning with a complete loss of hearing in his left ear. His primary care provider told him that a virus had invaded his auditory nerve, and that if he were any older, he would probably not regain any of his hearing. Being young and otherwise healthy, the doctor prescribed steroids and antibiotics, saying by following that regimen for between eight and twelve months, he could have up to 50 percent of his hearing restored. (Antibiotics do not treat viral infections, so that part of the treatment didn't make sense to me. I did not speak with his doctor directly, so it's possible Ethan was mistaken about that medication.)

Due to the seriousness of his condition, I said that I'd be willing to treat him if he would come for acupuncture every other day. I believed we would not make much progress with fewer treatments, and I did not want him to otherwise think Chinese medicine didn't work. He agreed, so I gave him a first treatment that day, on a Friday. He came back on Sunday, saying he already had some hearing return. On Monday, he called to tell me that by his estimation, he had at least 25 percent of his hearing back, and decided to go on a week's skiing vacation that he and his wife had planned but then cancelled to accommodate his treatment schedule.

Ethan came for his third treatment a week later on a Monday and told me he had an appointment with his audiologist the next day. On Tuesday, after seeing the audiologist he called to say he had 86 percent of his hearing restored and didn't feel he needed any further treatment! I never saw him again, so my assumption was that, subjectively at least, his hearing was fully back to normal.

I expected that Ethan would require at least two courses of ten treatments over five to six weeks, including an herbal prescription that we never got to. The rapidity of his recovery was a pleasant surprise but not implausible. His hearing loss was both of sudden onset and very recent, so the pathogenic factors did not have time to penetrate deeply and take a strong hold. He was smart to seek help as soon as he did. Being young and healthy, he had abundant Qi to work with, so the effects of the acupuncture were maximized even without the inclusion of herbs.

Severe Tendinitis/RSI

Barry, a man in his late twenties, lived in Los Angeles. During the summer, he bicycled from LA all the way across the country to Boston and developed a very painful, debilitating wrist tendinopathy from the continual stress of the ride. The doctors he consulted in Boston put him on anti-inflammatories, told him to rest his hands and apply ice, and said that in time it should improve but that surgery might become necessary. His doctors in LA continued the anti-inflammatories, prescribed physical therapy, and were adopting a wait-and-see approach before considering surgery. In late October it was still painful and difficult for him to use his hands.

Referred by a friend who was my patient, Barry came to see me in San Francisco while he was there on a months-long work assignment. After diagnosing him with Channel Obstruction (a type of localized Qi stagnation) with Blood Stasis and Heat, I recommended twice weekly acupuncture, and an herbal formula I'd have ready for him on his next visit. He agreed, and I gave him the acupuncture treatment that day.

The next night, Barry called and excitedly told me he'd been pain free since the previous evening, and asked me to hold off on picking up his herbs. The next day he called to cancel the treatment we scheduled for the following day, saying he'd reschedule if his pain returned. Weeks later, his friend who was my patient confirmed that Barry had remained pain free since his single acupuncture treatment.

Barry's amazingly rapid recovery was a big surprise to me. Even though he was young and healthy and followed all the conventional Western approaches to treat his condition, he'd been suffering unrelenting pain for months, so I expected it would take at least a few weeks for him to improve.

These examples illustrate that it is difficult to say with complete certainly how long a course of treatment will be necessary. In John's case, it took about as long as I'd expected. Although I let him know it would take significant time, he stuck with it, and we got the results I anticipated. Ethan improved much sooner than I thought likely, but there were circumstances that explained in part why that might have occurred. Barry's recovery was so rapid and complete that I concluded this was one instance where we got really lucky, that the treatment I gave him was perfectly targeted to his exact needs. It sometimes happens that way, but it's a rarity.

Adjunctive Therapies

Electroacupuncture

This involves attaching electrodes from an electroacupuncture device to the handle end of inserted acupuncture needles. A very low current is run through them to produce specific effects. The microampere range generally strengthens the main effect of the treatment. Microamp current is thought to closely duplicate the body's natural Qi and stimulates stronger Qi flow through the selected meridians. It typically produces a tonifying effect but can be used for sedation. The milliamp current range causes muscles to contract in a way similar to stimulation by a transcutaneous electrical nerve stimulation (TENS) device. This is a sedation effect, disperses Qi stagnation to reduce tension and pain, and is used in preoperative acupuncture anesthesia. The selection of microamp or milliamp stimulation depends upon the condition being treated and the therapeutically desired effect.

Moxibustion

This is an aspect of herbal medicine. It involves the burning of an herb called *Ai Ye* (Chinese mugwort) or "moxa" as a type of heat therapy or to add Yang Qi to specific points or to focused, relatively small regions of the body. The Qi of moxa is thought to be nearly identical to the Qi of a human and is especially beneficial for weaker patients or those with Cold conditions.

Moxa can be in the form of cigar-sized cylinders. One end is lit, and the hot tip is moved toward the patient's body to treat the desired regions, often in a pecking motion, although the lit tip never touches the patient's body. It may also be in loose form and rolled into rice-grain-shaped pellets, which are then placed on acupoints and lit. When the patient feels the heat, the pellet is removed. This may be repeated many times.

Moxa may also be placed in a small pile, usually on the navel, on a slice of ginger, *Fu Zi* (aconite, monkshood, wolfsbane), salt, or other substance and then lit. The therapeutic properties of the other substance are added to the moxa, which may be left in place or removed if the heat feels too strong for the patient.

Cupping

Involves creating a vacuum in small, thick glass cups and rapidly placing them on the patient's body to create a localized suction. This can be used to draw out pathogens, or when moving the cups along meridian pathways after lubricating the skin, to strongly open the affected meridian, moving both Qi and blood. This is commonly done on the back to open the Urinary Bladder meridian, which is useful for treating the onset of colds, fevers, and headache and for muscle tension from channel obstruction.

Western Perspectives on Acupuncture

Until recently, Western medical interest in acupuncture has largely been limited to pain management. In that context, gate control theory, discussed in Chapter 2, has been proposed as one possible mechanism. Another involves the release of endorphins, the body's "endogenous morphine." Endorphins are pain-relieving neuropeptides produced by the nervous system and pituitary gland and are believed to be stimulated by the needle insertions. This is also cited to account for acupuncture's effectiveness in addiction treatment. It fits the Western medical model nicely, but acupuncture's effects go far beyond pain management, so these are limited explanations.

Another posits that needling acupuncture points induces the nervous system to cause the release of other biochemicals beyond endorphin neuropeptides (neurotransmitters, neurohormones, endocrine and exocrine hormones) into the muscles, organs, spinal cord, and brain. They can influence the body's internal regulating systems or trigger the release of still other biochemicals. The improved biochemical balance supports the body's natural healing abilities, promoting physical and emotional health.

Since the mid-1990s, PET scans and fMRI technologies have demonstrated that parts of the brain light up corresponding to the traditional understanding of points used for specific purposes. For example, needling a point in the foot known to benefit the eyes lights up the optical region of brain.[19] Some of the most studied points have a wide range of clinical applications, including LI 4, St 36, P 6, Liv 3, and GB 34. These points influence large areas of the brain, including somatosensory, motor, auditory, and visual areas, the cerebellum, the limbic system, and higher cognitive area. Brain

---

19. Kathleen K. S. Hui, Jing Liu, and Kenneth K. Kwong, "Functional Mapping of the Human Brain during Acupuncture with Magnetic Resonance Imaging Somatosensory Cortex Activation," *World Journal of Acupuncture-Moxibustion* 7, no. 3 (1997): 44–49.

maps of acupuncture points belonging to different meridians vary considerably, while points belonging to a single meridian affect the same single region of the brain.

Imaging also corroborates the organs' ascendant times (see Chapter 5), showing a different level and type of brain activity when points are needled during the related organ's ascendant time than at other times of day. These and many other studies demonstrate that acupuncture affects the body in ways corresponding to thousands of years of traditional understanding. As of yet, there is no explanation for how it achieves those results within a Western medical paradigm.

Conditions Treated

For thousands of years, Chinese medicine has been used to treat virtually every medical condition that conventional Western medicine does. Each system has its relative strengths and weaknesses, which hopefully will one day make them truly complementary partners in the Western world as they are in China.

In a 2003 internal document titled *Acupuncture: Review and Analysis of Reports on Controlled Clinical Trials*, the World Health Organization published this updated list of conditions effectively treated by acupuncture. The full document is available for download from the WHO website. While far from exhaustive in regards to the benefits possible from the totality of Chinese medicine, it provides a credible foundation from a globally acknowledged source as a basis for Western understanding.

Upper Respiratory Tract

- Acute sinusitis
- Acute rhinitis
- Common cold
- Acute tonsillitis
- Sore throat

Respiratory System

- Acute bronchitis
- Allergies
- Bronchial asthma

- Emphysema
- Recurrent chest infections

Circulatory Disorders

- Hypertension
- Angina pectoris
- Arteriosclerosis
- Anemia

Disorders of the Eye

- Acute conjunctivitis
- Central retinitis
- Myopia
- Cataract

Disorders of the Mouth

- Toothache, postextraction pain
- Gingivitis
- Acute and chronic pharyngitis

Gastrointestinal Disorders

- Spasms of esophagus and cardia
- Hiccup
- Gastroptosis
- Acute and chronic gastritis
- Gastric hyperacidity
- Indigestion
- Anorexia
- Chronic duodenal ulcer (pain relief)
- Acute duodenal ulcer (without complications)

- Acute and chronic colitis
- Food allergies
- Acute bacillary dysentery
- Constipation
- Diarrhea
- Paralytic ileus
- Spastic colon
- Nausea and vomiting associated with chemotherapy

Neurological and Musculoskeletal Disorders

- Headache and migraine
- Trigeminal neuralgia
- Facial palsy
- Facial tics
- Pareses following a stroke
- Peripheral neuropathies
- Sequelae of poliomyelitis
- Meniere's disease
- Neuralgia
- Neurogenic bladder dysfunction
- Nocturnal enuresis
- Intercostal neuralgia
- Cervicobrachial syndrome
- Insomnia
- Dizziness
- Neck pain
- Various forms of tendinitis
- Frozen shoulder
- Tennis elbow

- Sciatica

- Low back pain

- Osteoarthritis

- Fibromyalgia

Emotional and Psychological Disorders

- Depression

- Anxiety

Addictions

- Alcohol, nicotine, and other drugs

Urinary, Menstrual, and Reproductive Problems

Herbal Medicine

Herbal medicine is Chinese pharmacology. Herbology is older than acupuncture and central to the practice of Chinese medicine. It can produce all of the effects of acupuncture, but its main strength is that it adds something to the body. While this is useful in all conditions, it may be especially valuable for Deficient conditions, since the substance of herbs can readily build Blood and Yin, along with Qi and Yang.

Although plant sources make up the largest part of its pharmacopoeia, animal and mineral substances are also employed. Oyster shell, earthworm, and mantis egg casing are commonly used. Tiger bone and other endangered-species animal parts were once commonly used but are now illegal and no longer included in contemporary Chinese pharmacies or patent medicines. (A patient can request no animal products. In that case, plant substitutes may be used.) Some minerals (like talc, gypsum, and hematite) can be found in "herbal" formulas.

Its meticulous detail and many well-defined treatment strategies make Chinese herbal medicine significantly different from its Western herbal counterparts. Those distinctions are discussed in Chapter 14. A Chinese herbalist will create a complex, balanced formula or possibly modify or combine any of thousands of established formulas. The herbalist takes the whole person into account and addresses the overt symptoms, secondary issues, underlying causes, and the constitutional needs of the individual, based on a detailed diagnosis. Used this way, herbal medicine is very safe, is very effective, and produces no side effects.

Chinese doctors continually expand their pharmacopoeia and have incorporated many Western and other nonlocal herbs over the millennia. They do this by analyzing the new substance according to its taste, temperature (or Qi), the channel or channels it enters, its compatibility with other herbs, and its potential toxicity. Only then do they include it in the Chinese pharmacopoeia. It's more about the way the herbs are applied, the rationale, rather than any intrinsic quality of the herb that makes it part of Chinese medicine. As an example, American ginseng, native to North America, is now a valued part of Chinese herbal medicine.

Forms of Chinese Herbs

Traditionally, herbal formulas were prepared by combining loose herbs and decocting them into very potent teas. This approach is still favored by most herbalists since it allows for precise customization of the formula content and dosages, which can be easily modified to accommodate changes in a patient's condition over time. This method produces the strongest and most predictably accurate therapeutic effect, since the effects of most of the formulas described in the Chinese pharmacopoeia were derived from decoction. Many herbalists contend that preparing a formula by decoction creates an interaction among herbs, modifying some of their actions to achieve the most desired results. Cooking them together alters their biochemistry.

The downsides of this approach include the amount of time spent brewing the decoction—a daily dose typically takes about forty-five minutes of cooking time—and the way they smell and taste, which many Westerners find unpleasant. There may also be more variability in the quality of the herbs used, since they are not standardized. Differences in soil composition, geography, length of the growing cycle, and the time of harvest, among other factors, all influence the potency of the herbs.

Chinese herbal formulas are available as patent medicines in tablet form, and varieties of herbal tablets or pills have existed for hundreds of years. Since these tablets are still whole herbs and not synthesized, concentrated pharmaceutical drugs, many more tablets must be consumed than most Westerners are used to. Depending on the form and size of the tablets, anywhere from nine to thirty-six tablets may be required daily. These are premade formulas and therefore not customizable, but there are literally hundreds of formulas available in tablet form. A close match may be readily found, and often two formulas may be used simultaneously for a more targeted outcome.

Pills were used historically most often in chronic conditions requiring an extended course of treatment. That may be one reason a physician might select tablets for US patients, but a more common reason is that Westerners are used to taking pills and are more likely to continue using herbs if given in that form.

Herbs are available as tinctures (usually an alcohol-based extract which may be added by dropper to a cup of hot water), granules (powders which are dissolved in a cup of hot water and then drunk), and as medicinal wines. Although granules are available as complete formulas, they are also available as single herbs. This makes granules a good compromise between loose herbs and tablets, since they are more readily customizable by adding one or two single herbs to a formula, don't make the house smell of herbs, and don't require any cooking time on the part of the patient. In the case of medicinal wines, the wine itself often supplies a part of the therapeutic effect and is used in a narrower range of applications than tablets, tincture, and granules.

After discussing the relative merits of the various forms of administering herbs and making recommendations, your physician will usually let you choose which form you prefer.

Western Understanding of Herbs

Western science exclusively views herbs in the context of their constituent components—that is, their vitamin, mineral, enzyme, and alkaloid content. This is a reductionist view, in keeping with much of Western medicine. Western pharmacology might try to isolate the "active ingredient" and extract it away from all the other parts of the herb that make it a whole, complete, natural substance. If it proves useful in a Western medical application, they will later synthesize that ingredient as a patentable drug, further distancing it from its natural origins.

To better understand why this is usually not a desirable approach, consider that when you extract the vitamin C from an orange, you do not get the bioflavinoids necessary for its most complete bioavailability and utilization, any of the fiber, nor any of the other minerals and enzymes that make it a whole, healthy food. When vitamin C is synthesized, even though touted as bioidentical to what is in the orange, your body is less able to absorb and utilize that concentrated synthetic substance.

In fact, in some well-known Western medical studies, synthetic versions of vitamins, notably vitamin E and beta-carotene, were shown to increase the risk of cancers and heart disease in some populations. This is similar to the occurrence of side effects in synthetic drugs, only more insidious since it raises doubts in the minds of some people about vitamins that are indispensable to good health in their natural forms.

Most Western doctors are woefully ignorant about herbs in any form, so they perhaps wisely tend to err on the side of caution, counseling their patients to avoid the use of herbs when taking pharmaceutical drugs to treat any condition. This is usually to avoid the risk of unwanted, potentially harmful interactions.

One of the most common examples is blood thinners. Patients on blood-thinning medications are routinely told to avoid garlic, ginger, aloe vera, and a few other common herbs and foods that thin the blood, to avoid excessive bleeding risks. From a holistic perspective, this is exactly backward thinking. Doesn't it make more sense to eat a lot of garlic, ginger, and aloe vera and stop taking medications? The same holds true for many other conditions, which most often can be safely and effectively treated through dietary changes and herbal (and other nutrient) supplementation. While they do have their place and can be lifesaving, all pharmaceutical interventions present the risk of unwanted side effects even when used as directed. Properly used, herbs and foods do not.

Physical Therapies

Physical therapies may be passive, as when a patient receives treatment in the form of acupressure, Tuina (a type of medical massage), bone-setting (Chinese chiropractic), or medical Qigong. (Bone-setting is not legally allowable in the United States under Chinese medical licensure, so it is not discussed here.) They may be active, as when a patient is taught to perform Chinese healing exercises, Qigong, or Taiji to address specific medical issues for themselves. Not every Chinese physician includes these in their practice. Some do, and many may refer patients to specialists in these practices.

Acupressure and Tuina

Acupressure follows the same principles as acupuncture, without needles. Its main strength is the same as for acupuncture, with the added benefit of more immediately opening areas of obstruction, thereby reducing pain, when direct pressure is applied to painful points. Acupressure is also suitable as a means of self-care for the general population, as taught in this book.

Physicians manually stimulate the acupoints with their fingertips, their knuckles, their palms, the edge of the hand, and, for some points, their elbows. There are many techniques used to tonify and sedate points. Some techniques are selected based on the part of the body being treated. For example, techniques on the face need to be finer and more delicate than those used on the glutes. This type of treatment is less likely to follow an acupuncture treatment on the same day, as it may be redundant. Treatments typically take between twenty and fifty minutes.

Tuina, meaning "to push and pinch," is another related type of bodywork, superficially resembling Western massage. It has its own techniques, many involving the pushing, lifting, and squeezing its name implies, along with rolling, grasping, shaking, and tapping and patting, among others. Its main strength lies in addressing acute and chronic pain, musculoskeletal disorders, and digestive or respiratory disorders that are caused by stress.

While acupressure's main focus is on the points, Tuina has a larger, whole-body focus. Joint mobilization is employed to free up joint restrictions. Tuina may contain a strong Qigong component, addressing the body in as much of, or possibly more of, an energetic way than purely physically. In that case it is sometimes distinguished as "Qigong Tuina." Tuina can include bone-setting in regions where that is legally allowed. Tuina may be employed directly after an acupuncture treatment, since it is not specifically a point-based therapy. Treatments typical take between thirty and sixty minutes.

There can be some overlap between acupressure and Tuina. Often a practitioner is equally accomplished in both modalities, and techniques from one practice may be beneficial for a patient being treated in the other. In China, specialists in these healing disciplines receive as much medical training as acupuncturists and are held in similarly high regard.

Medical Qigong

This term is sometimes used to mean a Qigong one practices oneself for a specific medical purpose, but here we are referring to a physician who uses Qigong to treat a patient. Since medical Qigong can be very draining and leave the physician open to the many pathogenic factors afflicting their patients, the Qigong doctor must first become a very adept Qigong practitioner for their personal cultivation.

All of the principles of Chinese medicine are followed in medical Qigong. The Qigong doctor directly manipulates the Qi of the patient, sometimes using some physical touch but most often involving no or minimal physical contact. Tonification is obtained by the physician directly infusing Qi into the patient. Sedation involves directly drawing the pathogenic Qi out of the patient. The physician directs Qi flow within the body of the patient to open channel obstruction or obtain harmonization. These things can only be done once the physician is able to tangibly perceive the Qi within the patient's body and primarily utilizes *Waiqi* (Wai Qi), or the externalization or projection of Qi.

These are the three main ways this projection of Qi is accomplished:

1. The doctor uses his own Qi to treat the patient. This is very demanding and can seriously deplete the doctor. I've known a few Qigong doctors who practice Qigong six to eight hours a day for their self-care for this very reason. One of my acupuncture teachers told me of Qigong doctors she knew in China who healed hundreds of patients but died young themselves due to such serious depletion of their own life force.

2. The doctor stores environmental Qi within himself, like a storage battery, and uses only that Qi to heal patients. While this is less draining than using one's own Qi, it can become tricky to distinguish between stored environmental Qi and one's own.

3. The doctor focuses celestial and terrestrial Qi, using only that and none of his own. This may be safest for the doctor, but there is some risk of becoming a perpetually "open circuit" for any external influence, which can be both physically and psychologically destabilizing.

Other more esoteric options such as induction into spiritual lineages are beyond the scope of this discussion.

Chinese Healing Exercises

Some physicians teach their patients Chinese self-healing exercises. Each of these simple exercises may be performed in just a minute or two. Some address the whole body at once, but most target small body regions to open localized restriction or obstruction, moving Qi to reduce pain and increase functionality. Since these are easy to learn and take little time, many can be learned quickly and combined prescriptively to address a wide range of specific medical concerns or to promote overall health. Like all active physical therapies, they can be performed daily to optimize their many health benefits. More information can be found in *Chinese Healing Exercises: A Personalized Practice for Health & Longevity*. (See Recommended Reading at the end of this book for more details.)

Qigong and Taiji

Qigong is discussed thoroughly in Chapter 16 and taught in Chapter 17, so it will only briefly be introduced here. Qigong involves working with Qi, the energy of life. It has hundreds, perhaps thousands, of forms, each with unique applications. They can improve health in a general way, target an individual Organ System to strengthen it or heal specific illnesses, help develop athletic or martial abilities, increase longevity, promote spiritual cultivation, or simply help one achieve excellence in secular endeavors. The type of Qigong you practice will make a difference in the results you experience, although there can be overlap among styles. For holistic healing purposes, practicing Qigongs that target Organ Systems, as are taught in this book, will give you the best outcomes, whether your goal is to maintain or improve upon your good health or to heal from illness, injury, or debility.

Taiji can work in similar ways to Qigong. It was developed as a martial art, although it can be modified to primarily access its healing qualities. There are many such variations available today. The single most significant difference is that even these modified forms are more lengthy and involved than most Qigongs. If your immediate needs are for healing, Qigong is likely a better option since you can learn it more quickly and access its healing benefits sooner. If you are healthy, learning Taiji is a great option for preventive maintenance, optimal health, physical strengthening, and self-defense if you're interested in that aspect. Then you will have it already available if you need to draw on it for healing at a later time.

As an important part of integrated natural healing, Qigong or Taiji specific to your health needs can and should be performed daily. With practice, both enable you to acquire more Qi. They enhance the effects of acupuncture/acupressure and herbs and support a healthy lifestyle.

Diet and Lifestyle

Diet and lifestyle are discussed extensively in Chapter 7. This brief summary of reminders may serve as a useful guide on your journey to better health.

Daily diet and lifestyle choices are among the things over which we have the most control. They often become ingrained habits and are not given much thought, which can make them difficult to change. The changes become easier if we first become mindful and then tackle them one at a time, replacing poor or careless habits with conscientious new ones that promote health and happiness.

There are very few things that will cause illness or injury unless done to excess or at the expense of other important elements of life. As in all other aspects of Chinese medical thought, balance is the key. Work must be balanced with recreation, activity with rest, wakefulness with adequate sleep.

When a person is in balanced good health, even exposure to external pathogenic factors will not cause illness unless the exposure is prolonged or intense. Strive for equanimity in all facets of emotional experience, and you'll reduce the possibility of imbalance due to internal pathogenic factors as well.

Regulate your daily schedule as much as possible by getting enough sleep (seven to eight hours) during the same hours each night and eating your meals at the same time each day. Balance your diet by including all of the Five Flavors each day. For most people, that means reducing sweet, salty, and spicy flavors and increasing bitter and sour flavors. In general, that involves cutting back on sugars and carbs and increasing vegetables and some fruits. While a simplification, this is at the core of most contemporary dietary recommendation. (See Appendix 2, Note 11.2.)

The best specific food advice for restoring health from a Chinese holistic perspective is found in the prescriptions in Chapter 18.

Try to eat organically and avoid genetically modified foods and ingredients. All traditional dietary advice precedes the advent of the now-common commercial methods of food production, including synthetic chemical pesticides, herbicides, fertilizers, and genetic modifications. The nutritional content and safety of commercial foods have altered dramatically since their traditional organic origins. As they are many steps removed from nature, they can no longer be considered part of a truly holistic lifestyle.

Avoid allowing yourself to become exhausted on a regular basis. This includes sexual exhaustion. You may want to include aspects of sexual regulation as previously discussed. Be mindful of the Five Exhaustions (see page 125). If you should exhaust yourself, do all you can to rest and replenish as soon as possible.

Diet and lifestyle are integral parts of creating or restoring and maintaining balance and harmony. This includes supporting the natural balance among all the Yin and Yang energies within us and harmonizing with and attuning to the hours of the day, the passage of the seasons, and the stages of our life. We are all products of nature and are optimally served by aligning ourselves with the rhythms of the natural world. This is the best way to avoid depletion, degeneration, and premature aging and is necessary to produce the abundant Qi and Blood required to maintain energy and good health throughout all of our years.

Chapter 12

Acupressure Self-Care: Your Healing Hands

In Chapter 11 you were introduced to Chinese massage therapy and some of its varieties. Acupressure is one of the easiest to apply to oneself. While there are many techniques that may be used by a professional, only a very few techniques are necessary for you to achieve a broad range of benefits. While acupressure is a gentler, milder therapy than acupuncture, it provides a significant advantage, since you can perform acupressure on yourself daily at no financial cost.

For the purposes of this book, acupressure is a necessary substitute for acupuncture. Acupuncture is not something you can learn to do safely and effectively from a book. Since the insertion of needles can cause serious harm if done incorrectly, acupuncture requires professional licensure to be legally performed, even on oneself. You can get many of the benefits of acupuncture through acupressure, which only requires directed pressure from your fingertips.

The points for acupressure self-care have been selected with a few purposes in mind:

1. Safety. Each point presented is safe for you to use. While acupressure is generally a very safe practice with little possibility of causing harm, it's wise to remember that anything that is powerful enough to cause healthful changes in your body if performed properly is powerful enough to cause harmful changes if done improperly.

(See Appendix 2, Note 12.1.) There's no danger of causing any harm to yourself with these points, and any cautions will be noted when necessary.

2. Ease of access. There are many points located on the back of your body, for example. They are difficult or impossible to reach by yourself, so they are not included here.

3. Easy to locate. Some points are very close together. They are easy enough to distinguish by the fine point of a needle but harder to separate by the much broader tip of a finger. Pressing on more than one adjacent point at a time is not harmful, but it may dilute the focus of the treatment. Conversely, some points are spread across your body away from convenient anatomical landmarks, so they are more difficult to find accurately. Again, it will not cause harm to apply pressure to a nonacupuncture point, but you will not be effectively addressing your purpose.

4. They must either have a broad range of effects or one or two very focused effects that can address a variety of common ailments and therefore benefit the greatest number of people. There are over 360 acupoints in common use by professionals and hundreds more that are less common. It would be overwhelming and impractical to include all those possibilities here. In fact, many acupuncturists select their everyday treatment points from a pool of about sixty points, since they can address the widest range of common patient complaints. The points selected here include most of those highly effective points. This is a useful, practical way to start your acupressure self-care. As you get more familiar with each point, you'll enjoy a wider, deeper range of benefits. Nearly one hundred points are included here, and you'll learn how to combine a few at a time in different ways. Each point has it primary effects, but the combination of points produces many different sets of effects, and it greatly expands the range of benefits to use the same points in different combinations.

Point combinations for common conditions are provided in Chapter 18. These are not the only possible prescriptions for those conditions, but they are among the most widely used. You may find points in Chapter 13 that seem useful for a condition that have been left out of the prescription. Feel free to experiment after you've acquired a little experience. That's why you have so many point options.

Methods of Locating the Points

Whenever possible, the simplest everyday language is used to help you identify the point location. Most of the time that will get you to exactly the place a physician would use when selecting that point. The precise anatomical location may also be provided. Sometimes more technical language may be necessary, and this is what you'll need to know.

The Chinese use an anatomical unit of measure called a *Cun*, roughly translated as a "body inch," in order to accurately locate points. As a body inch, a Cun is not a fixed distance but a relative distance, based on the size of any individual body. For example, on a person who is five feet tall, a vertical Cun would be a shorter objective distance than it would be on a person who is six feet tall.

There are two standard ways that Cun are measured. One is proportional distances, and the other is hand and finger measurements. Some points are located by anatomical landmarks only. We'll primarily be using hand and finger measurements and anatomical landmarks.

Proportional measurements require knowing the standardized, set number of Cun present in any body part and then dividing that body part in order to find the point location. For example, the distance between the elbow crease and the wrist crease is always 12 Cun. So if you wanted to find a point exactly 3 Cun above the wrist, you would need to mentally divide the forearm into four equal parts, 3 Cun each, and select the point a quarter of the way up from the wrist crease toward the elbow. Whether a person is four feet or six feet tall, that would be precisely 3 Cun, even though the objective inches would be different on each person. (See **Figure 12.1** on next page.)

Hand and finger measurements are a little easier to use, are still individualized units of measure, and are just about as accurate as proportional measurements. There are two commonly used hand measurements.

The first is the width of the knuckle joint closest to the tip of the thumb. This is a 1-Cun measurement (**Figure 12.2** on page 187). This is useful in measuring short distances between two points or between an anatomical landmark and a point.

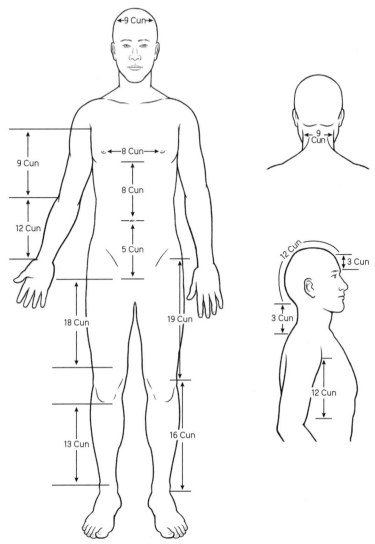

Figure 12.1 (Standard Cun Measurements)

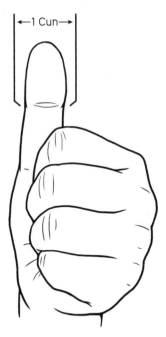

Figure 12.2 (1-Cun Measurement)

The second is the width of the four fingers held together. This measures 3 Cun. This measurement is taken at the proximal interphalangeal joint, the set of knuckles closest to the hand (**Figure 12.3** on next page). This is useful for measuring larger distances between two points or between an anatomical landmark and a point.

Anatomical landmarks are very obvious anatomical structures, such as nipples, the nose, the navel, kneecaps, and elbow tips. They are also slightly less obvious ones, such as bony protrusions like the greater trochanter (the large, bony prominence at the outside of your upper thigh) and the head of the ulna (the bony prominence on the little-finger side of the back of your wrist) or depressions in bones (like the depressions in your sacrum and in facial and skull bones). With just a little practice, even the less obvious ones will become easy to find, and they will be clearly described whenever they may be used.

Some Western anatomical language is used in describing a point's location. That will be kept to a minimum, and illustrations are provided to make it as easy for you as possible. Here are some simple terms that you will encounter, along with their meanings:

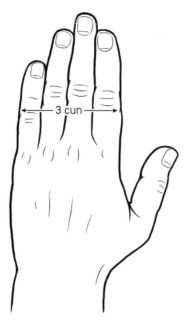

Figure 12.3 (3-Cun Measurement)

- *Lateral:* Lateral means away from the midline of the body or toward the sideward outside edge of the body. For example, the tip of each shoulder is lateral to the notch at the base of the throat. This is a relative term. The eyes are lateral to the bridge of the nose. The top of the right ear is lateral to the right eye. On an arm or leg, lateral may be relative to the midline of the arm or leg.

- *Medial:* Medial is the opposite of lateral and means toward the midline of the body. So the bridge of the nose is medial to the eyes or to either eye if only one eye is being discussed. This is also a relative term, requiring at least two body structures in relation to each other. The right eye is both lateral to the bridge of the nose and medial to the tip of the right ear. On an arm or leg, medial may be relative to the midline of the arm or leg.

- *Anterior:* Toward or at the front of the body or body part.

- *Posterior:* Toward or at the back of the body or body part.

- *Superior:* Above or upward, usually in the general direction of the top of the head. The navel is superior to the pubic bone.

- *Inferior:* Below or downward, usually in the general direction of the bottom of the feet. The anterior superior iliac spine (ASIS), or hip pointer, is inferior to the tip of the eleventh rib.
- *Distal:* This term relates to the four limbs: the arms (along with hands and fingers) and the legs (along with feet and toes). Distal means away from the torso and toward the fingertips or toe tips. The wrist is distal to the elbow; the knee is distal to the hip.
- *Proximal:* This relates to the four limbs, is the opposite of distal, and means toward the torso and away from the fingertips and toe tips. The shoulder is proximal to the elbow; the ankle is proximal to the toes.

These are relative terms, requiring at least two body structures in relation to each other. For example, the wrist is proximal to the fingers but distal to the elbow.

Acupressure Techniques

Chinese massage therapy has an extensive array of techniques, each intended for a specific therapeutic purpose. Acupressure techniques are less extensive, yet we can get an impressive variety of outcomes by learning to master just a couple.

Tonification

Tonification techniques are used to draw Qi to the targeted acupoint to strengthen its functions or to encourage Qi to flow in the appropriate direction within its meridian. In general terms, this is the best approach to take for a person who is weak, is recovering from an illness or injury, is usually tired or with little energy, tends to be very quiet, withdrawn, or depressed, catches colds frequently or is easily chilled, has poor digestion with loose stool, or is very elderly. Any or all of these presentations may apply.

To tonify a point, use relatively light pressure. You want to engage the point: use enough pressure so that you feel it, with enough depth that you may feel resistance from the muscle tissue below the skin, but you don't want to go deep into the muscle. There should be no discomfort (beyond what you might feel in a painful body part even if you were not touching the point) and definitely no pain.

You can enhance the tonification by maintaining that depth, that engagement of the point, and make very small clockwise circles with your fingertip. The only exception is if you are working on an abdominal point, in which case counterclockwise circles will be most effective for tonification.

An alternate method of tonification can be used anywhere on the body but may be especially useful in tight-spaced, narrow areas—between two very close tendons, for example. Here, place your fingertip on the acupoint firmly enough to engage the muscle under the skin, so your fingertip does not slide over the skin. Keeping on the point, move your fingertip back and forth along the line of the meridian. Use more force in the direction of normal Qi flow for that meridian and less force when moving your finger against the meridian flow. Remember that in Chinese anatomical position (hands above the head in an "I surrender" pose), Yang Qi normally flows downward, from the fingertips toward the toes, and Yin Qi flows upward, from the toes toward the fingertips.

Sedation

Sedation techniques are used to disperse Qi that is stuck around an acupoint or body region or to encourage Qi to flow counter to its normal direction for a brief period of time. (This is a little like unclogging a drain: you have to make the water flow opposite to its normal direction to dislodge the obstruction, after which it can freely return to its normal direction.) Generally, this is the best approach to take for a person who is fairly strong and robust, is excitable, is agitated or easy to anger, feels warm or hot much of the time, is suffering acute pain from an injury or other obstructive circumstance, or has a big appetite with frequent constipation. Any or all of these presentations may apply.

To sedate a point, use relatively deep pressure, going well into the muscle tissue below the skin, unless you are working on a bony area where that is not possible. You may feel some discomfort or mild to moderate pain that you recognize as beneficial—a "good kind of pain." You should not press so deeply that you feel a sharp or strong pain.

You can enhance the sedation by maintaining that depth and make very small counterclockwise circles with your fingertip. The only exception is if you are working on an abdominal point, in which case clockwise circles will be most effective.

An alternate method of sedation can be used anywhere on the body but may be especially useful in tight-spaced, narrow areas of the body, as between two very close tendons. Here, place your fingertip on the acupoint, firmly enough to engage the muscle under the skin, so your fingertip does not slide over the skin. Keeping on the point, move your fingertip back and forth along the line of the meridian. Use more force in the direction against normal Qi flow for that meridian and less force when moving your finger with the meridian flow.

The pressures and depths may seem counterintuitive at first glance, since a deep pressure seems strong, working at deep levels of the body, and so should be more tonifying, while a light touch is soothing and calming, the kind of touch you might use instinctively to comfort a troubled child. On a strictly physiological, neurological level, that makes sense and is sometimes appropriate. But on an energetic level, that is not the case. Think of what happens if you strongly push your hand into a basin of water. The water will splash over the side of the basin, dispersing. If you lightly place your hand on the surface of the water, though, and slightly lift your hand for an even lighter touch, the water's adhesive property will make it "stick" to your skin, and it will be drawn toward your hand. In this example, Qi behaves much like water.

Harmonization

Harmonization techniques are used to provide balance and clear communication among the points being treated and, by extension, throughout the entire body. They neither tonify nor sedate but may do both in equal measure. This is the best approach to use when a person has no particular health challenge but wants an energetic tune-up to facilitate optimal functioning, when someone may feel out of sorts or out of sync (emotionally a little off but with no obvious ailment), or when there is no clear need for either tonification or sedation.

To harmonize a point with the entire body or to harmonize a group of selected points, use moderate depth, clearly getting into the muscle tissue without going very deep. That pressure is maintained with little variation throughout the treatment.

You can enhance the harmonization by maintaining that depth and making an equal number of small clockwise and counterclockwise circles with your fingertip, first in one direction and then in the other. This technique is the same for abdominal points as for the rest of the body.

An alternate method of harmonization can be used anywhere on the body but may be especially useful in tight-spaced, narrow areas of the body. Here, place your fingertip on the acupoint, firmly enough to engage the muscle under the skin, so your fingertip does not slide over the skin. Keeping on the point, move your fingertip back and forth along the line of the meridian. Use equal force in both directions.

Since harmonization techniques are balancing, there is never a concern of harming yourself, and the treatments are always beneficial, if milder, in cases where tonification or sedation is best. Try to select the technique that closely matches your condition. Even if you select tonification when sedation is needed, for example, you won't do yourself any real harm. You may feel a little more stimulated, a pain or discomfort might be more noticeable, or you might feel a little more tired, but any such effect will pass within one to three days, leaving you about where you were before the treatment. Even among health professionals, these sorts of trial-and-error outcomes are typical when one is first learning and acquiring the necessary skill and sensitivity.

In the point prescription sections of Chapter 18, you'll find recommendations for tonification and sedation to fit the conditions being treated. These will guide you in the right direction, but because everyone is unique, some people may have a different cause of the condition from what is most typical, so some experimentation may be required. Again, you won't cause yourself any harm, but for greatest benefit and peace of mind, you may want to consult your acupuncturist for recommendations regarding technique selection.

Treatment Frequency

The effects of an acupressure treatment peak in about two days on average and then begin to decline. If you are trying to improve a specific health problem, self-treatment every two to three days is recommended, before much of a decline has occurred. If you want to treat yourself daily, that's optimal, as your improvements will accrue more quickly. For general health maintenance or a periodic boost in energy and performance, once a week is fine.

Selected Acupressure Points

The following Chapter contains some of the most potent and versatile acupoints, selected from among the 360 common meridian points and hundreds of other possible extra points, as well as their location, main functions, and conditions they commonly treat. They're arranged according to the meridian they're found on.

In addition to point number, the Chinese name is provided, along with an English translation. The point names are open to various interpretations. The ones given here are among the most commonly used. While many of the names are poetic, they either give clues to the point's location by referring to anatomical landmarks or clues to its function, although many of those functions may be obscured by cultural, historic, or alchemical metaphor. To more deeply explore the meaning behind the points' names, consult *Grasping the Wind* by Ellis, Wiseman, and Boss or *Acupuncture Points: Images and Functions* by Arnie Lade. (See Recommended Reading.)

After the point name, you'll find its location, described according to the methods outlined above. When necessary, alternative methods will be provided, along with illustrations, to make location as easy as possible.

After the location, you'll find its TCM function(s), the way the point is able to work in the way that it does. This will use the traditional terminology introduced to you in Chapter 7.

After the function, you'll find its indication(s), the symptoms for which it's commonly used. While these are presented in familiar Western terms, be careful not to assume they are a one-to-one correspondence with a Chinese diagnosis. For example, you'll find points with indications for headache on the Liver, Gall Bladder, Urinary Bladder, and Stomach meridians, but a headache can arise from many differing sources. If your headache is primarily related to a Urinary Bladder disharmony, selecting headache points from the Stomach meridian will likely not do you much good. The good news is it won't likely do you any harm either, as these are all safe points. So, if you're not clear on your diagnosis before you begin, some trial and error can be useful. Don't get discouraged. A little effort while you learn will pay off tremendously over time.

While most of these points have a wide range of effects and applications even beyond what is presented here, some are known to have an especially beneficial effect on just one or two of the many conditions they may treat. When applicable, those will be noted after the indications as "especially helps."

For the reader already familiar with Chinese medicine, you may freely combine these points according to your experience and understanding. For everyone else, it's fine to experiment by selecting points that address your needs. You will get the best results by selecting points that best match your condition or goals. The diagnostic methods introduced in Chapter 10 can help you with that.

Point prescriptions for common Western-defined diseases are provided in Chapter 18. In most cases, those prescriptions will be very helpful, since they are based on the most typical Chinese diagnoses for those conditions. If the prescription does not exactly match your condition, you will still get some beneficial results.

In all cases, spend some time familiarizing yourself with the locations of the points and the way they feel when you apply pressure to them using different techniques. Getting acquainted that way first will give you another advantage in your self-care.

All points are bilateral (located on both sides of the body) except where noted, specifically in the Du and Ren meridians.

Chapter 13

The Acupressure Points: Names, Locations, and Functions

Since we are using acupressure and not acupuncture, all of these points are generally safe. A few have cautions noted, mainly regarding pregnancy. Most of those are abdominal points and should not present any problems with light to moderate acupressure as long as they are not painful. All strong stimulation should be avoided during pregnancy. Let your feelings guide you. There are a couple of points that are contraindicated during pregnancy, as they may induce labor. They are clearly identified for you.

Throughout this book, abbreviations for organ/meridian point names are as follows:

Lung: Lu

Large Intestine: LI

Stomach: St

Spleen: Sp

Heart: H

Small Intestine: SI

Urinary Bladder: UB

Kidney: K

Pericardium: P

Sanjiao: SJ

Gall Bladder: GB

Liver: Liv

Each meridian with selected acupoints is shown at the beginning of the section devoted to that meridian. You can refer to that image as an aid to point location while reading through this chapter. You'll also find references to the same points in Appendix 1, indicated as "For alternate view, see Appendix 1, Figure A (image number)." There, the points are shown by body region, and it displays points from other meridians that are found on the same body region. This will help you see points in relation to one another, which may make point location even more clear, and it will provide you with a selection of points useful for treating problems local to that body part. For example, if you have wrist pain, seeing all possible points on the wrist will help you to find the ones that are most relevant to you.

Lungs, Hand Taiyin

Lu 1, Zhong Fu, Central Palace

Location: In the first intercostal space (between the first two ribs), 6 Cun lateral to the midline. Easiest way to find: Place the tip of your right index finger on the front tip of your left shoulder. Slowly slide your index finger toward your chest, just under the collarbone. As soon as you clear the shoulder bone, you'll feel a depression. Keep your index finger firmly pressed upward, touching your collarbone. Place your middle and ring fingers directly below your index finger, keeping all fingers touching. The point will be under the tip of your ring finger. For an alternate view of Lu 1, see Appendix 1, Figure A8.

Functions: Clears Heat and inflammation in the chest, regulates Lung Qi, tonifies Lung Qi and Yin.

Indications: Cough, wheeze, asthma, bronchitis, fullness in the chest, chest pain.

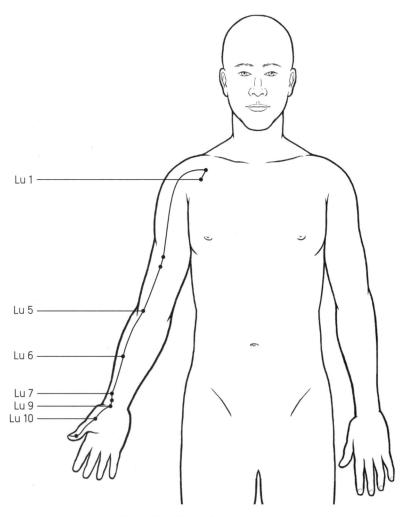

Figure 13.1 (Lung Acupressure Points)

Lu 5, Chi Ze, Cubit Marsh

Location: In the elbow crease, in a depression felt at the radial (thumb) side of the biceps tendon. For an alternate view of Lu 5, see Appendix 1, Figure A1.

Functions: Clears Heat in the Lungs, rectifies Lung Qi, nourishes Yin, moistens the Lungs.

Indications: Cough, asthma, pneumonia, sore throat, hemoptysis (coughing up blood).

Lu 6, Kong Zui, Collection Hole

Location: 5 Cun below Lu 5, 7 Cun above Lu 9 (at the wrist crease), on the line connecting those two points. For an alternate view of Lu 6, see Appendix 1, Figure A1.

Functions: Spreads and descends Lung Qi, cools and soothes the Blood. Especially useful when Heat has reached the Blood level, causing Lung-related bleeding disorders, like nosebleeds and coughing or spitting blood.

Indications: Cough, asthma, pneumonia, sore throat, hemoptysis, elbow and arm pain.

Especially helps: Nose bleed, coughing or spitting blood.

Lu 7, Lie Que, Broken Sequence

Location: 1.5 Cun above the wrist crease, in the depression superior to the styloid process of the radius. Easiest way to find: Cross your hands at the web between thumb and index finger. Place your left index finger on your right wrist, pointing toward your right elbow. The point is below the tip of your index finger (**Figure 13.2**). For an alternate view of Lu 7, see Appendix 1, Figure A1.

Functions: Regulates and rectifies Lung Qi, disperses external Wind, regulates the Ren meridian.

Indications: Common cold, headache, cough, sore throat, wrist pain and weakness.

Especially helps: Common cold.

Lu 9, Tai Yuan, Great Abyss

Location: In the depression at the radial (thumb) end of the wrist crease, at the lateral side of the radial artery. For an alternate view of Lu 9, see Appendix 1, Figure A1.

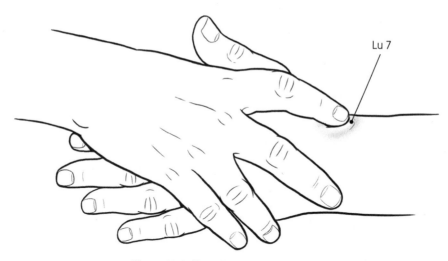

Figure 13.2 (Lu 7 Acupressure Point)

Functions: Clears Wind and transforms phlegm, regulates Lungs, tonifies Lung Qi and Yin. This is the best point to strengthen overall Lung function, especially useful in chronic or deficiency conditions.

Indications: Cough, asthma, pneumonia, sore throat, hemoptysis, pain in the chest, wrist, or hand.

Especially helps: Chronic deficiency or weakness, Phlegm.

Lu 10, Yu Ji, Fish Border

Location: Halfway between Lu 9 and the first thumb joint, at the border between the red and white skin. For an alternate view of Lu 10, see Appendix 1, Figure A1.

Functions: Clears Lung Heat, benefits the throat, regulates and rectifies Lung Qi, nourishes Yin.

Indications: Sore throat (important point for acute sore throat), cough, asthma, hemoptysis, fever (from respiratory tract infection).

Especially helps: Acute sore throat.

Large Intestine, Hand Yangming

LI 4, He Gu, Union Valley

Location: On the back of the hand, between the thumb and index finger, about halfway up the side of the second metacarpal bone (the bone in the hand that connects to the index finger).

Easiest way to find: Place the distal joint crease of the right thumb on the web of the left hand, between left thumb and index finger. The point is where the tip of the right thumb touches the left hand. For alternate views of LI 4, see Appendix 1, Figures A2 and A3.

Functions: Releases surface (exterior conditions), disperses Wind, clears Heat. A powerful Qi tonifying and regulating point, it influences almost everything from the neck up.

Indications: Common cold, headaches (especially frontal and sinus), diseases of the sensory organs, toothache, painful, red or watery eyes, allergies, painful swelling of the throat, sinus conditions, general pain. Strengthens the immune system.

Especially helps: Headaches.

LI 5, Yang Xi, Yang Ravine

Location: On the radial side of the crease at the back of the wrist, in the center of the "anatomical snuffbox," the depression formed between the tendons when spreading your thumb away from your index finger. For alternate views of LI 5, see Appendix 1, Figures A2 and A3.

Functions: Clears Wind and Heat.

Indications: Swollen eyes, toothache, sore throat, all local problems of the wrist joint. Useful in smoking withdrawal.

LI 10, Shou San Li, Arm Three Miles

Location: On the line joining LI 5 and LI 11, 2 Cun below LI 11. For an alternate view of LI 10, see Appendix 1, Figure A3.

Functions: Expels Internal Wind, harmonizes the Stomach, benefits the Intestines, invigorates the Qi and Blood.

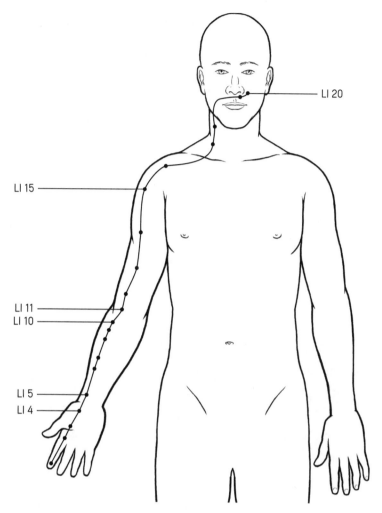

Figure 13.3 (Large Intestine Acupressure Points)

Indications: Tennis elbow, shoulder and arm pain, stomachache, abdominal pain. Helps in building energy by improving stomach and intestinal functions.

Especially helps: Stomachache.

LI 11, Qu Chi, Crooked Pool

Location: When the elbow is flexed, in the depression at the lateral end of the elbow crease. For an alternate view of LI 4 11, see Appendix 1, Figure A3.

Functions: Releases the surface, clears Wind and Heat, cools and regulates the Blood, resolves Damp.

Indications: High fever, skin conditions, high blood pressure, edema, abdominal pain, diarrhea, arm pain (including arthritic), upper arm paralysis.

Especially helps: High fevers.

LI 15, Jian Yu, Shoulder Bone

Location: When the arm is held straight out to the side, the point is in the depression slightly to the front of the very top of the shoulder. For an alternate view of LI 15, see Appendix 1, Figure A1.

Functions: Clears Wind, Heat, and Damp; regulates the channels.

Indications: Pain and inflammation in the shoulder joint, restricted shoulder movement, hives.

Especially helps: Shoulder problems.

LI 20, Ying Xiang, Welcome Fragrance

Location: In the nasolabial groove (the crease between the nostril and the corner of the mouth), just lateral to and slightly above the nostrils. For an alternate view of LI 20, see Appendix 1, Figure A5.

Functions: Clears Wind and Heat, opens the Lungs and nasal passages.

Indications: Nasal sinusitis, rhinitis, reduced sense of smell, facial paresis (muscle weakness with partial paralysis).

Especially helps: Sinuses.

Stomach, Foot Yangming

St 2, Si Bai, Four Whites

Location: Directly below the pupil, in the bony depression about .5 Cun below the infraorbital foramen (eye socket). For an alternate view of St 2, see Appendix 1, Figure A5.

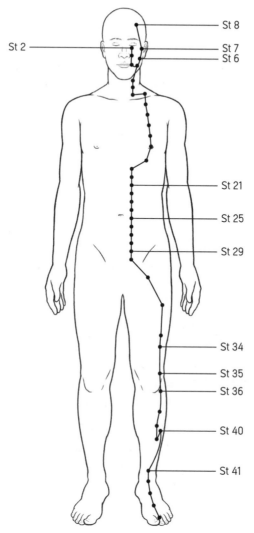

Figure 13.4 (Stomach Acupressure Points)

Functions: Clears Heat, brightens the eyes, smoothes Liver Qi, benefits the Gall Bladder.

Indications: All eye diseases (e.g. conjunctivitis, keratitis, night blindness, myopia), twitching eyelid, facial paralysis, second branch trigeminal neuralgia.

St 6, Jia Che, Jaw Chariot

Location: About 1 Cun anterior and superior to the lower angle of the mandible (jaw). When you clench your teeth, it is at the peak of the masseter, the muscle that bulges at that location. For an alternate view of St 6, see Appendix 1, Figure A6.

Functions: Clears Wind and Heat, opens the channels, benefits teeth and jaw.

Indications: Toothache, mumps, facial paralysis.

St 7, Xia Guan, Lower Hinge

Location: Place the tip of your index finger at the center of the tragus, the triangular skin flap at the front of your ear canal. Slowly move your finger forward, straight toward your nose. In about 1 Cun, it will slide over the jaw hinge, into a depression. That's the point. For an alternate view of St 7, see Appendix 1, Figure A6.

Functions: Clears Wind and Heat, opens the channels, sharpens hearing.

Indications: Tinnitus, deafness, toothache, facial paralysis, facial pain/trigeminal neuralgia, temporomandibular joint disorder (TMJ).

St 8, Tou Wei, Head Corner

Location: In the bony depression at the temple corner, .5 Cun within the ideal hairline (3 Cun above Yintang), 4.5 Cun lateral to the midline. For alternate views of St 8, see Appendix 1, Figures A5 and A6.

Functions: Opens the channels, clears Wind and Heat, relieves pain.

Indications: One-sided headache, eye pain.

St 21, Liang Men, Beam Gate

Location: 4 Cun above the navel, 4 Cun below the bottom of the breastbone, 2 Cun lateral to the midline. For an alternate view of St 21, see Appendix 1, Figure A8.

Functions: Regulates the Middle Jiao, harmonizes the Stomach and Intestines, disperses stagnation.

Indications: Stomachache, nausea, vomiting, lack of appetite, diarrhea.

St 25, Tian Shu, Celestial Axis

Location: 2 Cun lateral to the navel. For an alternate view of St 25, see Appendix 1, Figure A8.

Functions: Regulates and supports the function of the Intestines, regulates Qi and disperses stagnation.

Indications: Abdominal pain and distention, constipation, diarrhea, irregular menstruation.

Especially helps: Intestinal problems.

CAUTION: Contraindicated in pregnancy. This is primarily a concern with acupuncture, but strong stimulation should be avoided.

St 29, Gui Lai, Return

Location: 4 Cun below the navel (1 Cun above the pubic bone), 2 Cun lateral to the midline. For an alternate view of St 29, see Appendix 1, Figure A8.

Functions: Activates Qi, disperses Blood Stagnation and clears Damp Heat from the Lower Jiao, relieves pain, regulates menstruation.

Indications: Irregular menstruation, pelvic inflammatory disease (PID), leukorrhea, amenorrhea, hernia.

Especially helps: Reproductive organs.

CAUTION: Contraindicated in pregnancy. This is primarily a concern with acupuncture, but strong stimulation should be avoided.

St 34, Lian Que, Beam Mound

Location: 2 Cun above the lateral superior border of the kneecap. For alternate views of St 34, see Appendix 1, Figures A9 and A12.

Functions: Harmonizes the Stomach, clears the channels.

Indications: Numb or painful knee, stomachache, diarrhea, mastitis (swollen, painful, inflamed breasts).

St 35, Du Bi, Calf's Nose

Location: When the knee is flexed, in the depression at the lower border of the kneecap, lateral to the thick ligament (patellar ligament). For alternate views of St 35, see Appendix 1, Figures A9 and A12.

Functions: Dispels Wind and Cold, activates the channels, frees the joint, stops pain.

Indications: Pain, numbness, swelling, and motor impairment of the knee.

St 36, Zu San Li, Leg Three Miles

Location: 3 Cun inferior to St 35, 1 finger width lateral to the crest of the tibia bone.

Functions: Strengthens the Spleen, harmonizes the Stomach, regulates Qi and Blood, strengthens the entire body, boosts the immune system. For alternate views of St 36, see Appendix 1, Figures A9 and A12.

Indications: Stomach pain, diarrhea, constipation, knee joint and leg pain or numbness, mastitis, indigestion, dizziness, general weakness, anemia.

Especially helps: General body weakness and digestive deficiencies.

St 40, Feng Long, Abundant Bulge

Location: Halfway between the lateral center of the knee and the tip of the lateral ankle (or 8 Cun proximal to the tip of the lateral ankle), two fingers' width (1.5 Cun) lateral to the anterior crest of the tibia. For alternate views of St 40, see Appendix 1, Figures A9 and A12.

Functions: Regulates the Stomach and Intestines, transforms Phlegm and Damp, calms the spirit.

Indications: Cough with profuse phlegm, dizziness, headache, asthma, epilepsy, mania.

Especially helps: Phlegm.

St 41, Jie Xi, Divide Stream

Location: At the midpoint of the anterior ankle crease, between the two tendons. For an alternate view of St 41, see Appendix 1, Figure A12.

Functions: Supports the Spleen, clears Stomach Heat, calms the Spirit, provides general relaxation.

Indications: Paralysis and pain in lower leg and ankle, drop foot, headache, dizziness, vertigo, constipation.

Especially helps: All foot problems, facial edema.

Spleen, Foot Taiyin

Sp 3, Tai Bai, Supreme White

Location: At the inside (big-toe side) of the foot, just proximal to the ball of the foot (proximal and inferior to the first metatarsal-phalangeal joint), on the border between the red and white skin. For alternate views of Sp 3, see Appendix 1, Figures A10 and A13.

Functions: Strengthens the Spleen, resolves Damp, harmonizes the Stomach.

Indications: Stomach pain, abdominal distention, digestive disorders, sluggishness.

Especially helps: Spleen tonification.

Sp 4, Gong Sun, Ancestor and Descendant

Location: In the depression distal and inferior to the base of the first metatarsal bone, on the border between the red and white skin. For alternate views of Sp 4, see Appendix 1, Figures A10 and A13.

Functions: Strengthens the Spleen, harmonizes the Stomach, resolves Damp.

Indications: Acute or chronic stomachache, nausea, indigestion, diarrhea, foot and ankle pain, irregular menstruation.

Sp 6, San Yin Jiao, Three Yin Crossing

Location: 3 Cun above the tip of the inner ankle, on the posterior border of the tibia. For alternate views of Sp 6, see Appendix 1, Figures A10 and A13.

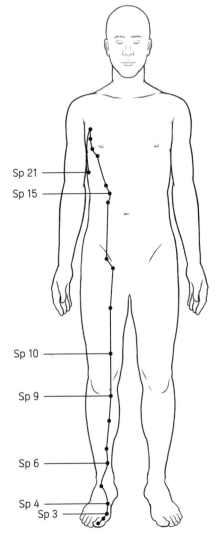

Sp 21

Sp 15

Sp 10

Sp 9

Sp 6

Sp 4
Sp 3

Figure 13.5 (Spleen Acupressure Points)

Functions: Strengthens the Spleen, harmonizes the Stomach, transforms Damp, smoothes the Liver Qi, nourishes the Kidneys.

Indications: Abdominal pain, distention, diarrhea, excessive urination or incontinence, impotence, premature ejaculation, menstrual irregularities, vaginal discharge, sterility, infertility, eczema, edema, insomnia. All diseases of the urogenital and digestive systems.

Especially helps: Build Yin and Blood, gynecological deficiencies.

CAUTION: Contraindicated in pregnancy. Strong stimulation may induce labor.

Sp 9, Yin Ling Quan, Yin Mound Spring

Location: On the medial side of the knee, in the depression just below the large bone at the bottom of the knee joint. (In the depression below the lower border of the medial condyle of the tibia.) For alternate views of Sp 9, see Appendix 1, Figures A9 and A10.

Functions: Strengthens the Spleen, clears Heat, drains Damp, disinhibits urination.

Indications: Abdominal distention, urinary incontinence or retention, menstrual irregularities, diarrhea, edema, pain in the external genitals, knee pain.

Especially helps: Urinary problems.

Sp 10, Xue Hai, Sea of Blood

Location: When the knee is flexed, 2 Cun above the medial superior corner of the kneecap. For alternate views of Sp 10, see Appendix 1, Figures A9 and A10.

Functions: Harmonizes Qi and Blood, clears Heat, cools and moves the Blood, regulates menstruation.

Indications: Irregular or painful menstruation, amenorrhea (no menses), anemia, eczema, hives.

Especially helps: Skin problems, excessive menstrual bleeding.

Sp 15, Da Peng, Great Horizontal

Location: 4 Cun lateral to the navel. For an alternate view of Sp 15, see Appendix 1, Figure A8.

Functions: Regulates Qi and alleviates pain, regulates Spleen Qi, moistens the Intestines, harmonizes the Large Intestines.

Indications: Diarrhea, constipation, abdominal distention and pain.

CAUTION: Light stimulation only during pregnancy. This is primarily a concern with acupuncture, but strong stimulation should be avoided.

Sp 21, Da Bao, Great Wrapping

Location: On the side of the chest, between the ribs, 6 Cun below the armpit, or midway between the armpit and that tip of the eleventh rib. (If you slide your finger down the front of your ribs, the eleventh rib is the first one that feels like a separate tip detached from the rest.) For an alternate view of Sp 21, see Appendix 1, Figure A8.

Functions: Regulates Qi and Blood, unbinds the chest and alleviates pain.

Indications: Asthma, pain in the chest or flanks, general ache and weakness throughout the body.

Heart, Hand Shaoyin

H 1, Ji Quan, Supreme Spring

Location: At the center of the armpit. For an alternate view of H 1, see Appendix 1, Figure A4.

Functions: Regulates the Qi, relaxes the chest, clears the meridians.

Indications: Palpitations, pain in the chest and heart region.

H 3, Shao Hai, Lesser Sea

Location: Flex your elbow. Place your fingertip on the bone at the inner elbow (the medial epicondyle of the humerus). Slide your finger toward the inner elbow crease. Just as it passes over the bone, it will fall into the depression where the point is located. For an alternate view of H 3, see Appendix 1, Figure A4.

Functions: Calms the Heart and spirit, rectifies Heart Qi, relaxes the chest, clears the channels.

Indications: Heart pain, pain in the arm and hand, depression, agitation, neurasthenia (fatigue, headache, and irritability associated with emotional disturbances).

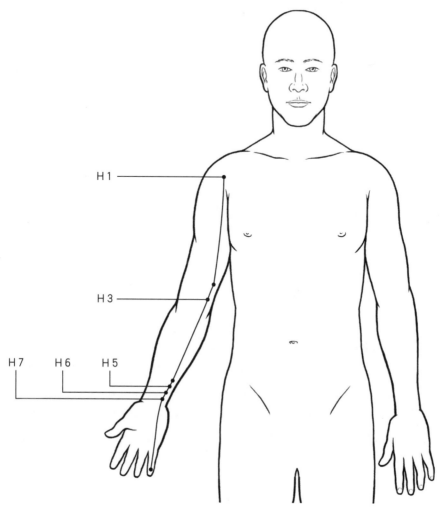

Figure 13.6 (Heart Acupressure Points)

H 5, Tong Li, Connecting Route

Location: 1 Cun proximal to the ulnar (little finger) side of the wrist crease, just medial to the tendon. For alternate views of H 5, see Appendix 1, Figures A1 and A4.

Functions: Calms the spirit, regulates Heart Qi and the mind, clears and invigorates the meridians.

Indications: Palpitations, sore throat, insomnia, sudden loss of voice, tongue rigidity, wrist strains.

Especially helps: Slow or irregular heartbeat, stuttering.

H 6, Yin Xi, Yin Accumulation

Location: .5 Cun proximal to the ulnar (little finger) side of the wrist crease, just medial to the tendon. For alternate views of H 6, see Appendix 1, Figures A1 and A4.

Functions: Calms the heart, clears Heat, cools the Blood, transforms phlegm.

Indications: Night sweats, palpitations, sudden loss of voice, coughing up blood, nose bleeds.

Especially helps: Night sweats.

H 7, Shen Men, Spirit Gate

Location: At the ulnar (little finger) side of the wrist crease, just medial to the tendon. For alternate views of H 7, see Appendix 1, Figures A1 and A4.

Functions: Clears and supports the Heart, calms the spirit, resolves depression.

Indications: Heart pain, neurasthenia, palpitations, insomnia, hysteria, irritability, mental restlessness or absent-mindedness, excessive dreaming.

Especially helps: Psychological problems—insomnia, depression, anxiety, nervousness.

Small Intestine, Hand Taiyang

SI 3, Hou Xi, Back Stream

Location: On the ulnar (little finger) side of the hand, about 1 Cun below where the little finger joins the hand. When making a soft fist, this is where the upper palm crease ends at the side of the hand, at the junction of the red and white skin. For an alternate view of SI 3, see Appendix 1, Figure A4.

Functions: Releases the surface, clears Wind, calms the spirit, relaxes the low back.

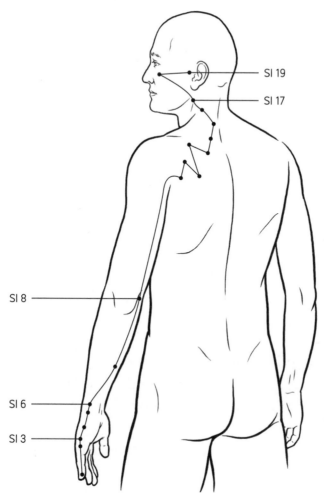

Figure 13.7 (Small Intestine Acupressure Points)

Indications: Low back pain, stiff neck, seizures, tinnitus, deafness, eye inflammation, pain in the lower arm and wrist.

Especially helps: Stiff neck and back, arthritis.

SI 6, Yang Lao, Nursing the Aged

• *Location:* In the depression just proximal and medial to the large bony bump below the little finger side of the back of the wrist. (On the radial side of the styloid process of the ulna.) For an alternate view of SI 6, see Appendix 1, Figure A2.

Functions: Relaxes muscles, clears and activates the meridians, brightens the eyes and benefits vision.

Indications: Eye problems, nearsightedness, blurred vision; low back, shoulder, elbow, and wrist pain.

SI 8, Xiao Hai, Small Sea

Location: With elbow flexed, at the little finger side of the elbow, in the depression between the elbow tip and the bony bump at the end of the humerus (the upper arm bone). The "funny bone" point. For an alternate view of SI 8, see Appendix 1, Figure A3.

Functions: Clears Wind, calms the mind, relaxes the tendons, relieves pain.

Indications: Ulnar nerve problems (neuralgia, paralysis), epilepsy, pain along the Small Intestine meridian.

SI 17, Tian Rong, Celestial Countenance

Location: In the depression just behind the angle of the jaw and in front of the sternocleidomastoid muscle. For an alternate view of SI 17, see Appendix 1, Figure A6.

Functions: Clears Heat and inflammation, sharpens hearing, relieves the throat, reduces edema.

Indications: Tonsillitis, sore throat, sore and swollen neck, tinnitus, deafness.

Especially helps: Sore throat, tonsillitis.

CAUTION: Light to moderate pressure only—the carotid artery and jugular vein are located here. This is primarily a concern with acupuncture, but strong stimulation should be avoided.

SI 19, Ting Gong, Auditory Palace

Location: Place your fingertip on the triangular flap of skin in front of your ear canal (the tragus), so that it also touches the hinge of your jaw. Open your mouth, and as your jaw hinge lowers, your fingertip will fall right into the opening of the point. For an alternate view of SI 19, see Appendix 1, Figure A6.

Functions: Calms the spirit, benefits hearing, opens the ear, improves vision.

Indications: Tinnitus, deafness, inflammation of the ear canal, trigeminal neuralgia.

Especially helps: Ears.

Urinary Bladder, Foot Taiyang

UB 1, Jing Ming, Eye Brightness

Location: .5 Cun medial to the inner corner of the eye. Point your finger toward your nose to feel the depression. For an alternate view of UB 1, see Appendix 1, Figure A5.

Functions: Clears Wind and Heat, opens the meridians, brightens the eyes.

Indications: All eye diseases, conjunctivitis, night blindness, itchy, tearing eyes, color blindness, nearsightedness, blurred vision, early stage cataracts, glaucoma.

Especially helps: Eyes.

UB 2, Zan Zhu, Collecting Bamboo

Location: At the medial tip of the eyebrow, directly above UB 1. For an alternate view of UB 2, see Appendix 1, Figure A5.

Functions: Clears Wind and Heat, sharpens vision.

Indications: Headache, blurred and failing vision, facial paralysis, eye pain.

Especially helps: Eyes, headache.

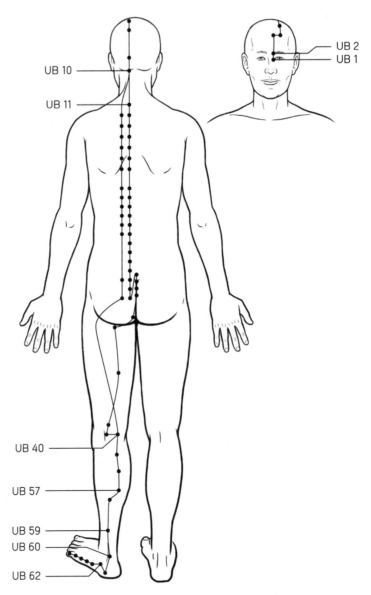

Figure 13.8 (Urinary Bladder Acupressure Points)

UB 10, Tian Zhu, Celestial Pillar

Location: .5 Cun within the posterior hairline, 1.3 Cun lateral to the midline, in the depression on the lateral edge of the trapezius muscle. For an alternate view of UB 10, see Appendix 1, Figure A7.

Functions: Clears Wind and Heat, frees meridian flow and reduces pain, opens the senses, restores consciousness.

Indications: Occipital (base of the head) headache, sore and stiff neck, shoulder and back pain.

Especially helps: Neck, mental and emotional issues.

UB 11, Da Zhu, Great Shuttle

Location: Feel for the large bony spine bump at the back of your neck, where your neck joins your back. This is the spinous process of your first thoracic vertebra, T1. Feel for the depression just below T1. The point is 1.5 Cun lateral to the midline at the level of that depression. For an alternate view of UB 11, see Appendix 1, Figure A7.

Functions: Clears Heat, releases the surface, rectifies Lung Qi, regulates the joints, strengthens bones, reduces pain.

Indications: Common cold, cough, bronchitis, pneumonia, neck and back pain, fever, stiff neck.

Especially helps: Bones.

UB 40, Wei Zhong, Bend Middle

Location: At the center of the crease at the back of the knee. For an alternate view of UB 40, see Appendix 1, Figures A11.

Functions: Clears Summer Heat, benefits the low back and knees.

Indications: Low back pain, tight muscles at the back of the knee, acute stomach and intestinal pain especially due to Heat, vomiting, diarrhea, heat exhaustion, heat stroke.

Especially helps: Low back pain, heat stroke.

UB 57, Cheng Shan, Supporting Mountain

Location: At the tip of the depression formed between the twin bellies of the calf muscle (gastrocnemius), 8 Cun below UB 40. For alternate views of UB 57, see Appendix 1, Figures A11 and A12.

Functions: Clears Heat, relaxes the muscle meridians, reduces pain, benefits hemorrhoids.

Indications: Sciatica, cramping and pain in the lower back and calf, constipation, hemorrhoids.

Especially helps: Hemorrhoids.

UB 59, Fu Yang, Instep Yang

Location: 3 Cun directly above (proximal to) UB 60. For an alternate view of UB 59, see Appendix 1, Figure A12.

Functions: Clears Wind, activates the meridians, moves Qi, reduces pain.

Indications: Headache, low back pain, pain and numbness in the lower leg.

UB 60, Kun Lun, Kunlun Mountains

Location: In the depression directly between the lateral tip of the ankle and the Achilles tendon. For alternate views of UB 60 see Appendix 1, Figures A11 and A12.

Functions: Clears Wind and Heat, opens the meridians, relaxes the muscles and tendons, reduces pain.

Indications: Headache, blurred vision, stiff neck, low back pain, sciatica, ankle and heel pain.

Especially helps: Headache, stiff neck.

CAUTION: Mild to moderate stimulation only during pregnancy. This is primarily a concern with acupuncture, but strong stimulation should be avoided.

UB 62, Shen Mai, Extending Vessel

Location: In the depression directly below the lateral tip of the ankle. For an alternate view of UB, see Appendix 1, Figure A12.

Functions: Calms the spirit, relaxes the muscles, clears Wind, reduces pain.

Indications: Headache, dizziness, insomnia, backache, heel pain, epilepsy.

Especially helps: Headaches, insomnia.

Kidney, Foot Shaoyin

K 1, Yong Quan, Bubbling Well

Location: On the midline of the sole of the foot. From where the toes join the foot, approximately one-third the distance toward the heel.

Functions: Replenishes the Kidneys, nourishes Yin, calms the spirit, soothes the Liver, clears Wind.

Indications: Headache, dizziness, sore throat, insomnia, loss of voice, painful or difficult urination.

Especially helps: Shock (a strong revival point).

K 3, Tai Xi, Great Stream

Location: In the depression between the medial tip of the ankle and the Achilles tendon; the opposite side from UB 60. For alternate views of K 3, see Appendix 1, Figures A10, A11, and A 13.

Functions: Replenishes the Kidneys, nourishes Yin, cools Heat, strengthens the low back and knees.

Indications: Sore throat (from prolonged Yin Deficiency), deafness, tinnitus, toothache, low back pain, male sexual dysfunction, irregular menstruation, insomnia, excessive urination or incontinence.

Especially helps: Provide balance in all Kidney disharmonies; building Kidney Yin, Yang, and Qi.

K 6, Zhao Hai, Luminous Sea

Location: In the depression directly below the medial tip of the ankle. For alternate views of K 6, see Appendix 1, Figures A10 and A13.

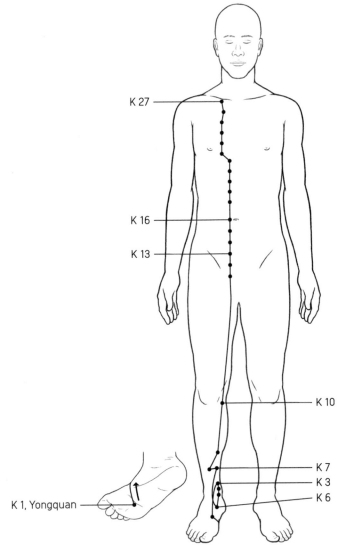

Figure 13.9 (Kidney Acupressure Points)

Functions: Replenishes the Kidneys, nourishes Yin, clears Heat, calms the spirit, regulates menstruation.

Indications: Irregular or painful menstruation, leukorrhea (vaginal discharge), urinary frequency or retention, insomnia, sore throat.

Especially helps: Build Kidney Yin, sore throat.

K 7, Fu Liu, Recover Flow

Location: 2 Cun directly above K 3, on the anterior border of the Achilles tendon. For alternate views of K 7, see Appendix 1, Figures A10 and A13.

Functions: Replenishes the Kidneys, tonifies Kidney Yang, consolidates the surface (Weiqi), and regulates sweating.

Indications: Inflammation of the Kidneys or testes, urinary tract infection, edema, insufficient or excess sweating, spontaneous sweats, night sweats, back pain, abdominal distention.

K 10, Yin Gu, Yin Valley

Location: With knee flexed, at the medial side of the back of the knee crease, between the tendons found there. For alternate views of K 6, see Appendix 1, Figures A10 and A11.

Functions: Benefits the Kidneys, nourishes Yin, regulates menstruation.

Indications: Impotence, hernia, urogenital disorders, dysfunctional uterine bleeding, knee pain.

K 13, Qi Xue, Qi Hole

Location: 3 Cun below the navel, .5 Cun lateral to the midline (.5 Cun lateral to Ren 4). For an alternate view of K 13, see Appendix 1, Figure A8.

Functions: Supplements Kidney Qi, regulates the Chong and Ren meridians.

Indications: Gynecological disorders, painful urination, abdominal pain.

CAUTION: Mild to moderate stimulation only during pregnancy. This is primarily a concern with acupuncture, but strong stimulation should be avoided.

K 16, Huang Shu, Vital Transport Point

Location: .5 Cun lateral to the navel. For an alternate view of K 16, see Appendix 1, Figure A8.

Functions: Harmonizes the Stomach, regulates Large Intestine Qi.

Indications: Hernia, constipation, abdominal pain.

CAUTION: Mild to moderate stimulation only during pregnancy. This is primarily a concern with acupuncture, but strong stimulation should be avoided.

K 27, Shu Fu, Transport Mansion

Location: On the lower border of the collarbone, 2 Cun lateral to the midline. For an alternate view of K 27, see Appendix 1, Figure A8.

Functions: Supports Kidney Yang, opens the Lungs, descends rebellious Qi.

Indications: Cough, asthma, chest pain, bronchitis.

Pericardium, Hand Jueyin

P 3, Qu Ze, Marsh at the Bend

Location: At the midpoint of the elbow crease, just to the ulnar (little finger) side of the biceps tendon. For an alternate view of P 3, see Appendix 1, Figure A1.

Functions: Rectifies Heart Qi, clears Heat from the Blood, harmonizes the Stomach, calms the spirit.

Indications: Heart pain, palpitations, stomachache, fevers and associated diseases (e.g., fever causing a seizure), vomiting, pain in the arm and elbow.

P 6, Nei Guan, Inner Gate

Location: 2 Cun above the wrist crease, between the tendons. For an alternate view of P 6, see Appendix 1, Figure A1.

Functions: Regulates Heart Qi, calms the Heart and spirit, clarifies the mind, strengthens the Spleen, regulates the Liver, benefits abdominal organs, suppresses pain.

Indications: Heart pain, palpitations, pain below the ribs, stuffy chest, stomachache, nausea, vomiting, mental disorders, epilepsy, insomnia, irritability.

Especially helps: Nausea (motion sickness, morning sickness).

P 7, Da Ling, Big Mound

Location: In the middle of the wrist crease, between the tendons. For an alternate view of P 7, see Appendix 1, Figure A1.

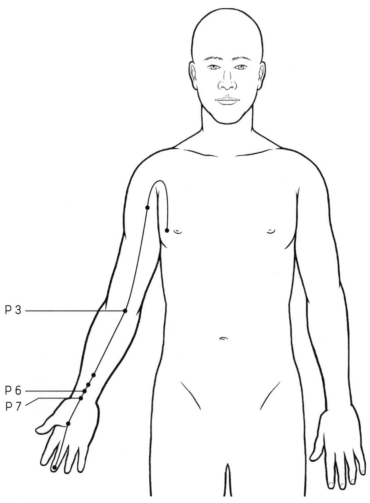

P 3

P 6
P 7

Figure 13.10 (Pericardium Acupressure Points)

Functions: Clears the Heart, calms the spirit, harmonizes the Stomach, clears Heat, relaxes the joint.

Indications: Heart pain, palpitations, stomachache, chest and wrist pain, insomnia, irritability.

Especially helps: Carpal tunnel syndrome.

Sanjiao, Hand Shaoyang

SJ 3, Zhong Shu, Middle Islet

Location: On the back of the hand, in the depression proximal to the knuckles of the little and ring fingers. For alternate views of SJ 3, see Appendix 1, Figures A2 and A3.

Functions: Clears Heat, activates the channels, benefits eyesight and hearing, opens the throat.

Indications: Tinnitus, deafness, headache, sore throat, fevers, elbow and arm pain.

Especially helps: Ears.

SJ 5, Wai Guan, Outer Gate

Location: 2 Cun proximal to the back of the wrist crease, between the two bones.

Functions: Clears Heat, releases the surface, benefits eyesight and hearing, facilitates Qi circulation. For alternate views of SJ 5, see Appendix 1, Figures A2 and A3.

Indications: Common cold, fevers, pneumonia, headache, deafness, tinnitus, stiff neck, pain in the arm and elbow.

Especially helps: Immune system.

SJ 6, Zhi Gao, Branch Ditch

Location: 3 Cun proximal to the back of the wrist crease, between the two bones. For alternate views of SJ 6, see Appendix 1, Figures A2 and A3.

Functions: Smoothes the Liver, spreads the Qi, opens the Intestines, sharpens hearing.

Indications: Deafness, tinnitus, constipation, chest and rib pain.

Especially helps: Constipation.

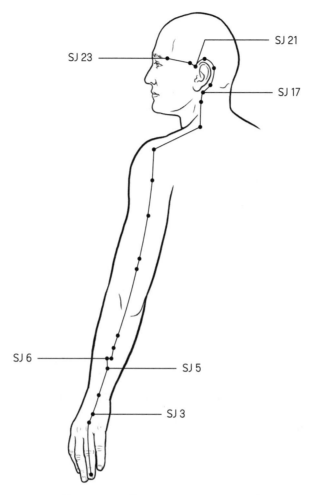

Figure 13.11 (Sanjiao Acupressure Points)

SJ 17, Yi Feng, Wind Screen

Location: Directly behind the earlobe, in the depression behind the mid-jaw (between the mandible and the mastoid process). For an alternate view of SJ 17, see Appendix 1, Figure A6.

Functions: Benefits hearing and vision, frees Qi flow in the channels, opens and relaxes the throat.

Indications: Tinnitus, deafness, facial paralysis, toothache, inflamed parotid glands (mumps), painful or locked jaw.

Especially helps: Ears.

SJ 21, Er Men, Ear Gate

Location: In the bony depression just in front of the top of the tragus (the triangular flap of skin at the front of the ear canal.) For an alternate view of SJ 21, see Appendix 1, Figure A6.

Functions: Clears Heat, opens the ear, sharpens hearing.

Indications: Tinnitus, deafness, toothache.

SJ 23, Si Zhu Kong, Silk Bamboo Hole

Location: In the depression at the lateral end of the eyebrow. For an alternate view of SJ 23, see Appendix 1, Figure A6.

Functions: Clears Wind and Heat, opens the channels, sharpens eyesight.

Indications: Headache, red and painful eyes (conjunctivitis), eyelid twitch, blurred vision.

Gall Bladder, Foot Shaoyang

GB 1, Tong Zi Liao, Pupil Bone Hole

Location: In the depression .5 Cun lateral to the outer corner of the eye. For alternate views of GB 1, see Appendix 1, Figures A5 and A6.

Functions: Clears Wind and Heat, opens the channels, improves vision.

Indications: Headache, failing vision, excessive tearing, night blindness.

Especially helps: Eyes.

GB 2, Ting Hui, Auditory Convergence

Location: In the depression just below the lower corner of the tragus (the triangular flap of skin in front of the ear canal). For an alternate view of GB 2, see Appendix 1, Figure A6.

Functions: Clears Wind, smoothes Liver and Gall Bladder Qi, frees and activates channel Qi, sharpens hearing, benefits the eyes.

Indications: Deafness, tinnitus, toothache, mumps, locked jaw.

Especially helps: Ears, jaw.

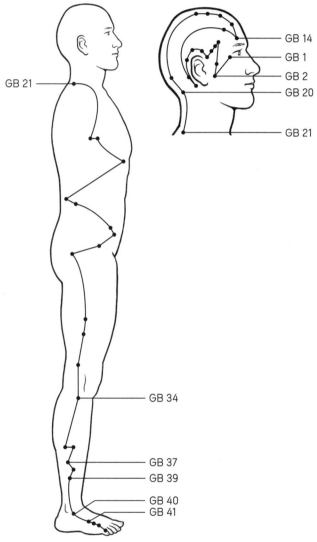

Figure 13.12 (Gall Bladder Acupressure Points)

GB 14, Yang Bai, Yang White

Location: Directly above the pupil, 1 Cun above the eyebrow. For alternate views of GB 14, see Appendix 1, Figures A5 and A6.

Functions: Clears Wind and Heat, reduces pain, improves vision.

Indications: Headache, eye pain, eye twitch, droopy eyelid, excessive tearing, night blindness, glaucoma.

GB 20, Feng Chi, Wind Pool

Location: Just below the base of the skull, 1 Cun within the posterior hairline, in the depression between the trapezius and sternocleidomastoid muscles. About 2 Cun lateral to the midline. For an alternate view of GB 20, see Appendix 1, Figure A7.

Functions: Clears Wind and Heat, releases the surface, soothes the Liver, benefits hearing and vision, reduces pain.

Indications: Common cold, headache, dizziness, stiff neck, insomnia, blurred vision, glaucoma, tinnitus, deafness, nasal obstruction.

Especially helps: Headache, hypertension.

GB 21, Jian Jing, Shoulder Well

Location: At the highest point of the trapezius muscle, halfway between the center of the base of the neck (C 7) and the bony prominence at the top of the shoulder (the acromion process). For an alternate view of GB 21, see Appendix 1, Figure A8.

Functions: Clears Wind and Heat, clears and invigorates the channels, descends rebellious Qi, smoothes Liver Qi, benefits the shoulders, reduces pain.

Indications: Painful and stiff neck, shoulder and back pain, mastitis, insufficient lactation, difficult labor.

Especially helps: Descend the Qi, neck and shoulder pain.

CAUTION: Mild stimulation only during pregnancy. *Strong stimulation may induce labor.* This is primarily a concern with acupuncture treatments, but strong stimulation should be avoided.

GB 34, Yang Ling Quan, Yang Mound Spring

Location: In the depression inferior and anterior to the bony prominence found about 2 Cun below the lateral knee (the head of the fibula). For an alternate view of GB 34, see Appendix 1, Figure A12.

Functions: Smoothes Liver and Gall Bladder Qi, clears Heat and Damp, frees the channels, benefits the tendons and ligaments.

Indications: One-sided paralysis, weakness, numbness or pain in the lower leg, swollen or painful knee, hepatitis, jaundice, gall bladder diseases (cholecystitis and cholelithiasis), low back pain, acid regurgitation, vomiting.

Especially helps: Tendons and ligaments (throughout the body).

GB 37, Guang Ming, Bright Light

Location: 5 Cun above the tip of the lateral ankle, on the anterior border of the bone (fibula). For an alternate view of GB 37, see Appendix 1, Figure A12.

Functions: Regulates the Liver, sharpens eyesight.

Indications: Knee pain, eye pain, blurred vision, night blindness, cataract, glaucoma, early stage mastitis.

Especially helps: Eyes and calf.

GB 39, Xuan Zhong, Suspended Bell

Location: 3 Cun above the tip of the lateral ankle, on the anterior border of the bone (fibula). For an alternate view of GB 39, see Appendix 1, Figure A12.

Functions: Clears Wind and Damp, cools Gall Bladder Heat, activates the channels.

Indications: One-sided paralysis, stiff and painful neck, knee, lower leg and ankle pain or weakness.

Especially helps: Neck pain, immune system.

GB 40, Qiu Xu, Hill Ruins

Location: Anterior and inferior to the lateral ankle, in the depression on the lateral side of the tendon (extensor digitorum longus). For an alternate view of GB 40, see Appendix 1, Figure A12.

Functions: Clears Heat, smoothes the Liver Qi, benefits the Gall Bladder, sharpens eyesight.

Indications: Eye inflammation, neck pain, acid regurgitation, inflamed gall bladder, outer ankle pain and swelling.

GB 41, Zu Lin Qi, Foot Falling Tears

Location: Place your fingertip on GB 40. Slowly slide it toward the space between your little toe and the toe next to it. Just past the halfway point, your fingertip will drop into a depression between the bones of your foot, where the point is located (distal to the juncture of the fourth and fifth metatarsal). See figure 14.19. For alternate views of GB 41, see Appendix 1, Figures A12 and A14.

Functions: Clears Wind and Heat, rectifies the Liver and Gall Bladder, reduces pain.

Indications: Headache, dizziness, tinnitus, deafness, conjunctivitis, outer eye pain, breast pain, pain below the ribs, irregular menstruation, foot swelling and pain.

Especially helps: Painful menses.

Liver, Foot Jueyin

Liv 3, Tai Chong, Great Surge

Location: On the top of the foot, in the depression between the tendons, 1.5 Cun proximal to the margin of the web between the first and second toes. For an alternate view of Liv 3, see Appendix 1, Figure A14.

Functions: Calms the Liver, clears Wind, smoothes and regulates Liver Qi, harmonizes the Liver and Spleen, transforms Damp.

Indications: Headache, dizziness, insomnia, eye pain, depression, high blood pressure, hernia, irregular or painful menstruation, urinary incontinence or retention.

Especially helps: Headaches, calms the nervous system.

Liv 7, Xi Guan, Knee Gate

Location: On the medial side of the knee, in the depression just below the large bone at the bottom of the knee joint, 1 Cun posterior to Sp 9 (posterior to the depression below the lower border of the medial condyle of the tibia.) For an alternate view of Liv 7, see Appendix 1, Figure A10.

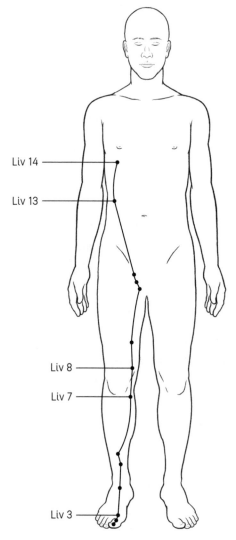

Figure 13.13 (Liver Acupressure Points)

Functions: Clears Wind and Damp, benefits the knee, reduces pain.

Indications: Headache, knee pain.

Liv 8, Qu Chuan, Spring at the Bend

Location: Seated with the knee flexed, the point is in the depression at the medial end of the crease at the back of the knee, above the tendon. For an alternate view of Liv 8, see Appendix 1, Figure A10.

Functions: Clears Damp Heat, regulates the Liver, benefits the Kidneys and Urinary Bladder, relaxes the muscle and knee joint.

Indications: Vaginitis, prostatitis, kidney pain, hernia, genital pain, impotence, nocturnal emission, knee and thigh pain.

Liv 13, Zhang Men, Order Gate

Location: Just below the tip of the eleventh rib. If you slide your finger down your rib cage from your breastbone (sternum), the eleventh rib is the first separate rib tip you'll find, near the bottom of your ribcage. For an alternate view of Liv 13, see Appendix 1, Figure A8.

Functions: Clears Cold and Damp, tonifies the Spleen, harmonizes the Stomach, smoothes Liver Qi, benefits the Gall Bladder.

Indications: Abdominal distention (enlarged liver and spleen), hepatitis, pain below the ribs, indigestion, vomiting, diarrhea.

Liv 14, Qi Men, Cycle Gate

Location: Directly below the nipple, in the sixth intercostal space (the space between the ribs). For an alternate view of Liv 14, see Appendix 1, Figure A8.

Functions: Regulates and rectifies the Liver and Gall Bladder, tonifies the Spleen, harmonizes the Stomach, disperses Blood Stagnation, promotes lactation.

Indications: Hepatitis, enlarged liver, pain below the ribs, inflamed gall bladder, mastitis, depression.

Du, Governing Vessel

Du 1, Chang Qiang, Long Strong

Location: Midway between the tip of the coccyx (tailbone) and the anus.

Functions: Opens the Ren and Du meridians, regulates the Intestines.

Indications: Constipation, diarrhea, hemorrhoids, low back pain, impotence, scrotal eczema, urinary incontinence.

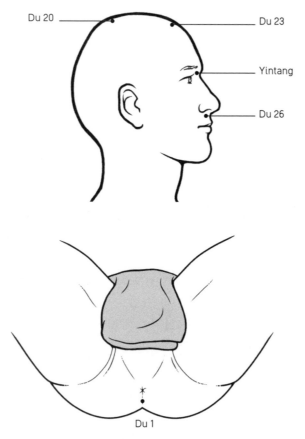

Figure 13.14 (Du Acupressure Points)

Du 20, Bai Hui, One Hundred Convergences

Location: On the midline of the head, 5 Cun above the natural anterior hairline (or 7 Cun above the posterior hairline), intersecting the line that can be drawn above the head between the tips of each ear.

Functions: Smoothes the Liver, clears Wind, opens the senses, calms the spirit.

Indications: Headache, dizziness, tinnitus, nasal obstruction, high blood pressure, insomnia, mental disorders, prolapse (dropping) of the anus, rectum, and uterus.

Especially helps: Headache, dizziness, high blood pressure.

Du 23, Shang Xing, Upper Star

Location: On the midline of the head, 1 Cun within the middle of the natural anterior hairline. For an alternate view of Du 23, see Appendix 1, Figure A5.

Functions: Clears Wind Heat, opens the nose, sharpens vision, strengthens the mind, calms the spirit.

Indications: Headache, nosebleed, sinusitis, runny nose, eye pain, mental restlessness.

Especially helps: Sinuses.

Yintang, Seal Hall

Note: This is not a Du point but a very useful extra point that lies directly on the Du meridian.

Location: Midway between the medial ends of the eyebrows. For an alternate view of Yintang, see Appendix 1, Figure A5.

Functions: Clears Wind, sharpens eyesight, calms the spirit, opens the nose.

Indications: Headache, dizziness, eye diseases, sinusitis, insomnia, agitation.

Du 26, Ren Zhong, Person's Center

Location: On the midline, just below the base of the nose, two-thirds of the way up from the upper lip. For an alternate view of Du 26, see Appendix 1, Figure A5.

Functions: Clears the brain, opens the senses, cools Heat, calms the spirit.

Indications: Shock, motion sickness, seizures, epilepsy, mental disorders, loss of consciousness, deviation of the mouth, low back pain.

Especially helps: Shock (revival point).

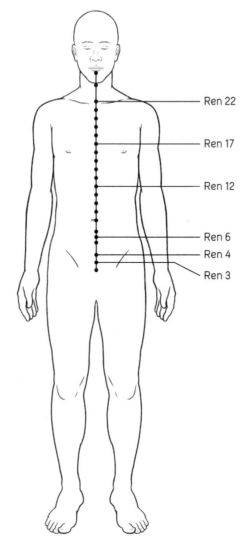

Figure 13.15 (Ren Acupressure Points)

Ren, Conception Vessel

Ren 1, Hui Yin, Meeting of Yin

Location: On the midline, halfway between the anus and the external genitals (scrotum and labia).

Functions: Clears Damp Heat, regulates menstruation, benefits the Urinary Bladder, clears the mind, opens the senses.

Indications: Urinary retention or incontinence, vaginitis, hemorrhoids, urethritis, prostatitis, irregular menstruation, nocturnal emission, mental disorders.

Ren 3, Zhong Ji, Central Pole

Location: On the midline of the abdomen, 4 Cun below the navel, 1 Cun above the pubic bone. For an alternate view of Ren 3, see Appendix 1, Figure A8.

Functions: Clears Heat and Damp, regulates menstruation, benefits the Urinary Bladders, frees urination.

Indications: Urinary retention or incontinence, nocturnal emission, impotence, premature ejaculation, hernia, irregular or painful menstruation, lower abdominal pain, urethritis, urinary tract infection.

CAUTION: Mild stimulation only during pregnancy. This is primarily a concern with acupuncture, but strong stimulation should be avoided.

Ren 4, Guan Yuan, Origin Pass

Location: On the midline of the abdomen, 3 Cun below the navel, 2 Cun above the pubic bone. For an alternate view of Ren 4, see Appendix 1, Figure A8.

Functions: Nourishes the Kidneys, replenishes source (Yuan) Qi, regulates menstruation, promotes urination.

Indications: Urinary incontinence or retention, nocturnal emission, impotence, infertility, sterility, irregular menstruation, hernia, lower abdominal pain, diarrhea, all conditions of general weakness. (This point strengthens the body and improves overall health.)

Especially helps: Fatigue (tonifies Yang).

CAUTION: Mild stimulation only during pregnancy. This is primarily a concern with acupuncture, but strong stimulation should be avoided.

Ren 6, Qi Hai, Sea of Qi

Location: On the midline of the abdomen, 1.5 Cun below the navel. For an alternate view of Ren 6, see Appendix 1, Figure A8.

Functions: Tonifies and regulates Qi, tonifies the Kidneys, supplements essence, regulates menstruation.

Indications: Abdominal pain, incontinence, frequent nighttime urination, nocturnal emission, impotence, hernia, irregular, painful, or absent menstruation, constipation, asthma, all conditions of general weakness. (This point strengthens the body and improves overall health.)

Especially helps: Tonify Qi.

CAUTION: Mild stimulation only during pregnancy. This is primarily a concern with acupuncture, but strong stimulation should be avoided.

Ren 12, Zhong Wan, Central Venter

Location: On the midline of the abdomen, 4 Cun above the navel. For an alternate view of Ren 12, see Appendix 1, Figure A8.

Functions: Tonifies the Spleen, harmonizes the stomach, transforms Damp, descends Rebellious Stomach Qi.

Indications: Stomachache, abdominal distention, nausea, vomiting, indigestion, hiccups, diarrhea, constipation, jaundice, insomnia.

Especially helps: Stomach, digestive disorders.

Ren 17, Dan Zhong, Center of the Chest

Location: On the anterior midline in the fourth intercostal space (the space between the ribs), usually midway between the nipples. Note: The position of the nipples change as a person ages or gains weight, so try your best for the fourth intercostal space, which always remains constant. For an alternate view of Ren 17, see Appendix 1, Figure A8.

Functions: Regulates and rectifies the Qi of the whole body, relaxes and expands the chest, benefits the diaphragm, soothes difficult breathing.

Indications: Asthma, bronchitis, chest pain, cough, hiccup, mastitis, palpitations, insufficient lactation.

Ren 22, Tian Tu, Celestial Chimney

Location: In the depression just above the notch at the base of the throat (the suprasternal fossa). For an alternate view of Ren 22, see Appendix 1, Figure A8.

Functions: Regulates and rectifies Lung Qi, subdues rebellious Qi, opens and cools the throat, clears the voice.

Indications: Asthma, bronchitis, cough, sore throat, dry throat, hiccup, nervous vomiting, esophagus spasm (difficulty swallowing), sudden loss of voice.

Chapter 14

Chinese Herbs: Nature's Healing Allies

Herbology is the oldest and arguably the most comprehensive branch of Chinese medicine. When Westerners consider taking herbs, most will go to their local nutritional supplement or natural foods store and ask for help from the staff. They might be given echinacea for a cold, St. John's wort for depression, ginger for an upset stomach, black cohosh for a menstrual difficulty, or valerian for insomnia. This isn't a bad thing, as those herbs are often a better choice than a drug alternative. Many Western herbalists and naturopathic doctors (NDs) use this approach, even when creating herb formulas. However, results can vary considerably, and the desired improvement might not occur, possibly leading one to believe that herbs are ineffective. This is not due to a problem with the herb itself but with the rationale behind how it was selected and administered.

That approach follows the Western pharmaceutical/allopathic model, where one drug is used to treat one symptom or disease. That is, it's the disease that is being addressed, not the individual who has the disease. Even though a natural substance is being substituted for a drug, this is not really a holistic approach. As you've seen, there are many possible root causes for any symptom. If the root imbalance, the pattern of disharmony, isn't addressed, the person is not brought back into balance. Some symptoms may improve, some may not, and others could get worse (see Appendix 2, Note 14.1), while the pattern remains unchanged, setting the stage for future occurrences of the same problem.

The following introduction provides insight into the main criteria and methods used in Chinese herbology, from analyzing and categorizing individual herbs to constructing herbal formulas. This is a completely holistic application of herbs as medicine.

Main Attributes of Chinese Herbs: Temperature and Taste

There are two primary characteristics that define Chinese herbal properties. They are temperature, also referred to as Qi, and taste.

All herbs, and in fact all ingestible substances, can be analyzed according to temperature. In common experience, everyone understands that pepper is hot and mint is cool. Chinese pharmacology recognizes five temperatures along the hot-cold spectrum: hot, warm, neutral, cool, and cold. Sometime qualifiers are noted to hone degree, such as slightly cold or slightly hot. The most obvious use of this understanding is that hot herbs are used to treat cold diseases, and cold herbs are used to treat hot ones. (See Appendix 2, Note 14.2.)

The second characteristic all herbs and consumables have is taste. Herbal medicine recognizes five primary tastes that correspond to the Five Element tastes—spicy (acrid), sweet, bitter, sour, and salty—along with a neutral taste, bland. An herb may have more than one taste.

The tastes may indicate the organ or organs that the herb most readily influences, and each has additional therapeutic effects. Spicy has an affinity for the Lungs and Large Intestine and makes Qi scatter and move. That Qi movement can direct various accumulations to scatter or can direct fluids like blood and sweat to move. Sweet has an affinity for the Spleen and Stomach, tonifies Qi, and harmonizes and sometimes tonifies Yin to promote moistening. Sweet also slows and moderates the effects of harsh herbs. (See Appendix 2, Note 14.3.) Bitter has an affinity for the Heart and Small Intestine and produces drying and draining effects. Sour has an affinity for the Liver and Gall Bladder, is astringent, and restrains or prevents leakage of fluids or Qi. Salty has an affinity for the Kidneys and Urinary Bladder, softens hardness (such as cysts), and purges. Bland does not have a definitive organ affinity, although based on its function, which is to leech out Damp and promote urination, some sources say it has an affinity for the Spleen, the organ most sensitive to Damp.

Directionality

Some herbs have specific directional qualities and are able to address targeted locations in the body through differing means.

Some physically heavier substances are not herbs at all but bones, shells, and rock-like minerals that are part of the Chinese pharmacopoeia. Their heaviness imparts a weighty, descending quality that is used to subdue inappropriately rising Qi, Yang, or Heat, which can disturb the Heart and cause anxiety, palpitations, and insomnia. Accordingly, many of these heavier substances are found in the category "Settles and Calms the Spirit."

Light and aromatic herbs can produce an upward and outward dispersing effect. Both physically light and aromatic, *Bo He* (peppermint) has an upward movement that helps clear the Lungs, throat, head, and eyes, and it directs Qi outward to the body's surface to fight off external invading Wind Heat pathogens.

Still other herbs have the ability to direct Qi through no discernible means. *Huang Qi* (*Astragulus*) directs Qi upward (notably Stomach and Spleen Yang Qi), which can be overstimulating if taken in large doses. *Jie Geng* (*Platycodon grandiflorus*) directs the effects of other herbs upward, primarily to the chest, useful in formulas treating any type of constriction or accumulation in the chest or lungs. *Niu Xi* (*Achyranthes bidentata*) directs the effects of other herbs downward, useful in formulas treating any type of pain below the waist.

Channels Entered

Every Chinese herb is said to enter an acupuncture channel or channels. This means that the effects of an herb most strongly influence the organ or organs of the related channel, so if an herb enters the Lung channel, it will most strongly affect the Lungs or the Lung channel itself, in cases of a channel pathology.

There is often a correspondence with taste, so a spicy herb is likely to enter the Lung channel, for example. There are many exceptions, especially in herbs with complex tastes, so this is not always the case. The channels entered have largely been determined empirically, through careful observation of an herb's therapeutic effects over time.

Categorizing Herbs

Chinese herbs are classified into categories with herbs that share similar functions and attributes. While primarily addressing its category designation, each herb has its own individual qualities that allow it to function slightly differently from others within the same category. This provides a great deal of versatility in selecting the herbs that best match the patient's presentation, helping address various symptoms related to the primary concern. Secondary symptoms or concerns may be addressed by herbs from other categories, creating a highly individualized formula for each patient's needs.

What follows is a list of the most commonly recognized herb categories, along with a short description of its purpose. Below each description you'll find the following:

- *Representative Herbs:* These may not always be the most commonly used herbs in the category, but they are ones that most Westerners will recognize. Their common name is followed by their Chinese name. (Many Chinese herbs only have Chinese names and botanical name counterparts.) You will note that not every substance is an herb; some are animal and mineral substances. They are all loosely called "herbs" as a matter of convenience among many herbalists, so there is no distinction made to point those out when they occur.

   The herbs presented in this chapter are intended to provide some common representative examples only. Only an experienced herbalist should attempt to include these individual herbs in their self-care. Each herb can produce a variety of effects or target only one set of symptoms from its category. When used improperly, the results may be unpredictable and in some rare cases harmful.

- *Common Symptoms Treated:* These are some of the symptoms most commonly treated by the category of herbs. Not every symptom needs to be present in order to beneficially use these herbs. Not every herb in its category will treat all of the common symptoms. Determining which herbs within a category may best treat the patient is part of the art of constructing an effective Chinese formula.

- *Related Western Diseases:.* These are the disease or condition names commonly used in Western medicine where some, most, or all of the symptoms imply a Chinese diagnosis may be present. Remember there are no one-to-one correspondences between Chinese and Western diagnoses. The Western disease name implies one set of symptoms a Chinese physician may take into consideration when making a diagnosis.

- *Similar Western Drug Actions:* The herbs within a category will have actions similar to, or in some cases identical to, these Western-defined drug actions. Not every herb in its category will provide all of these actions. Some of the actions are only a secondary effect of an herb and may not directly relate to its category. In some cases, herbs produce effects that have no clear Western pharmacological counterpart, as when tonifying Qi, Yang, or Yin.

Herb Categories

1. Spicy (Acrid) Warm

These herbs treat superficial conditions that are cool or cold in nature. Those conditions are usually caused by Wind alone or a Wind Cold combination, sometimes additionally combined with Damp. Most of these herbs are diaphoretic, causing sweat to assist in releasing the external pathogens.

- Representative Herbs: Cinnamon twig (*Gui Zhi*), ginger root (*Sheng Jiang*).
- Common Symptoms Treated: Chills more than fever, headache, body ache, sinus congestion.
- Related Western Diseases: Common cold, flu.
- Similar Western Drug Actions: Antimicrobial, analgesic, antipyretic, decongestant, diaphoretic.

2. Spicy (Acrid) Cool

These herbs treat superficial conditions that are warm or hot in nature. Those conditions are usually caused by Wind alone or a Wind Heat combination and include common colds and flus. They are also used to treat early stages of Wind Damp and Summer Heat.

- Representative Herbs: Peppermint (*Bo He*), white mulberry leaf (*Sang Ye*), chrysanthemum flower (*Ju Hua*).
- Common Symptoms Treated: Fever more than chills, sore throat, itchy red eyes, headache, sinus congestion.
- Related Western Diseases: Common cold, flu.

- Similar Western Drug Actions: Antimicrobial/antibiotic, analgesic, antipyretic, decongestant, diaphoretic.

3. Clears Heat, Purges Fire

These are among the coldest herbs in the Chinese materia medica. They are used to treat all conditions that present internal Heat signs and high fevers.

- Representative Herbs: Gypsum (*Shi Gao*), gardenia fruit (*Zhi Zi*), bamboo stem and leaves (*Dan Zhu Ye*).
- Common Symptoms Treated: High fevers, irritability, thirst, fever-induced delirium.
- Related Western Diseases: Most diseases involving high fever.
- Similar Western Drug Actions: Anti-inflammatory, antipyretic, antimicrobial.

4. Clears Heat, Cools Blood

These cold herbs are used to treat conditions that exhibit signs of Heat in the Blood. This presents as Heat signs combined with bleeding disorders that are attributable to internal Heat.

- Representative Herbs: Rhinoceros horn (*Xi Jiao*), wolfberry root (*Di Gu Pi*), Chinese foxglove root (*Sheng Di Huang*). Note that rhinoceros horn is from an endangered species and is no longer used. It is mentioned here for historical reference and as a substance that is more familiar to most readers than others in this category.
- Common Symptoms Treated: Fever (often worse at night), dry throat, nosebleeds, coughing or spitting up blood, blood in the urine or stool, fever-induced delirium, rashes.
- Related Western Diseases: Diseases involving high fever with bleeding symptoms/hemorrhage.
- Similar Western Drug Actions: Anti-inflammatory, antipyretic, antimicrobial, hemostatic.

5. Clears Heat, Dries Damp

These cold herbs are also drying, used primarily in Damp Heat patterns. This includes things such as dysentery, painful, burning urination, and weeping, hot skin conditions.

- Representative Herbs: Skullcap root (*Huang Qin*), cork tree bark (*Huang Bai*).
- Common Symptoms Treated: Severe diarrhea, painful, burning urination, inflamed sores, swelling.
- Related Western Diseases: Jaundice, eczema, boils, encephalitis, diphtheria.
- Similar Western Drug Actions: Anti-inflammatory, antipyretic, antimicrobial, antifungal, possibly anticholinergic.

6. Clears Heat Toxin

These cold herbs are used to treat Heat patterns causing fever along with other signs of infectious or internal disease, indicative of toxins or purulent infection that must be cleared from the body.

- Representative Herbs: Honeysuckle flower (*Jin Yin Hua*), forsythia fruit (*Lian Qiao*), dandelion (*Pu Gong Ying*).
- Common Symptoms Treated: Fever, hot, painful swellings usually containing pus, lethargy, generalized malaise.
- Related Western Diseases: Shingles, abscesses, appendicitis, mastitis, dysentery.
- Similar Western Drug Actions: Anti-inflammatory, antibiotic, antiviral, diuretic.

7. Clears Summer Heat

These herbs can be cold, cool, or neutral and treat Summer Heat patterns of Damp combined with high Heat. Heat pathogens can be drying and create thirst, so these herbs both drain pathogenic Damp and generate healthy fluids while clearing Heat.

- Representative Herbs: Mung bean (*Lu Dou*), watermelon (*Xi Gua*), hyacinth bean (*Bai Bian Dou*).
- Common Symptoms Treated: Fever, profuse sweat, thirst, diarrhea, scant and dark urination.

- Related Western Diseases: Most febrile conditions that occur during summertime.
- Similar Western Drug Actions: Antibiotic, antipyretic, diuretic.

Downward Draining (for 8, 9, and 10)

All of the downward draining herbs either stimulate intestinal movement (peristalsis), moisten the intestines, or cause a strong diarrhea, in order to evacuate intestinal accumulations. They are used in different circumstances and produce their effects in different ways, described in the categories list.

8. Downward Draining, Purgative

These bitter, cold herbs clear Heat and are used either in cases of constipation caused by internal Heat, which dries intestinal fluids and usually present with high fever, or cases of constipation from internal Cold, which weakens peristalsis. In the latter case, other herbs are added to warm the interior in order to relieve internal Cold symptoms at the same time.

- Representative Herbs: Rhubarb rhizome (*Da Huang*), senna leaf (*Fan Xie Ye*), aloe juice, dried (*Lu Hui*).
- Common Symptoms Treated: Constipation, fever, dizziness, irritability, red and painful eyes.
- Related Western Diseases: Chronic constipation, jaundice, amenorrhea.
- Similar Western Drug Actions: Cathartic, laxative.

9. Downward Draining, Moist Laxative

These relatively mild herbs are nuts and seeds, primarily used to moisten and lubricate the intestines of the very weak or elderly suffering from a Blood or Yin Deficiency.

- Representative Herbs: Marijuana seeds (*Huo Ma Ren*).
- Common Symptom Treated: Constipation.
- Related Western Diseases: Constipation, edema.
- Similar Western Drug Actions: Laxative, diuretic.

10. Downward Draining, Harsh Expellant

These cold, bitter herbs induce strong diarrhea and possibly excess urination. They are used to treat constipation due to various disruptions of fluid metabolism, presenting with an inflammation of and fluid accumulation in the membranes around the lungs or with a fluid accumulation in the abdomen caused by cirrhosis of the liver. As these conditions are very serious, the herbs are accordingly very harsh, in order to produce their desired effects rapidly. They must be used with extreme care, as they can deplete and harm both Yin and Qi.

- Representative Herbs: Morning glory seeds (*Qian Niu Xi*), poke root (*Shang Lu*).
- Common Symptoms Treated: Constipation with thoracic or abdominal edema, difficult urination.
- Related Western Diseases: Pleurisy, ascites and cirrhosis.
- Similar Western Drug Actions: Cathartic, diuretic.

11. Drains Damp

These cool or cold herbs help drain accumulated fluids anywhere in the body, including the respiratory and digestive systems, and below the waist. They may also be combined with herbs that clear Heat in Damp Heat conditions.

- Representative Herbs: Talcum (*Hua Shi*), Job's tears/pearled barley (*Yi Yi Ren*), winter melon seed (*Dong Gua Ren*).
- Common Symptoms Treated: Fluid accumulation in the chest, abdomen, or below the waist, painful urination, rashes.
- Related Western Disease: Edema.
- Similar Western Drug Action: Diuretic.

12. Expels Wind Damp

These herbs treat various painful obstruction syndromes of the joints, muscles, or channels, characteristic of Wind Damp patterns. They are also useful in Cold and Hot painful obstruction syndromes, typically found in various types of arthritis.

- Representative Herbs: Chinese clematis root (*Wei Ling Xian*), Chinese quince fruit (*Mu Gua*).

- Common Symptoms Treated: Joint pain, back pain, painful, cramped muscles.
- Related Western Disease: Arthritis.
- Similar Western Drug Actions: Analgesic, anti-inflammatory, antipyretic.

Transforms Phlegm (for 13, 14, and 15)

In Chinese medicine, the term "Phlegm" can have many meanings. One is the same as is used in Western medicine: phlegm is the thick, sticky fluid that often accumulates in the lungs due to a cold, the flu, or allergies. This causes the familiar cough and wheeze associated with those conditions.

The Spleen both dislikes Damp and generates Damp when it is not functioning well. Some generated Damp can congeal into Phlegm and be sent to the Lungs, but some is readily sent to the Stomach, where it can cause nausea, poor appetite, distension, and other digestive disorders. Another aspect of Phlegm accumulates in the channels and muscles, forming Phlegm nodules. These can be simple lipomas or cysts, goiters, inflamed lymph glands, or the glandular swelling found in tuberculosis when Phlegm is combined with Fire. Insubstantial Phlegm, which is not an obvious physical fluid, can obstruct the Heart orifice, leading to various perceptual disorders, some types of seizures, stroke, and coma.

The three herb categories that address these manifestations of Phlegm are Dissolves (or Transforms) Hot Phlegm, Dissolves (or Transforms) Cold Phlegm, and Relieves Cough and Wheeze. Depending upon the presentation, herbs from each category may be used to treat any of the above Phlegm disorders.

13. Dissolves (or Transforms) Hot Phlegm

These cold herbs are used to treat Hot and Dry Phlegm disorders.

- Representative Herbs: Dried bamboo sap (*Zhu Li*), bamboo shavings (*Zhu Ru*), pumice (*Fu Hai Shi*), seaweed (*Hai Zao*).
- Common Symptoms Treated: Cough and wheeze with thick sputum, lung and breast abscess, chest pain, distension or constriction.
- Related Western Diseases: Lymphadenopathy, goiter.
- Similar Western Drug Actions: Expectorant, antitussive, anti-inflammatory, sedative.

14. Dissolves (or Transforms) Cold Phlegm

These warm herbs are used to treat Cold Phlegm conditions.

- Representative Herbs: White mustard seed (*Bai Jie Zi*), jack-in-the-pulpit rhizome (*Tian Nan Xing*).
- Common Symptoms Treated: Nausea, vomiting, chest pain, distension or constriction, nodules, facial paralysis, seizure, stroke.
- Related Western Diseases: Bell's palsy, lymphoma, opisthotonos, lockjaw, tuberculosis.
- Similar Western Drug Actions: Expectorant, antitussive, antiemetic.

15. Relieves Cough and Wheeze

These herbs are used to reduce coughing and wheezing and are the mildest of the herbs that transform Phlegm. They can be combined with other categories of herbs to facilitate a wider range of effects, clearing Heat, Cold, or Phlegm.

- Representative Herbs: Almond kernel (*Xing Ren*), bark of mulberry root (*Sang Bai Pi*).
- Common Symptoms Treated: Cough, wheeze, chest constriction, nausea, sore throat, hoarseness.
- Related Western Disease: Chronic bronchitis.
- Similar Western Drug Actions: Expectorant, antitussive, bronchodilator, antibiotic, diuretic, laxative.

16. Aromatic, Transforms Damp

Most of these herbs are spicy, warm, and aromatic, awakening the Spleen to transform Damp in the Middle Jiao. Primarily they are used for acute digestive disorders. Their warm, aromatic nature makes many of these herbs drying, potentially damaging Yin. They should be used carefully, and short-term use is recommended.

- Representative Herbs: Patchouli (*Huo Xiang*), magnolia bark (*Hou Po*).
- Common Symptoms Treated: Nausea, vomiting, abdominal distension, diarrhea, poor appetite.
- Related Western Diseases: Food poisoning, gastroenteritis, amoebic dysentery.
- Similar Western Drug Actions: Antibiotic, antiviral, antiemetic.

17. Relieves Food Stagnation

Most of these herbs are warm or neutral with a slightly sweet taste that guides their effects to the Spleen and Stomach. They work to dissolve food stagnation and guide that accumulation out of the body through the intestines. They can be combined with Heat-clearing herbs in cases of Hot Stagnation, with Warms the Interior herbs in cases of Cold Stagnation, or with purgative herbs if stronger evacuation is required.

- Representative Herbs: Hawthorn fruit (*Shan Zha*), barley sprout (*Mai Ya*), radish seed (*Lai Fu Zi*).
- Common Symptoms Treated: Poor digestion, abdominal distension, belching, acid regurgitation, diarrhea.
- Related Western Diseases: All digestive problems from poor digestive functions or overeating.
- Similar Western Drug Actions: Enzymatic, antimicrobial.

18. Regulates Qi

These herbs are primarily spicy and warm, and each herb possesses additional qualities. Regulating Qi means moving Qi, required in cases of Qi stagnation. This commonly manifests as discomfort or pain and sometimes as emotional distress, along with symptoms that vary according to the organ most involved.

- Representative Herbs: Tangerine peel (*Chen Pi*), sandalwood (*Tan Xiang*), Chinese rose (*Mei Gui Hua*).
- Common Symptoms Treated: Abdomen and chest pain, breathing difficulties, bloating, poor appetite, nausea, indigestion, food stagnation, constipation or diarrhea, depression, irritability.
- Related Western Diseases: Various discomforts and pain syndromes in the chest or abdomen. Many of these are not definitively diagnosable by Western methods, since the root cause is often a Qi obstruction, which is outside the province of Western medicine.
- Similar Western Drug Actions: Cholinergic agonists, prokinetic agents, laxatives or antidiarrheals (depending on presentation), analgesic, antimicrobial.

19. Stops Bleeding

These herbs are used to stop bleeding from any cause. Trauma is one clear cause of bleeding, but other bleeding disorders can be caused by Heat, Deficiencies of Qi or Yin, or other causes. The underlying cause must be addressed by other types of herbs added to these. Blood loss itself usually creates Blood Deficiency, which must be addressed once the acute bleeding has stopped.

- Representative Herbs: Cattail pollen (*Pu Huang*), pseudoginseng root (*San Qi*), charred human hair (*Xue Yu Tan*).
- Common Symptoms Treated: Blood in the stool, urine, or vomit, nosebleeds, excessive menstrual bleeding, coughing blood, trauma.
- Related Western Diseases: Any diseases involving excessive or abnormal bleeding, hemorrhagic disorders.
- Similar Western Drug Actions: Hemostatic, anti-inflammatory, antibiotic, anti-emetic.

20. Invigorates Blood

These herbs are used to move the Blood in cases of Blood Stasis. Presentations can include acute onset of localized sharp pain from a known injury, ulcerations and abscesses in skin, muscles, or internal organs, enlarged liver or spleen, or abdominal or pelvic tumors. Herbs of varying strength are used in differing types of presentations.

- Representative Herbs: Turmeric (*Yu Jin*), peony root (*Chi Shao*), peach kernel (*Tao Ren*), safflower (*Hong Hua*).
- Common Symptoms Treated: Sharp focal pain, inflammation, masses, painful or absent menstruation.
- Related Western Diseases: Appendicitis, hepatomegaly, splenomegaly, thrombosis, abdominal tumors and cysts, ulcers, abscesses, ischemia, some gynecological disorders.
- Similar Western Drug Actions: Anticoagulant, analgesic, antibiotic, anti-inflammatory.

21. Warms Interior, Expels Cold

These warm herbs treat Interior Cold patterns, whether caused by external or internal pathogenic factors.

- Representative Herbs: Dried ginger (*Gan Jiang*), cinnamon bark (*Rou Gui*), fennel (*Xiao Hui Xiang*), black pepper (*Hu Jiao*).
- Common Symptoms Treated: Generalized cold, absent thirst, loose stool, excessive urination, weakness and fatigue. More serious symptoms: profuse sweating, watery diarrhea, frigid extremities.
- Related Western Diseases: Shock, some cardiovascular events, impotence, gastroenteritis.
- Similar Western Drug Actions: Cardiotonic, anti-inflammatory, antiparasitic, antibiotic.

22. Tonifies Qi

These herbs are generally warm or neutral and are sweet. They are used in Deficient Qi patterns, where the functional energy of an organ or organs is low.

- Representative Herbs: Ginseng (*Ren Shen*), astragalus (*Huang Qi*), licorice root (*Gan Cao*)
- Common Symptoms Treated: Shortness of breath, spontaneous sweating, weak voice, weak limbs, poor appetite, diarrhea, fatigue.
- Related Western Diseases: Any diseases involving generalized weakness or low energy, especially when involving the lungs or digestive system. Many of these are not definitively diagnosable by Western methods, since the root cause is often Qi Deficiency, which is outside the province of Western medicine.
- Similar Western Drug Actions: Some of the herbs in this category have antibiotic, antineoplastic, blood pressure regulatory, endocrine, cardiovascular, and other effects as secondary attributes. Primarily, they are highest-quality nutrition targeted toward specific organs, improving the efficiency and functional energy of those organs.

23. Tonifies Blood

These sweet herbs treat all types of Deficient Blood patterns and are used to nourish and build the Blood both in quality and quantity. They are not limited to treating the Western diagnosis of anemia, a common misperception.

- Representative Herbs: Goji berries (*Gou Qi Zi*), peony root (*Bai Shao*).
- Common Symptoms Treated: Dizziness, insomnia, poor vision, heart palpitations, menstrual disorders, dry hair and skin, sore back and legs.
- Related Western Diseases: Cardiovascular disorders, amenorrhea, dysmenorrhea.
- Similar Western Drug Actions: Some of the herbs in this category are antibiotic, sedative, or analgesic, lower blood pressure and cholesterol, improve glucose metabolism, and have cardiovascular and other effects as secondary attributes. Primarily they are highest-quality nutrition targeted toward building the quality of Blood, and they contain many vitamins, amino acids, sterols, lecithin, small amounts of healthy sugars, and other nutrients.

24. Tonifies Yang

These herbs are used to treat Deficient Yang patterns, primarily of the Heart, Spleen, and Kidneys. Common symptoms include very low energy and a strong aversion to cold.

- Representative Herbs: Horny goat weed (*Yin Yang Huo*), fenugreek seed (*Hu Lu Ba*), walnut (*Hu Tao Ren*).
- Common Symptoms Treated: Sexual (impotence, spermatorrhea) and urogenital (incontinence, profuse urination) disorders, low back pain, pallor, shortness of breath, diarrhea.
- Related Western Diseases: Possibly endocrine disorders. Many of these diseases are not definitively diagnosable by Western methods, since the root cause is often Yang Deficiency, which is outside the province of Western medicine.
- Similar Western Drug Action: Androgenergic.

25. Tonifies Yin

These primarily sweet and cool herbs are used to treat Deficient Yin patterns. They are nourishing and moistening, generate fluids, and mainly address Lung, Liver, Kidney, and Stomach Yin. The presentations vary some based on the organs or organs most in-volved.

- Representative Herbs: American ginseng (*Xi Yang Shen*), black sesame seed (*Hei Zhi Ma*), tortoise shell (*Gui Ban*). Note that endangered species are not used in contemporary Chinese medicine.
- Common Symptoms Treated: Thirst, dry throat, dry cough, dry skin, insomnia, vertigo, tinnitus, constipation, poor appetite, weak low back and knees, low sexual energy.
- Related Western Diseases: Various respiratory, digestive, gynecological, and pain disorders. Many of these diseases are not definitively diagnosable by Western methods, since the root cause is often Yin Deficiency, which is outside the province of Western medicine.
- Similar Western Drug Actions: Laxative, diuretic, anti-inflammatory, antibiotic, analgesic. Some lower blood pressure and serum cholesterol.

26. Astringent

These primarily sour herbs restrain the leakage of fluids and help hold organs in their proper positions.

- Representative Herbs: Nutmeg seed (*Rou Dou Kou*), pomegranate husk (*Shi Liu Pi*), lotus seed (*Lian Zi*).
- Common Symptoms Treated: Profuse sweating, excessive urination or incontinence, diarrhea, some types of bleeding disorders, nocturnal emission, premature ejaculation, prolapse of the uterus and rectum.
- Related Western Diseases: Some autonomic nervous system disorders.
- Similar Western Drug Actions: Astringent, hemostatic, antidiarrheal.

27. Settles Heart, Calms Spirit

These minerals and shells settle the Heart to calm the spirit, in large part by their heaviness. Their weight causes settling of Qi that rises inappropriately to disturb the Heart. When other organ patterns cause Qi to rise (as in Liver Yang Rising, for example), their influence is also subdued.

- Representative Herbs: Oyster shell (*Mu Li*), pearl (*Zhen Zhu*), amber (*Hu Po*).
- Common Symptoms Treated: Anxiety, insomnia, restlessness, palpitations, headaches, tinnitus, dizziness, coughing, vomiting, belching.
- Related Western Diseases: Insomnia, some psychological and emotional disorders.
- Similar Western Drug Actions: Sedative, tranquilizing.

28. Nurtures Heart, Calms Spirit

Similar but milder in effect than the minerals and shells in the previous category, these primarily sweet herbs nourish the Heart. They treat similar problems caused by Heart Blood Deficiency and Liver Yin Deficiency patterns.

- Representative Herbs: Sour jujube seed (*Suan Zao Ren*), mimosa tree bark (*He Huan Pi*).
- Common Symptoms Treated: Insomnia, anxiety, irritability, confusion, and palpitations.
- Related Western Diseases: Insomnia, some psychological and emotional disorders.
- Similar Western Drug Actions: Sedative, hypnotic, tranquilizing.

29. Aromatic, Opens Orifices

These herbs are used for changes in or loss of consciousness, usually associated with Hot or Cold Closed syndromes. The orifices that require opening are internal, always associated with the Heart in its role of housing the mind, and roughly correlate with the Western idea of sensory and motor neural pathways. The Spleen and Liver are two other frequently involved organs.

- Representative Herbs: Gall stone from cattle (*Niu Huang*), musk deer navel gland secretion (*She Xiang*). Note that musk is from an endangered species and no longer used. It is mentioned here for historical reference and as a substance that is more familiar to most readers than others in this category.
- Common Symptoms Treated: Coma, tetany or other seizure disorders, convulsions, delirium, fainting.

- Related Western Diseases: Meningitis, encephalitis, heat stroke, coronary artery disease, cerebrovascular events.
- Similar Western Drug Actions: Central nervous system stimulant, tranquilizing.

30. Extinguish Wind, Stop Tremors

These herbs and animal substances treat internal Wind, usually arising from Liver or Kidney Yin Deficiency, Blood Deficiency, or strong internal Heat.

- Representative Herbs: Antelope horn (*Ling Yang Jiao*), abalone shell (*Shi Jue Ming*), earthworm (*Di Long*). Note that antelope horn and abalone shell are from endangered species and are no longer used. They are mentioned here for historical reference and as substances that are more familiar to most readers than others in this category.
- Common Symptoms Treated: Headache, dizziness, blurred vision, palpitations, insomnia, anxiety, muscle twitch or spasm, facial paralysis, hemiplegia, high fever, convulsions, loss of consciousness.
- Related Western Diseases: Hypertension, atherosclerosis, anemia, opisthotonos, epilepsy, some psychological disorders, some nervous system disorders.
- Similar Western Drug Actions: Antihypertensive, sedative, anticonvulsant.

31. Expels Parasites

Herbs in this category are used to kill and expel many types of parasites, including tapeworm, roundworm, hookworm, pinworm, ringworm, trichomonas, and others.

- Representative Herbs: Garlic (*Da Suan*), pumpkin seed (*Nan Gua Zi*), betel nut (*Bing Lang*).
- Common Symptoms Treated: Abdominal distension, pain, poor appetite, lethargy, weakness, and diarrhea, all when caused by parasites.
- Related Western Disease: Parasitic infestation.
- Similar Western Drug Action: Antiparasitic.

32. External Application/Miscellaneous

These substances are used topically to treat bleeding and various types of infection or inflammation and to accelerate the healing of skin lesions. Some of these substances may be used internally, but most are too toxic for anything other than topical application as plasters, ointments, and soaks.

- Representative Herbs: Alum (*Ming Fan*), calamine (*Lu Gan Shi*), sulfur (*Liu Huang*).
- Common Symptoms Treated: Itch, open sores and ulcerations, superficial parasites (scabies), bleeding, swelling.
- Related Western Diseases: Eczema, parasites, syphilis (chancres), leukoderma, tinea/ringworm, dermatomycoses, neurodermatitis.
- Similar Western Drug Actions: Antiparasitic, antifungal, anti-inflammatory, antimicrobial.

Formula Basics

A Chinese herbalist will rarely prescribe a single herb to treat a patient. It's much more common to formulate a detailed prescription to treat multiple facets of a pattern of disharmony, addressing the root cause as well as the expression of symptoms and often addressing related side concerns and the patient's constitutional needs. Typical formulas contain between four and twelve herbs, although formulas with fewer or more herbs are not uncommon. Over many weeks or months of treatment, a prescribed formula may be modified slightly or significantly to accommodate changes in the patient as their health improves.

According to You-Ping Zhu's *Chinese Materia Medica,* there are approximately 8,000 herbs in the Chinese pharmacopoeia.[20] However, most herb shops and clinics in the United States stock between two and three hundred loose herbs, which are more than adequate to handle most patient needs. These are augmented by Chinese patent medicines, commonly used herbal formulas primarily in pill form. Since there is no set number of herbs in a formula and new ones are continually created, there is nearly an infinite number of formulas possible.

A competent herbalist may know a hundred or so classic formulas, understanding how and why they are constructed, along with two or three hundred single herbs, most of which may be contained within those formulas. The effects of a classic prescription

---

20. You-Ping Zhu, *Chinese Materia Medica: Chemistry, Pharmacology and Applications* (Boca Raton, FL: CRC Press, 1998), 33.

can change considerably simply by subtracting or adding a couple of herbs, modifying it to best meet the patient's individual health challenges. Many herbal texts include a number of such modifications to base formulas, so they can address a wide range of variations patients may present.

Formulas follow a basic template (principles used for combining herbs), with each herb filling one of four roles within the formula. Traditionally, these roles are the following:

1. *Chief/Lord:* The primary herbs or herbs in a formula, addressing the main complaint and providing the main therapeutic focus.

2. *Deputy/Minister/Associate:* These herbs have similar effects to the chief herb, strengthening or enhancing the main therapeutic focus.

3. *Assistant/Adjutant:* These herbs may address a secondary health issue, serve to attenuate harsh or unwanted effects of other herbs, or provide symptomatic relief without necessarily addressing the root disharmony.

4. *Envoy/Messenger:* These herbs may provide directionality to the other herbs, guiding them to specific parts of the body, or they may harmonize the effects of the other herbs, which is especially important in larger formulas or those containing herbs of diverse and possibly conflicting attributes.

This template is followed most often, but liberties are taken as needed. There can be more than one herb fulfilling each role or one herb fulfilling more than one role. Not every formula will necessarily include all four roles. Small formulas may have just two or three herbs, and even some larger formulas may only have herbs functioning as chief and deputy. It always comes down to what will make the best formula for the needs of each individual patient.

There are many other factors that an herbal physician must take into account when constructing formulas, such as knowing which herbs are incompatible and may become toxic when combined, which enhance each other's functions in specific settings, and which counteract or suppress each other. Contemporary herbal physicians also know what herbs may interact with specific Western medications, for good or ill. These are professional-level concerns and won't be covered here.

Chapter 15

Chinese Herbal Formulas

The fifty-six herbal formulas included in this chapter have been selected for their safety, effectiveness, broad range of application, and relative availability. Patent medicines (that is, traditional herbal formulas in pill form) are given here to make this easiest for the most people. Loose raw herbs are the strongest and most customizable option, but they can be more costly and require significantly greater commitment in both acquiring and learning how to properly combine and prepare them.

These are common formulas that are useful for a wide range of ailments. If you do not live near a Chinese herbs shop, the patent medicines can be found online. The name of each patent is given in pinyin, the current standard of romanization for the Mandarin Chinese language. This is done because whether you order online or visit an herbs shop, the pinyin name is the one most easily recognized, so you'll get the exact formula you want. Also, there are many English-language herbs companies that have their own versions of the traditional formulas, with many different English names possible for the nearly identical formula. (The formulas are "nearly identical" because many companies have modified the original formula according to their idea of improving it or by replacing an expensive or harder-to-get herb with a more common one with similar functions.) If you give those companies the pinyin name, they will be able to provide you with their version of the appropriate formula.

English translations are provided when possible and helpful. In cases where the translation only states the names of the formula's primary herbs, those are not included. The common name is sometimes given when that is most widely used. For example,

Bao Xin An You translates to "Maintain Peaceful Heart Oil," but it is best known by its common Cantonese name, *Po Sum On*.

Patent groupings given here are based on traditional formula categories but have been simplified for your convenience and to accommodate this select number of formulas. They are grouped according to either the general conditions they treat along with the organ or organs most commonly involved or according to their primary purpose, such as the tonics for Qi, Yang, Yin, and Blood. Some formulas include common variations, modifications to the main formula that have become standardized in order to address a different but related range of symptoms.

Most conditions are treated by more than one formula. This is because there can be many underlying patterns of disharmony that present with similar symptoms. Selecting the formula that most matches your pattern will always yield the best results. The category, functions, and typical symptoms information will help with your selection, and in Chapter 18 you'll find additional guidance.

Note that while all the formulas are generally safe, there are a very few instances where cautions are given, primarily regarding pregnancy. In those cases, there is still no inherent toxicity in the herbs. Those formulas contain herbs that move the blood, which is very useful in pain conditions. However, those herbs will consider the fetus as a type of Blood Stasis that needs to be moved, which may result in a miscarriage.

Lungs: Common Cold with Variations

1. Yin Qiao Jie Du Pian

Category: Releases the Surface

Function: Releases External Wind Heat.

Typical Symptoms: Common cold with fever more than chills, sore throat, headache, body ache. Can help with tonsillitis, measles.

Special Instructions: Best taken within the first day of onset of symptoms; use for three days only. Because it releases the surface and dispels Heat, it can be used off-label for some skin conditions, such as poison ivy, poison oak, or hives.

Additional Note: This is a "medicine chest" formula that everyone should keep on hand.

2. Xiao Feng San

Translation: Eliminate Wind Powder

Category: Releases Wind from Skin and Channels

Functions: Disperses Wind and Damp, clears Heat and cools Blood.

Typical Symptoms: Eczema, hives, acne, dermatitis, itchy, red skin lesions with pus.

3. Bi Yan Pian

Translation: Nasal Inflammation Pills

Category: Releases the Surface

Function: Releases External Wind Heat or Wind Cold.

Typical Symptoms: Common cold with nasal symptoms, sinus pain, sinusitis, facial sinus, and nasal congestion.

4. Gan Mao Ling

Category: Releases the Surface

Function: Releases External Wind Heat or Wind Cold.

Typical Symptoms: Common cold and flu, swollen lymph glands, headache, sore throat, body aches.

5. Yu Ping Feng San

Translation: Jade Windscreen Powder

Category: Stabilizes the Exterior

Functions: Tonifies Weiqi, stops sweating.

Typical Symptoms: Frequent colds, aversion to wind, spontaneous sweat.

Additional Notes: Boosts immune system, increases resistance to disease, prevents colds.

6. Chuan Xiong Cha Tiao Tang

Category: Releases the Surface (for head and neck)

Functions: Disperses External Wind Cold, alleviates pain.

Typical Symptoms: Common cold with pain, headache, nasal congestion, sinus infection.

7. Zhi Ke Chuan Bei Pi Pa Lu

Category: Releases Surface

Functions: Dispels Wind, tonifies Lungs.

Typical Symptoms: Cough from many causes, such as external Wind, Lung Qi deficiency, and Lung Yin deficiency with hot phlegm.

Additional Note: This is a cough syrup.

8. Lo Han Guo Zhi Ke Lu or Lo Han Guo Chong Ji

Category: Nourishes Yin

Function: Moistens and cools Lungs.

Typical Symptoms: Cough with Heat (sore throat or fever), especially with Lung Yin deficiency.

Additional Notes: Lo Han Guo Zhi Ke Lu is a syrup and may be stronger for deep cough with yellow phlegm. Lo Han Guo Chong Ji is a powder pressed into cubes for tea.

9. Superior Sore Throat Powder Spray

Function: Clears external Wind Heat or internal Heat toxin.

Typical Symptoms: Sore throat, inflammation, sinus and ear infections, open sores in mouth or skin.

Additional Note: This is used topically in throat or on skin.

CAUTION: In throat application, use for short term only. Stop use once throat is better.

10. Watermelon Frost

Typical Symptoms: Sore throat, toothache, mouth sores/ulcerations.

Additional Note: Similar to Superior Sore Throat Powder Spray but milder.

Lungs: Asthma, Emphysema, Bronchitis

11. Qing Qi Hua Tan Wan

Translation: Clear Qi, Expel Phlegm Pill

Categories: Clears Heat, Transforms Phlegm

Functions: Clears Heat, expels Phlegm, descends Qi, stops cough.

Typical Symptoms: Cough with thick, yellow, sticky phlegm, fullness in the chest and diaphragm, sinus congestion, asthma, emphysema, bronchitis. Possible nausea.

Additional Note: Best used for Spleen deficiency generating internal phlegm.

12. Ping Chuan Wan

Translation: Calm Asthma Pill

Categories: Tonifies Qi, Transforms Phlegm

Functions: Tonifies Qi, Lungs, and Kidneys; resolves Phlegm.

Typical Symptoms: Chronic cough, difficult breathing, asthma, emphysema, bronchitis.

Additional Note: Best used for Kidneys failing to grasp Lung Qi.

Stomach/Spleen: Digestive Disorders

13. Ping Wei Pian

Translation: Peaceful Stomach Tablets

Category: Transforms Damp

Functions: Dries Damp, benefits Spleen, harmonizes the Middle Jiao (primarily Stomach and Spleen), moves and regulates Qi.

Typical Symptoms: Loss of taste and appetite, stomachache, fatigue, nausea, vomiting, diarrhea, abdominal distension.

Additional Note: A classic formula for most types of stomach distress.

14. Kang Ning Wan

Translation: Pill Curing

Common Name: Stomach Curing Pills

Category: Transforms Damp Phlegm

Functions: Disperses Wind Damp, resolves Spleen Damp.

Typical Symptoms: Stomach flu, nausea, cramping, abdominal pain, constipation or diarrhea, food poisoning. Also used for motion sickness and morning sickness.

Additional Notes: Most widely known as Stomach Curing Pills. This is a "medicine chest" formula that everyone should keep on hand for stomach first aid.

15. Bao He Wan

Translation: Preserve Harmony Pill

Category: Reduce Food Stagnation

Functions: Disperses food stagnation and accumulations of Phlegm or Hot Phlegm in the Stomach, invigorates Stomach Qi.

Typical Symptoms: Abdominal and epigastric distension and pain, belching, abdominal gas, constipation, diarrhea, high blood pressure.

Additional Note: Can lower cholesterol.

16. Shen Ling Bai Zhu Pian

Category: Tonifies Qi

Functions: Builds Qi, strengthens the Spleen, resolves Damp.

Typical Symptoms: Fatigue, poor digestion, poor appetite, indigestion, belching, abdominal bloating, weight loss, diarrhea, morning sickness.

17. Liu Jun Zi Tang

Translation: Six Gentlemen Formula

Category: Tonifies Qi

Functions: Tonifies Spleen Qi, transforms Damp and Phlegm, stops vomit.

Typical Symptoms: Poor appetite, indigestion, diarrhea, nausea, vomiting.

18. Xiang Xia Liu Jun Zi Tang

Category: Tonifies Qi

Functions: Tonifies and regulates Spleen Qi, harmonizes Stomach and Spleen, transforms Cold Damp, stops pain.

Typical Symptoms: Poor appetite, abdominal distension with pain, diarrhea, nausea, vomiting. Used for morning sickness.

Additional Note: This builds on Liu Jun Zi Tang, adding two herbs for a stronger effect, and also warms the center.

19. Ban Xia Huo Po Tang

Category: Moves Qi

Function: Clears Stomach Damp and constrained Stomach Qi.

Typical Symptoms: Nausea, vomiting, poor appetite, food stagnation or poisoning, morning sickness, cough with profuse phlegm, and a sense of having a plum-pit stuck in the throat (plum-pit Qi).

Heart: Insomnia, Anxiety

20. An Mian Pian

Translation: Peaceful Sleep Tablet

Categories: Nourishes Heart, Calms Spirit

Functions: Cools Liver Heat, smoothes Liver Qi, calms spirit.

Typical Symptoms: Insomnia, anxiety, restlessness, eye irritation, dream-disturbed sleep.

Additional Note: This is a "medicine chest" formula that everyone should keep on hand.

21. Tian Wang Bu Xing Dan

Translation: Celestial Emperor's Tonify the Heart Pill

Categories: Nourishes Heart, Calms Spirit

Functions: Nourishes Heart Blood and Yin, nourishes Kidney Yin, clears Yin-deficient Heat, calms spirit.

Typical Symptoms: Insomnia, irritability, anxiety, vivid dreams, fatigue, constipation, poor concentration, forgetfulness, nocturnal emission.

22. Gui Pi Wan

Translation: Restore the Spleen Pill

Category: Tonifies Blood

Functions: Nourishes Heart Yin and Blood, tonifies Heart and Spleen Qi, calms spirit.

Typical Symptoms: Insomnia, fatigue, night sweats, palpitations, restlessness, dream-disturbed sleep, anxiety, forgetfulness, poor digestion, abdominal distension.

23. Suan Zao Ren Tang

Translation: Sour Jujube Decoction

Categories: Nourishes Heart, Calms Spirit

Functions: Nurtures the Heart, nourishes Blood, calms spirit, clears Heat.

Typical Symptoms: Insomnia, irritability, palpitations, night sweats, dizziness, dry throat and mouth.

Liver: Detox, Stress

24. Xiao Yao Wan

Translation: Free and Easy Wanderer Pill

Category: Regulates and Harmonizes Liver and Spleen

Functions: Spreads constrained Liver Qi, tonifies the Spleen, nourishes Blood, harmonizes Liver and Spleen.

Typical Symptoms: Digestive disorders, menstrual disorders, pain below the ribs, emotional upset, dizziness, headache, fatigue, blurred vision.

Additional Notes: May also be helpful with food and airborne allergies. It is a calming formula.

25. Shu Gan Wan

Translation: Soothe the Liver Pills

Category: Regulates and Harmonizes Liver and Spleen

Functions: Spreads constrained Liver Qi, regulates the Spleen, nourishes Blood, stops pain.

Typical Symptoms: Abdominal distension and pain, gas, belching, diarrhea, poor digestion, poor appetite.

Additional Notes: May be helpful for hepatitis.

CAUTION: Contraindicated during pregnancy.

26. Long Dan Xie Gan Wan

Category: Clears Heat from the Liver

Functions: Clears Fire from the Liver and Gall Bladder, clears and drains Damp Heat from the Lower Jiao.

Typical Symptoms: Headache, dizziness, pain below the ribs, red and sore eyes, reduced hearing or tinnitus, easy to anger, difficult or painful urination, herpes.

27. Dan Zhi Xiao Yao Wan

Category: Regulates and Harmonizes Liver and Spleen

Functions: Spreads constrained Liver Qi, clears Liver Heat, tonifies the Spleen, nourishes Blood, harmonizes Liver and Spleen.

Typical Symptoms: Premenstrual syndrome (PMS), abdominal and breast distension, headache, irritability, poor appetite, restlessness, menopausal hot flashes.

Additional Note: For menstrual disorders with Liver Heat signs.

28. Xiao Chai Hu Tang

Category: Regulates and Harmonizes Liver and Spleen

Functions: Spreads constrained Liver Qi, clears Liver Heat, tonifies the Spleen, nourishes Blood, harmonizes Liver and Spleen, regulates the Gall Bladder.

Typical Symptoms: Poor appetite, poor sleep, neck and shoulder tension, full sensation in the chest and below the ribs, headache, anxiety, alternating fever and chills.

Kidneys: Low Energy, Urinary and Sexual Dysfunction, Arthritis

29. Ba Zheng Tang

Translation: Eight Rectifying Powder

Category: Clears Damp Heat

Function: Clears Damp Heat in the Kidneys and Urinary Bladder.

Typical Symptoms: Urinary tract infections, painful urination, prostatitis, bladder stones, dry mouth and throat, abdominal distension and pain.

CAUTION: Contraindicated during pregnancy.

30. Wu Ling San

Categories: Promotes Urination, Drains Damp

Functions: Tonifies Spleen, warms Yang, promotes urination and drains Damp.

Typical Symptoms: Headache, irritability, fever, edema, ascites, urinary frequency and retention, diarrhea and other digestive disturbances, dizziness, shortness of breath.

31. Du Huo Ji Sheng Wan

Category: Dispels Wind Damp

Functions: Dispels Wind Damp, disperses painful obstruction in the channels and joints, tonifies Liver Kidneys, Qi, and Blood.

Typical Symptoms: Arthritis, rheumatism, low back and knee pain, sciatica, shortness of breath, aversion to cold, possible numbness.

CAUTION during pregnancy.

32. Kang Gu Zheng Sheng Pian

Translation: Counters Bone Hyperplasia Pill

Category: Tonifies Yang

Functions: Tonifies Qi, Yang, Kidneys, and Liver; benefits marrow, tendon, and bone.

Typical Symptoms: General back pain, vertebral bone spurs, subluxation, spondylitis, spinal inflammation.

33. Te Xiao Bai Shi Wan

Translation: Special Effective Discharge (Kidney) Stone Pill

Common Name: Passwan Formula

Category: Clears Damp Heat

Functions: Clears Damp Heat in Kidneys and Urinary Bladder; benefits Kidneys, Bladder, Spleen, and Intestines.

Typical Symptoms: Kidney, bladder, and ureter stones, kidney infection or inflammation, blood in the urine.

Qi Tonics

34. Ba Zhen Wan

Translation: Eight Treasures Pill

Category: Tonifies Qi and Blood

Function: Tonifies Qi and blood.

Typical Symptoms: Fatigue, poor appetite, loose stool, heart palpitations, anxiety, shortness of breath, menstrual irregularities.

Additional Notes: It promotes tissue regeneration after surgery or prolonged illness. This formula is a blend of the Qi tonic Si Jun Zi Tang and the Blood-nourishing formula Si Wu Tang. Combining the benefits of both, it's a great all-purpose tonic. One of my herbs teachers called this "Chinese vitamin pills," in that it's a formula that has something to benefit just about everyone. This is a "medicine chest" formula that everyone should keep on hand.

35. Si Jun Zi Tang

Translation: Four Gentlemen Decoction

Category: Tonifies Qi

Function: Tonifies Spleen Qi.

Typical Symptoms: Low energy, poor appetite, loose stool, abdominal gas.

36. Bu Zhong Yi Qi Wan

Translation: Tonifies the Middle (Jiao) and Supplements the Qi Pill

Category: Tonifies Qi

Functions: Tonifies the Qi of the Middle Jiao, raises Yang Qi (primarily Spleen Yang).

Typical Symptoms: Abdominal distension and gas, loose stool, spontaneous sweat, aversion to cold, all types of prolapse/sinking Qi from Spleen Qi and Yang deficiency. Prolapse symptoms include prolapsed rectum, colon, and uterus, varicose veins, hemorrhoids, frequent miscarriage, hernia, chronic diarrhea.

37. Shen Qi Da Bu Wan

Translation: Ginseng and Astragalus Great Tonifying Pill

Category: Tonifies Qi

Functions: Tonifies Qi and Weiqi, strengthens the immune system.

Typical Symptoms: General weakness, low energy, debility, fatigue, digestive disorders due to Spleen Qi deficiency.

Additional Notes: This formula has only two ingredients, ginseng (Ren Shen) and astragalus (Huang Qi). It may be used effectively by itself and may be taken with other tonic formulas when the presentation is appropriate.

Blood Tonics

38. Si Wu Tang

Translation: Four Substance Decoction

Category: Nourishes Blood

Function: Nourishes Blood, regulates the Liver.

Typical Symptoms: Anemia, fatigue, dizziness, muscle tension, numerous dry symptoms like dry hair, dry skin, dry nails, constipation, and delayed or absent menses.

39. Shou Wu Zhi/Pian

Categories: Nourishes Blood, Tonifies Jing

Functions: Nourishes Liver Blood, Jing, and Yin; moves Blood.

Typical Symptoms: Fatigue, delayed or absent menses, dry hair, skin, throat, and lungs, premature gray hair, insomnia, blurred vision, floaters (spots in the visual field, male sexual depletion.

Additional Note: Helps lower cholesterol.

Yang Tonics

40. Jin Gui Shen Qi Wan

Translation: Kidney Qi Pill from the Golden Cabinet

Category: Tonifies Yang

Function: Warms and tonifies Kidney Yang.

Typical Symptoms: Cold hands and feet, low back pain, frequent or profuse urination, incontinence, edema, impotence, infertility, other sexual dysfunction.

Additional Note: Based on the Yin tonic Liu Wei Di Huang Wan, with herbs added to address Kidney Yang.

41. Ba Wei Di Huang Wan

Category: Tonifies Yang

Functions: Tonifies and warms Kidney and Spleen Qi and Yang.

Typical Symptoms: Poor digestion, cold hands and feet, low back pain, frequent or profuse urination, incontinence, edema.

Additional Notes: Useful for diabetes and to prevent senility. Based on the Yin tonic Liu Wei Di Huang Wan, with herbs added to address Kidney and Spleen Yang. There are at least two formulas with this name; the formula intended here contains cinnamon bark (Rou Gui) and aconite (Fu Zi) as Yang tonics.

42. You Gui Wan

Translation: Restores the Right (Kidney) Pill

Category: Tonifies Yang

Functions: Tonifies and warms Kidney Yang, nourishes Jing and Blood.

Typical Symptoms: Debility from chronic illness, cold limbs, hands, and feet, low back pain, diarrhea, spermatorrhea, impotence, infertility, incontinence, edema.

Yin Tonics

43. Liu Wei Di Huang Wan

Category: Nourishes Yin

Functions: Nourishes Kidney, Liver, and Spleen Yin.

Typical Symptoms: Low back pain, dizziness, restlessness, insomnia, tinnitus, reduced hearing, night sweats, sore throat, impotence.

44. Qi Ju Di Huang Wan

Category: Nourishes Yin

Functions: Nourishes Kidney Yin and Liver Yin and Blood.

Typical Symptoms: Night blindness, dry or painful eyes, blurred vision, reduced visual acuity, light sensitivity.

Additional Note: This is a variation of Liu Wei Di Huang Wan with two herbs added to enhance benefits for the eyes.

45. Ming Mu Di Huang Wan

Translation: Improves Vision Pill (with Rehmannia)

Category: Nourishes Yin

Functions: Nourishes Kidney Yin and Liver Yin and Blood.

Typical Symptoms: Night blindness, dry or painful eyes, blurred vision, reduced visual acuity, light sensitivity, glaucoma and cataracts.

Additional Notes: This is a variation of Qi Ju Di Huang Wan, with herbs added to clear Liver Internal Heat and Wind, and treats eye disorders more strongly than the principal formula.

46. Zhi Bai Di Huang Wan

Category: Nourishes Yin

Functions: Nourishes Kidney Yin, clears Heat.

Typical Symptoms: Night sweats, intermittent low-grade fever, restlessness, poor sleep, high blood pressure, urinary difficulty, low back pain.

Additional Notes: This is a variation of Liu Wei Di Huang Wan, with two added herbs to clear strong Kidney Yin Deficiency Heat consuming Lung, Liver, and Heart Yin fluids.

47. Da Bu Yin Wan

Translation: Great Tonify the Yin Pill

Category: Nourishes Yin

Functions: Nourishes Yin, descends Fire.

Typical Symptoms: Night sweats, insomnia, menopausal hot flashes, spontaneous emission, irritability, knee and leg pain with heat.

Pain: General, Traumatic, Arthritis

48. Yi Yi Ren Tang

Category: Dispels Wind Damp

Functions: Dispels Wind Damp from the surface and channels, nourishes and moistens Blood.

Typical Symptoms: Swollen and painful joints primarily in the hands, feet, arms, and neck, neuritis, arthritis, rheumatism, fever.

49. Yan Hu Suo Zhi Tong Pian

Categories: Moves Blood, Dispels Blood Stasis

Functions: Moves Qi and blood in the channels, dispels Wind Damp.

Typical Symptoms: Headache, sinus pain, stomachache, menstrual cramps, toothache, most pain disorders.

Additional Notes: Zhi Tong Pian means "Stops Pain Tablets." One of my herbs teachers called the herb *Yan Hu Suo* "Chinese aspirin."

50. Yunnan Te Chuan Tian Qi Pian

Categories: Moves Blood, Stops Bleeding

Functions: Warms and moves Blood, breaks up Blood Stasis, stops bleeding, reduces swelling and pain.

Typical Symptoms: Nosebleeds, blood in urine, bleeding from trauma, bruising, menstrual cramps.

Additional Note: Helps lower blood pressure and serum cholesterol. This is a single-herb tablet of Tienqi ginseng.

CAUTION: Contraindicated during pregnancy.

51. Yunnan Bai Yao

Translation: Yunnan (Province) White Medicine

Categories: Moves Blood, Stops Bleeding

Functions: Moves Blood, stops bleeding and pain.

Typical Symptoms: Pain, internal or external bleeding (may be applied topically for external bleeding), swelling and pain from injury, severe menstrual bleeding, bleeding ulcers.

Additional Notes: This is a "medicine chest" formula that everyone should keep on hand. It is a powerful first-aid remedy for most pain and bleeding conditions. Not a traditional formula, this is available in powder or capsule form only. The main known ingredient is Tienqi ginseng, but it contains other proprietary secret ingredients.

CAUTION: Contraindicated during pregnancy.

52. Jin Gu Die Shang Wan

Translation: Muscle and Bone Traumatic Injury Pill

Categories: Moves Blood, Stops Bleeding and Pain

Functions: Moves the Blood, stops bleeding, strengthens tendons, promotes healing.

Typical Symptoms: Acute traumatic injuries of all sorts, including fractures, strains, and sprains, with swelling and pain.

CAUTION: Contraindicated during pregnancy.

53. Dan Shen Yin

Category: Moves Blood, Stops Bleeding

Functions: Moves Blood and Qi, disperses Blood Stasis, stops pain.

Typical Symptoms: Chest pain, angina, heart attack, stroke, abdominal pain radiating to the back and shoulder blades.

Additional Notes: Helps lower blood pressure and serum cholesterol. The classic formula has just three ingredients and generally addresses the Middle Jiao while still addressing Heart and Liver Blood Stasis. Contemporary pill forms contain fourteen ingredients, more strongly addressing the Heart and Liver. Both have *Dan Shen* as the main herb. The listed symptoms are more fully addressed by the pill form.

CAUTION: Contraindicated during pregnancy.

54. Chuan Bi Tang

Translation: Relieves Painful Obstruction Decoction

Categories: Releases Wind Cold Damp, Moves Blood

Functions: Clears Wind Cold Damp in the channels, breaks up Blood Stasis.

Typical Symptoms: Arthritis, bursitis, rheumatism, and other joint pain, especially in the upper body.

Topicals for Pain

55. Bao Xin An You

Translation: Maintain Peaceful Heart Oil

Common Name: Po Sum On

Category: Topical to Move Blood

Function: Clears Wind Cold, warms and moves Blood.

Typical Symptoms: Pain syndromes, rheumatism, chronic pain, acute injury.

Additional Notes: This is best known as *Po Sum On*. It is a "medicine chest" formula that everyone should keep on hand.

56. Zhen Gu Shui

Translation: Rectify Bone Liquid

Category: Topical to Move Qi and Blood

Functions: Moves Qi and Blood, relaxes muscles and tendons.

Typical Symptoms: Traumatic injuries of all sorts, fractures, sprains, torn muscles and ligaments.

Additional Notes: Promotes healing and stops pain. Popular among athletes and martial artists.

Chapter 16

Introduction to Qigong:
Harnessing the Energy of Life

Defining Qigong

The word "Qigong" is made from two syllables that are discrete words. *Qi* means vital life energy or life force, often translated just as "energy." *Gong* means cultivation, practice, or work. Implicit in the word "Gong" are the concepts of effort, time, and purpose. So, while the simplest translation is "energy work" or "energy cultivation," a fuller definition is "effort over time put into the cultivation of life force, for the purpose of being able to sense it, increase it, and direct its use." Those uses can vary considerably, depending on each individual's goals.

If we look at the five philosophical bases of Qigong, we can get a general understanding of possible purposes or uses.

1. Daoist Qigongs are most concerned with aligning with the natural world, primarily for better health and longer life.

2. Buddhist Qigongs are most concerned with spiritual cultivation according to Buddhist principles.

3. Medical Qigongs are most concerned with healing illness and preserving health.

4. Martial Qigongs are most concerned with facilitating martial ability and healing related injuries.

5. Confucian Qigongs are most concerned with intellectual development, primarily in service to the culture, community, and government.

There is substantial overlap among these philosophies and their consequent practices. Although all the Qigongs taught here are medical, some have their roots in Daoist and Buddhist practices as well. There is no religious content or overtones to be found here. These are entirely secular medical practices.

The Three Regulations

In order for any practice to truly be a Qigong, it must adhere to the principle of the Three Regulations: the regulation of the body, whether in a moving or stationary practice; the regulation of the breath; and the regulation of the mind, which includes thinking and understanding but is more about the most subtle ways of perceiving Qi and related aspects of one's being. When all three are combined, you have the most effective means of regulating the Qi.

Other types of exercise may have two of the three, but Qigong must have all three. Energy moves differently once you begin to modify your breath, thoughts, and movements. When combined conscientiously, they produce many different effects.

The Basic Standing Posture: The Side Channel Stance

In many Qigong practices and in many styles of Taiji, the student is often given this instruction, or a very similar variation, in order to get into the proper standing posture: "Stand straight, with your feet parallel at shoulder to hip width apart, your knees slightly bent, and weight evenly distributed across the bottoms of your feet." This gets you into the general ballpark of what is known as the Side Channel Stance, also known as *Zhan Zhuang*, but in practice most students stand with their feet too wide with this instruction. This is because, in addition to possibly not having sufficient body awareness, they are not told exactly what is meant by "shoulder" and "hip" and how those body parts relate to the side channels.

The left and right side channels run through both legs, the torso, both arms, and the head. All of the twelve regular meridians and half of the extraordinary meridians grew out of the core side channels meridians, and the side channels continue to influence Qi flow through all of those meridians.

Within the torso, the upper portion is delimited by the shoulder's nest and the lower portion by the *Kwa*, which is roughly the center of the inguinal groove (points A and B on **Figure 16.1**, respectively) If you draw your shoulders forward, toward the center of your chest, you'll feel a hollow form just to the chest side of your shoulders. That depression indicates the front portion of the shoulder's nest and is the only landmark you'll need to identify its location. That location is what is meant by "shoulder" in the instruction, considerably narrower than the outer tip of the shoulders that most beginners assume.

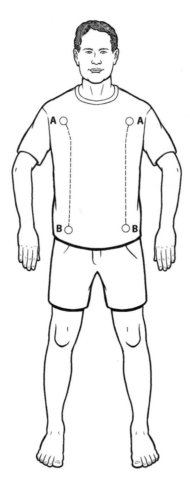

Figure 16.1 (Shoulder's Nest [A] and Kwa [B])

To locate the Kwa, squat slightly, as though you are about to sit on a stool. Try to not let your knees move forward as you do this, although slight knee movement is fine. In the center of your inguinal fold, where your legs join your torso, you'll feel a depression form that is similar to what you felt at the shoulder's nest. That depression indicates the lower front portion of the Kwa, which is all you need to identify its location. The Kwa is really what is meant by "hip" in the stance instruction.

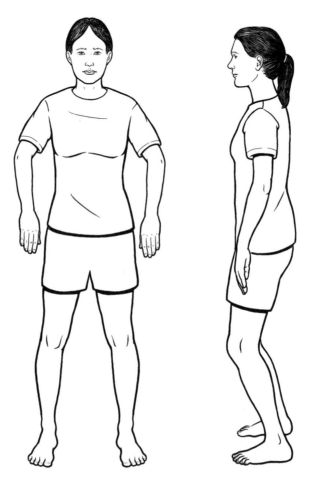

Figure 16.2 (Side Channel Stance)

By standing with your feet parallel and on the side channels, you are automatically minimizing physical obstruction in those channels and maximizing the potential to move Qi effectively through them. That's important in this practice and in most styles of Qigong. If your shoulders are wider than your hips, place your feet at shoulder width; if your hips are wider, place your feet at hip width, to give you the most stable stance. Allow your arms to hang comfortably at your sides (**Figure 16.2**). Practice this by itself until you get the clear feeling you can get into a Side Channel Stance without having to check yourself. You've now learned the Side Channel Stance.

General Breathing Guidelines

If you are already trained in Daoist natural breathing, you should use that in this practice. Otherwise, simply keep your breath comfortably long and full. Breathe in and out through your nose only (unless your sinuses are too congested to allow that), and try to breathe into your belly more than into your chest. The most important thing is to keep your breathing relaxed. It should never feel forced or strained. That would increase tension in your nervous system, which is counterproductive in these practices and bad for your health in general.

Before adding the breathing component to any practice, it's a good idea to check your breathing alone first. Get in your Side Channel Stance, arms relaxed at your sides, and breathe comfortably in and out through your nose. See if you can get your belly to expand a bit on each inhalation and retract back to its starting point on each exhalation. Try to keep your chest relaxed, with a sense of sinking, so that it doesn't move or moves very little with each breath. Let your breathing become slower and fuller, maintaining a sense of relaxed comfort. Once you've found your longest comfortable breath, note how that feels and approximately how long it takes.

In each Qigong practice your breath will link to your movement in slightly different ways. Sometimes one breathing cycle will match the entire movement, and sometimes it will only include part of a movement. In either case, the length of your comfortable breath will determine the speed of your movement. You can always adjust the speed of your movement to match your breath, but you never want to force your breath to match the speed of a movement that you may set arbitrarily. Once you are clear about that, you can add the breathing to the practice.

In all cases, keep your breathing circular. That is, continue to inhale all the way through to the time to exhale, and then continue to exhale all the way through to the time to inhale. There should be no held breath at any time in these practices, no gaps between inhalation and exhalation.

Working with Your Qi

Learning to work with your Qi can be the most difficult yet the most rewarding part of your practice. You are learning to sense and influence the subtlest parts of yourself, things of which most people remain completely unaware and so never attend to. While you will learn to feel your Qi kinesthetically, it's the focus of a quiet mind that allows the kinesthetic sense to develop. This is the first big difficulty. So much of contemporary life seems designed to distract and overstimulate the mind, so, especially in the earlier stages of your practice, it's important to find a peaceful environment free of all distraction to help you quiet your mind and feel for various Qi sensations.

Some people feel Qi fairly soon in their practice, but most take longer to develop that sensitivity. Don't try to rush things; allow yourself to grow at your own pace. If you are one of those who take longer, the second big difficulty is not succumbing to frustration, disappointment, or a sense of hopelessness or failure. Remember that gong (practice) contains the meaning "effort over time." For those wanting more guidance in cultivating Qi sensitivity, my first book, *Chinese Healing Exercises*, contains an exercise called Waking the Qi: Dragon Playing with a Pearl that will help you quickly develop a sense of Qi between your hands, a very useful first step in any Qigong practice.

Along the same lines, remember that learning how to do Qigong is not the same thing as doing Qigong. Consider that if you want to play a musical instrument, you wouldn't expect to pick it up one day and master it the next. Even if your goal were simply to entertain yourself or a few friends and family at home, you'd expect to practice for months at least, learning what you need in order to do that. If you have greater ambitions, you'd expect to invest more practice time and effort in order to meet your goals. It's exactly the same with Qigong. The more you practice, the better you'll get, and when you are actually doing Qigong, you have the greatest potential for continued improvement.

If you are less sensitive to Qi sensations, it may be encouraging to know that long before you feel Qi, you will still positively influence it and even feel its effects if you know what to look for, just by carefully practicing the Three Regulations. Here's why:

1. Our bodies are "wired" with nerves and meridians, both of which conduct subtle energies. The movements of Qigong in part are intended to move your body in specific ways, through the earth's electromagnetic and gravity fields. Moving conductive wiring through energy fields generates a current. The sum of all bioelectrical energies is Qi. Regulating the body helps generate those healing bioelectric energies and amplifies Qi.

2. If you are able to get breath into your belly with minimal movement of your chest, you'll be drawing in more atmospheric Qi (Qingqi). That imbues your blood with more Qi, and as belly breathing massages your internal organs, more Qi-infused blood is delivered there, increasing organ health and functionality.

3. The mind directs the Qi. If you keep your mind focused on those parts of the practice included in the instructions, your Qi will be directed there by your mental focus, even if you don't feel it.

4. After practicing for a few weeks, you may notice that your mood is better, you're sleeping better, you have more energy throughout the day, and you don't get sick as often as you did. If you do get sick, you may notice that your symptoms are milder and don't last very long. These are all signs that your practice is having a positive effect, regardless of whether you feel Qi.

Practice Times

Generally, practicing Qigong between 5 a.m. and 7 a.m. is considered ideal. The air is often the cleanest it will be throughout the day, and the Yang Qi is strong and still growing. When you are practicing an organ-specific Qigong (as all of these are) for the purpose of healing a medical problem or for optimizing organ function to maximize health and increase longevity, practicing at the organ's ascendant time of day will provide the very best results. Those times are given at the end of each Qigong instruction. With contemporary time constraints this may be impossible, but it's important to know those constraints are not the schedule of nature. When trying to heal a significant illness or to cultivate longevity, follow nature's schedule as much as you can for greatest benefit.

If you are unable to practice between 5 a.m. and 7 a.m. or at the organ's ascendant time, you can practice anytime you can fit it into your day. Any practice is better than none, and you'll get substantial benefits regardless.

Length of Practice

Some Qigongs are composed of a single movement or stationary posture. Most practices taught here have been extracted from longer medical Qigong sets. Some of those sets have specific medical goals—Dragon and Tiger Qigong is used extensively in China as a cancer treatment protocol, for example—while others are intended to benefit health in general ways, still giving each Organ System its necessary attention. Whether a single-movement Qigong or a full set, each practice takes approximately twenty minutes to perform, which is often all that's required to maintain health if you are in good health. When trying to heal a particular illness, it's recommended to perform the entire practice two or more times a day to more rapidly and effectively build up a body's healing energies and reserves.

Here, we are not performing Qigong sets. Rather we're using a single Qigong exercise to address a specific condition and combining it with acupressure and herbs in order to provide an integrated approach to holistic healing, as it is usually practiced in China.

For a single Qigong, twenty minutes of daily practice is a reasonable goal to work toward and is the minimum required to maintain good health. If you are working to heal a medical problem, longer is better, but never practice to exhaustion. You can practice a number of times a day if you can't do more than twenty minutes at a time. Don't be discouraged if you can't manage twenty minutes. Practice as long as you comfortably can, and as your health improves, you'll gradually become able to add more time.

You may include more than one Qigong practice from this book in your daily routine, but do not try to link them into a set. They were not designed to be used that way. Ideally, practice each Qigong during its ascendant time of day. Alternatively, practicing different Qigongs at different times of day also works fine. If including more than one Qigong in a single practice session, be sure to fully conclude the first before beginning the next one. Doing a Qi storage after each Qigong is a good way to ensure that separation.

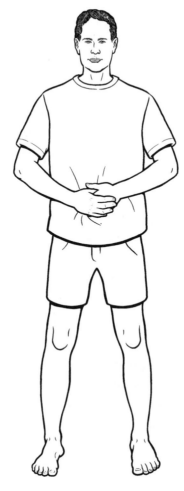

Figure 16.3 (Man Storing Qi in the Dantian)

Ending a Practice Session: Storing Qi in the Dantian

At the end of each practice session, you want to store the Qi you've just acquired so that you build up your reserves rather than allow it to dissipate. The easiest way to do this is by bringing your hands to your Dantian. Men should place their left hand directly on their Dantian and then place their right hand over their left (**Figure 16.3**). Women should place their right hand directly on their Dantian and place their left hand over their right. You may want to close your eyes, although that's not a requirement. Feel the warmth of your hands and any sense of Qi you have penetrate into your Dantian. Place your mental focus on your Dantian, and gather the Qi you feel throughout your body there. This should not require any force or effort. With your mind being present at your Dantian, Qi will be drawn there and absorbed in much the same way as water is absorbed by a sponge. Allow any sense of activity to become quiet and still, as your mind becomes quiet and still.

You can stay in this posture as long as you'd like. When everything becomes quiet and it feels as though you've absorbed whatever Qi you can, you've completed Qi storage at the Dantian. Then simply lower your hands, open your eyes, and do whatever comes next in your day.

Final Practice Guidelines

Do not practice when you are very hungry or very tired. Your Qi body is not well consolidated during those times, and it will be difficult for you to move, acquire, or store Qi. Have a light snack if you are hungry, take a nap if you are tired, and then practice.

Do not practice when you are very full. Much of your body's energy is being taken up by the process of digestion, and there may be additional discomfort if you have eaten too much.

Do not practice when you are very emotional. Your Qi will be scattered or otherwise directed away from its normal course and therefore much more difficult to access and control. If you are upset, it is beneficial either to stand in the basic standing posture, breathe as instructed, and wait for your emotions to calm or to follow the exercise prescription for emotional distress on page 271 of *Chinese Healing Exercises*.

Do not practice in a toxic environment. This can be something as obvious as a room that has been freshly painted or recently smoked in or as subtle as a place just not feeling right to you, even if you can't figure out exactly how or why that is. Toxic environments also include hospitals, where there is a lot of sick Qi, and cemeteries, which may seem peaceful but are considered by the Chinese to be full of dead Qi. When you practice Qigong, you are interfacing with the energy of your immediate environment and are particularly susceptible to whatever energies may be present.

Do practice in the healthiest environments you can find. Traditionally, the Chinese prefer places on mountaintops, by the ocean, or in forests. Clean outdoor environments provide the most abundant source of healthy Qi, which will be most supportive of your goals.

Do not practice within one to two hours of sexual activity. When practicing before sex, much of the Qi you may acquire will be lost during sex. When practicing after sex, you will not be able to store any Qi you've acquired until after your Qi body is once again stable and consolidated. Neither instance is dangerous; it's just a waste of your practice time. This is most relevant to men, but some women may experience similar effects.

Women should be careful during menstruation. For some women this is not a problem, but Qigong does move Qi, and Qi moves blood. If you notice that your bleeding becomes heavier or prolonged, do not practice during menstruation.

Chapter 17

Qigong Practices for Each Organ

Qigong for the Lungs and Large Intestines

The Lungs are the first organs in the meridian system, so we'll begin the Qigong practices with one that focuses on them. I learned this practice from Master Hong Liu in 2000, as part of his Awakening Healing Energy Qigong set. Master Hong is uniquely qualified to teach healing Qigong practices. He is an acknowledged Qigong Grandmaster, having studied for over thirty years with many of the highest level Daoist and Shaolin masters in China; is an MD (China) specializing in oncology; and has advanced degrees in Chinese herbal medicine, working with the NIH National Cancer Institute in formulating Chinese herbal adjunctive cancer treatments.

While a wide range of healing benefits will result from learning the whole Awakening Healing Energy set, this practice works well as a stand-alone Lung and Large Intestine Qigong. Master Hong recounted the story of one of his elderly students, a woman who only remembered how to do this first practice from the entire Awakening Healing Energy system. She practiced it for twenty minutes every day, and in one year, she cured herself of liver tumors and back pain and improved the appearance of her skin and hair.

Preparation: The Tiger's Claw

In this practice, your hands will frequently be in a Tiger's Claw position. You make a Tiger's Claw by spreading your fingers wide and then curling them like hooks, like you are trying to hold a large hockey puck (**Figure 17.1** on next page). Your wrist should be held straight, not bent forward or backward. (Note: A backward-bent wrist creates a Dragon's Claw, which is useful but with its own purpose and not a part of this practice.)

The Tiger's Claw restrains the Yin Qi. In this exercise it pushes energy from the fingers to the internal organs related to each finger. At different times throughout this Qigong, the claw either opens or closes the organs related to the fingers. Breathing will also be used to influence the opening and closing of those meridian endpoints and related internal organs.

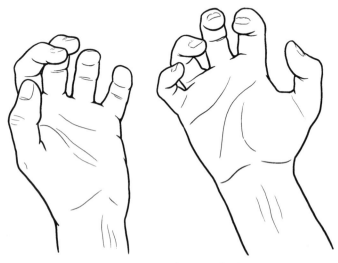

Figure 17.1 (Tiger's Claw)

The thumb contains the Lung meridian endpoint, but the entire thumb also influences and reflects the Spleen (Earth) anatomically/energetically in a Five Element context. The finger area is different from the meridian. The index finger contains the Large Intestine meridian endpoint but reflects the Liver (Wood) anatomically/energetically in a Five Element context. The middle finger contains the Pericardium meridian endpoint and reflects the Heart (Fire) anatomically/energetically. The ring finger contains the Sanjiao meridian endpoint but reflects the Lungs (Metal) anatomically/energetically. The little finger contains the Heart and Small Intestine meridian endpoints but reflects the Kidneys (Water) anatomically/energetically.

Using the Tiger's Claw, the meridian endpoints and finger areas can balance the whole body. Toes have similar correspondences to the finger areas, although those will not be directly addressed in this practice.

Physical Instructions

Stand in a Side Channel Stance, following the instructions in Chapter 16. Your eyes can be closed or kept "soft" (open but relaxed, slightly downcast, and with no specific focus). Throughout the first few instructions, your hands are kept open and relaxed with your fingertips pointing to the ground.

Inhaling, roll your shoulders forward so that your shoulder blades spread from your spine, while slightly rotating your arms so that the backs of your hands come together in front of you on your midline. Keep your shoulders' nests relaxed and soft. Feel for a moderate stretch in the area between shoulder blades. This opens the backs of your lungs horizontally (**Figure 17.2**).

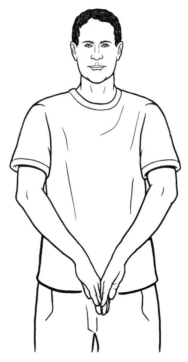

Figure 17.2 (Qigong for Lungs and Large Intestines)

Continuing your inhalation, sequentially raise your shoulders as high as possible, followed by raising your elbows as high as possible. Next, keeping your fingertips pointing toward the ground for as long as you can, raise your hands (**Figure 17.3** on next page).

Somewhere around the height of your forehead your hands will gradually rotate so that your fingertips ultimately point toward the sky directly above your head with your palms facing out toward your sides (**Figure 17.4**). The backs of your hands remain together throughout. Keep your fingers relaxed, especially the thumb and index finger. (A modification to Master Hong's original instructions: While your arms are rising, slightly shift your weight to the balls of your feet without lifting your heels from the ground. This will stimulate K 1, *Yongquan*, near the ball of your foot and biomechanically facilitate the rising of Qi.)

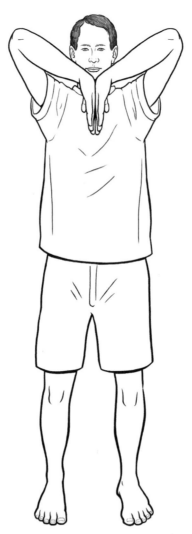

Figure 17.3 (Qigong for Lungs and Large Intestines)

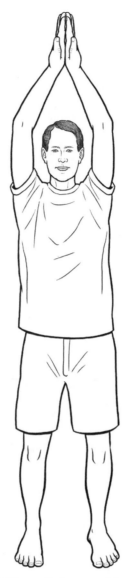

Figure 17.4 (Qigong for Lungs and Large Intestines)

Exhaling, spread your arms and palms out laterally, slowly lowering your arms to your sides. Your palms face outward and then down as your arms lower farther down the sides of your body (**Figure 17.5** on next page). Just before your fingertips once again point toward the ground, draw your shoulder blades together while moving your arms slightly rearward, bringing the backs of your hands to rest at the top of your buttocks with your fingertips down (**Figure 17.6**). (A modification to Master Hong's original instructions: While your arms are lowering, slightly shift your weight to your heels without lifting your toes from the ground. This will stimulate the *Shimian* point near the center of your heel and biomechanically facilitate the descending of Qi.)

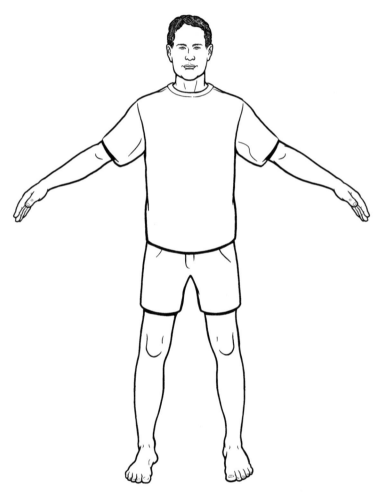

Figure 17.5 (Qigong for Lungs and Large Intestines)

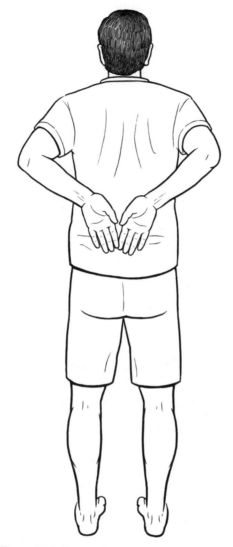

Figure 17.6 (Qigong for Lungs and Large Intestines)

Inhaling, slightly shift your weight to the balls of your feet, and slide the backs of your hands straight up your back to just above your kidneys. Your shoulders remain down, not hunched, while you gradually increase the bend in your elbows out to your sides as your hands rise up your back. Once above your kidneys, move the backs of your hands up to your armpits, led by your wrists. With your hands curled, wrists in your armpits (or as near as you can get) with fingertips pointing rearward, bring your elbows toward one another, as though they were magnetically attracted behind your back (**Figure. 17.7**). This opens the front of the chest and lungs horizontally.

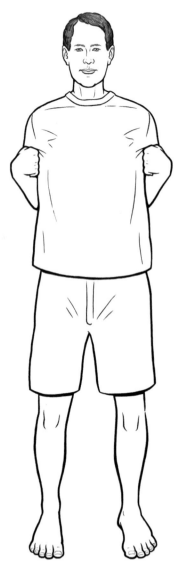

Figure 17.7 (Qigong for Lungs and Large Intestines)

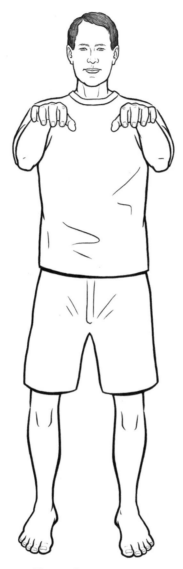

Figure 17.8 (Qigong for Lungs and Large Intestines)

Exhaling, draw your wrists forward from under armpits, and extend your arms forward, palms up. At full arm extension, your elbows should be slightly bent, not locked, and your pectoral muscles (across the top of your chest and inner shoulders) should be relaxed. That is, your shoulder's nests should remain soft and open. Then turn your palms down and form a Tiger's Claw as described earlier (**Figure 17.8** on previous page). There should be some tension in your fingers and hands at this point, securely holding in the Yin Qi. Be sure to keep your wrists flat, not bent in either direction. The line from your forearm to your hand should be completely straight.

Inhaling, shift your weight toward your heels while keeping your arms fully extended with Tiger's Claw, and squat as low as you comfortably can—but not below where your thighs are parallel to the ground!—without losing your balance or hurting your knees. In Master Hong's original instructions, it's okay to move your knees forward and your butt rearward while squatting. If you already know how to do a kwa squat, I'd recommend doing that, as I've found it to be even more beneficial in my practice.

Exhaling, slightly shift your weight to the balls of your feet and relax your fingers, releasing the Tiger's Claw as you rise from your squat.

Repeat the squat two more times, following the instructions in the previous two paragraphs from where you form the Tiger's Claw. After rising from the third squat, continue to exhale as you lower your arms and hands in front of you until they are relaxed at your sides.

Breathing Instructions

Inhalations and exhalations are included in the physical instructions above. Also follow the general breathing guidelines included in Chapter 16.

The first inhalation and exhalation facilitates opening the lower and upper Lung meridian and muscle-tendon regions upward vertically. When your hands slide up the back of your body, with elbows moving backward, the inhalation facilitates opening the lung region horizontally. Additional breathing aspects are included next.

Mind/Qi Instructions

There are two primary components addressed here. The first is that Qi is directed by the physical and breathing practices, and the second involves specific mental focus on Qi sensations, acupoints, and meridians.

When raising your shoulders in the opening movement, Qi is released down the Lung and Large Intestine channels of the arms. When the arms are extended above your head, Qi is released down the flanks. Breath is used to increase Qi flow here.

The moderate tension in the Tiger's Claw locks the Yin Qi in at the fingers, while the squat presses Qi to the Large Intestine. When rising from the squat, the relaxing and opening of the Tiger's Claw releases stagnant Qi. The simultaneous exhalation facilitates that release. If you are performing a Kwa squat, the opening of the Kwa further increases the release. The tension and relaxation need to be appropriate during each phase of the exercise in order to promote the most beneficial Qi flows.

In addition to the energetics of Yongquan and Shimian, in acupressure different areas of the bottom of feet represent different organs. Putting pressure at the bottom of the feet influences those organs, whether you maintain even pressure or shift your weight if performing the modified version of this practice. Either way, don't let your heels or toes rise off the floor when doing the squat. Inhale when squatting. Exhale when rising.

As a useful place to start, keep some of your mental focus on your hands. Notice what feelings and sensations you may have on the surface of arms and hands. Over time, accurate practice will cause sensations of cold, heat, tenderness, numbness, tingling, electricity, a watery or wind-like flowing sensation, or other possible sensations. Once you are comfortable with that, if you want deeper benefits, focus on the acupoints Lu 1, Lu 7, and LI 4. (See **Figures 13.1, 13.3, A1, A2, A3,** and **A8.**) Feel for the same or similar sensations you had generally in your hands and arms. Finally, if you are a Chinese physician, focus on the length of the Lung and Large Intestine meridians. As this is more mentally demanding, it should only be attempted after the physical and breathing aspects have become second nature, no longer requiring much thought. Even if you limit yourself to Qi regulation through physical movement and breath, you will get substantial benefits.

Conclude your practice with Qi storage at the Dantian.

If you are trying to heal a significant illness, the best time to practice this is at Lung or Large Intestine time, between 3 a.m. and 7 a.m., when the energy of those organs is ascendant.

Qigong for the Spleen and Stomach

I learned this practice from Dr. Deguang He as part of the Organ Harmony Qigong set he developed. (That set is available on DVD directly from him.) Dr. He is the first person in China to earn master's degrees in both medical Qigong and acupuncture. He practiced as a medical doctor in China and has over twenty-five years of clinical experience. Currently, he practices acupuncture at the Massachusetts General Hospital Cancer Center in Boston, is on the faculty of the New England School of Acupuncture, and has a private office called Gold Living Acupuncture in Waltham, Massachusetts, where he offers medical Qigong treatments.

Preparation: The Horse Stance

In order to do this Qigong, you'll need to learn Horse Stance. Horse Stance is commonly used in Taiji and some forms of Qigong, with a few slight variations. Here is the version we'll use for this Qigong.

To begin, stand with your heels together and toes slightly apart, forming an angle between 20 and 30 degrees. Your arms can remain at your sides. Shift all your weight to your right leg, keep your body perpendicular to the ground, and move your left leg directly to the left. Try to keep all your weight on your right leg while you do this, so that when you place your left foot down, it feels like a normal step and not like you are falling onto your left leg. Your left foot should be angled slightly outward as it was when your heels were together, with your left toes slightly farther left than your heel. You will step into and out of Horse Stance in this way during this practice. In Horse Stance your feet are wider apart than shoulder or hip width by whatever distance is a comfortable and secure sideways step for you. Once you've placed your left foot down, return your weight to the center, so that you are evenly double weighted (both feet are bearing equal amounts of your total body weight). Keep your back straight and squat just a bit, dropping your tailbone closer to the ground without letting your knees move forward. This is a basic Horse Stance (**Figure 17.9**).

Physical Instructions

Stand as in the preparation for Horse Stance, with your heels together and toes slightly apart. Raise your arms in front of you, with your palms facing your shoulders' nests, as though encircling a large ball (**Figure 17.10** on page 302). Turn your body slightly to the right, facing the same direction as your right foot, and hold the ball to the right.

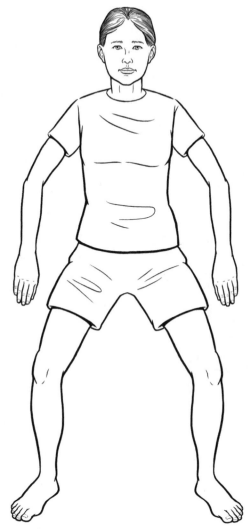

Figure 17.9 (Basic Horse Stance)

Inhaling, shift all your weight to your right leg. Lift your left leg in front of you, bending it at the knee and hip, so that your upper leg is parallel to the ground while your lower leg is perpendicular to the ground (**Figure 17.11**). Hold it there for one or two seconds.

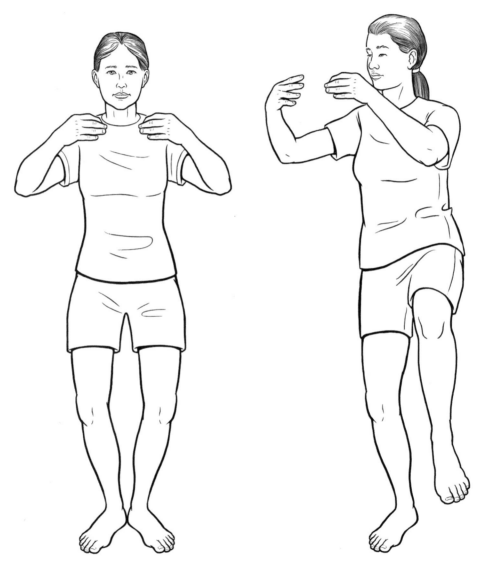

Figures 17.10 and 17.11 (Qigong for the Spleen and Stomach)

Swing your left leg wide to the left and place your left foot on the ground in a Horse Stance. Simultaneously turn your body straight forward, hold the ball directly in front of you, and double weight your legs.

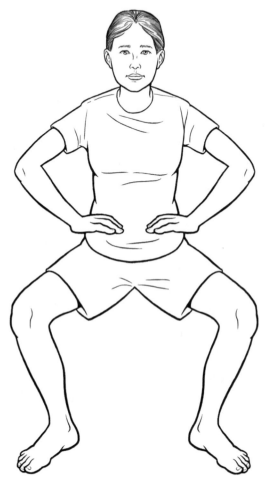

Figure 17.12 (Qigong for the Spleen and Stomach)

Exhaling, turn your palms to face the ground and squat deeply, pushing the ball down as you squat. Try to not let your knees move forward while you squat, and do not let your knees bend more than 90 degrees so that your thigh does not lower past parallel to the ground (**Figure 17.12**). It's fine if you are unable to get that low; just squat as deeply as you comfortably can with minimal forward movement of your knees.

While rising from the squat, shift your weight to your left leg and bring your right foot to the left so that your heels are once again touching and your toes are angled out. While rising, simultaneously circle your arms outward while rotating them outward so that your palms face outward slightly; continue to circle your arms upward while rotating them inward so that your palms face down; and then circle your arms inward, continually rotating them inward so that your palms face your shoulders' nests as you are once again holding a large ball in front of you. Turn your body and the ball to face slightly to your left, in line with your left foot.

Inhaling, lift your right leg in front of you, bending it at the knee and hip so that your upper leg is parallel to the ground while your lower leg is perpendicular to the ground. Hold it there for one or two seconds.

Swing your right leg wide to the right and place your right foot on the ground in a Horse Stance. Simultaneously turn your body straight forward, hold the ball directly in front of you, and double weight your legs.

Exhaling, turn your palms to face the ground and squat deeply, pushing the ball down as you squat. Follow the instructions for the squat above.

While rising from the squat, shift your weight to your right leg and bring your left foot to the right so that your heels are once again touching and your toes are angled out. Follow the earlier instructions for raising your arms until you are once again holding a large ball in front of you.

Breathing Instructions

Follow the breathing pattern provided in the physical instructions and the general breathing guidelines given at the beginning of Chapter 16. Parts of the breathing strongly link with the mental guidance of Qi, and they are described below.

Mind/Qi Instructions

Qi is moved biomechanically from one physical part of this Qigong. As you continually shift your weight from side to side, the weighted leg is full of weight, and the other leg is full of Qi. This back-and-forth alternation harmonizes the Qi of your entire body.

Inhalation brings Qi into the body and is often used to increase the drawing in of Qi through mental guidance. At the beginning of this movement, with weight shifted right and the left leg raised, the weighted right leg anchors Qi through it to ground and provide stability (grounding is a function of the Spleen and Stomach, as Earth element organs), while Qi is bought in through the left leg, guided by the mind and facilitated by the breath. With palms facing the side channels at the shoulders' nests, the side channels are most directly affected and opened here. The spleen is entirely on the left channel, and most of the stomach is also on the left channel. Qi is most strongly brought in through the left side channel during the opening movement, energizing the Spleen and Stomach and setting the stage for the most significant Qi flows in this Spleen Qigong.

When squatting, palms face downward and push Qi down near the centerline, enhancing the Stomach's function of descending Qi while also clearing out stagnant Stomach Qi. This is facilitated by the simultaneous exhalation. Use your mind to guide the Qi down your centerline here. A broad swath of two to three inches on either side of your midline is fine. The deep squat works the thigh muscles, some of the largest muscles in the body. The Spleen dominates the muscles. A strong Spleen creates strong and supple muscles, and anything that strengthens the muscles, such as this squat, will likewise benefit the Spleen.

When rising from the squat, the way in which the arms raise further opens the side channels, moving more Qi through them, and physically moves the spleen, gently massaging it. The liver receives a secondary benefit here too. Use your mind to guide your Qi up through the side channels here.

After your last repetition, remember to store your Qi at your Dantian to close your session.

If you are trying to heal a Spleen or Stomach problem, the best time to practice this exercise is between 7 a.m. and 11 a.m., when the energy of those organs is ascendant.

Qigong for the Heart: Tiger Separates Her Cubs

Dragon and Tiger is a comprehensive, extremely versatile medical Qigong set of seven movements. Although 1,500 years old, it was first introduced to the United States in the 1980s by my primary Qigong teacher, Master B. K. Frantzis. As a full Qigong system, Dragon and Tiger may be practiced to greatest advantage by performing all seven movements. However, each movement provides its own unique benefits, and the fourth movement, Tiger Separates Her Cubs, is specific for the Heart.

The version presented here is simplified just enough so that it can be effectively learned from a book yet will substantially improve Heart functioning. If you enjoy this movement and feel its results, I encourage you to learn the full Dragon and Tiger set from a qualified instructor. It will be time well spent.

To begin, there are two new considerations that must first be learned in order to optimize your practice. These are shoulder blade awareness and movement, and Beak Hands. The Side Channel Stance is also essential to this Qigong.

Shoulder Blade Awareness and Movement

Most people have little awareness of their shoulder blades. B. K. Frantzis has referred to them as "the forgotten joint"; people tend to disregard things that are not directly in front of them, literally or figuratively. In the case of the shoulder blades, this is a crucial oversight.

On both physical and energetic levels, the region between the shoulder blades contains important structures specific to heart health and the health of the Upper Jiao in general. At the level of the fifth thoracic vertebra, the spinal nerve that innervates the heart exits the spine. About one and one-half inches on either side of that vertebra are the back *Shu* (transporting) acupoints that strengthen Heart functions. At about three inches on either side, practically at the inner border of the shoulder blades, are acupoints related to the heart on an emotional level. At the level of the fourth thoracic vertebra, there are identical structures related to the Pericardium, which protects the heart.

Other Upper Jiao correspondences include related structures for the Lungs at the level of the third thoracic vertebra and for the diaphragm at the level of the seventh thoracic vertebra. The seventh thoracic is at the same level as the apex of the shoulder blades, its lowest tip. It's extremely important to keep the region between the shoulder blades soft and supple so that both Qi and nerve energy can move freely and abundantly to the Heart and its allied organs.

The easiest way to develop shoulder blade awareness is to enlist the aid of a friend, who will place their hands on your shoulder blades so you can tangibly feel them. Then, move both shoulder blades as close to your spine as you can. Ask your friend to report your shoulder blade movement to make sure you are objectively doing what you think you are doing. Next, move both shoulder blades as far away from your spine as you can. This should be wider apart than your neutral, natural starting posture and may be more difficult than moving your shoulder blades toward your spine.

Once you are able to do both of those movements repeatably well, try moving just one shoulder blade toward, and then away from, your spine. Have your friend report your progress. Then repeat with the other shoulder.

The last and most challenging step is to move your left shoulder blade toward your spine while simultaneously moving your right shoulder blade away from your spine. Then reverse, moving your right shoulder blade toward your spine and your left away. Do not get discouraged if this does not come easily. It really is more challenging than most people think at first, especially if the muscles between and beneath your shoulder blades are tighter than you know. It also takes a level of muscular control to which most people are unaccustomed.

If you do not have a friend to practice with, you can do these initial exercises most easily by yourself if you stand with your back very close to a wall so that your shoulder blades touch the wall. Do all of the shoulder blade awareness exercises and feel for the movement of your shoulder blades across the wall. If needed, to further loosen your shoulder blades and related muscles, practice all of the shoulder exercises in my book *Chinese Healing Exercises*. With practice over time, your shoulder blade movement will increase and feel more comfortable.

Beak Hands

Beak Hands is so named because when formed properly, it resembles a bird's beak. If you practice Taiji, this is identical to the Whip Hand, the hand posture used in Single Whip.

Beak Hand is formed by wrapping the tips of all four fingers around the tip of the thumb (**Figure 17.13** on next page). This requires a little suppleness in your hands and fingers, which allows for unimpeded Qi flow through your hands. This is important because there are two separate yet parallel energetic constructs that come into play.

At the tips of each finger are the end points of six of the twelve main acupuncture meridians. From thumb to little finger, these include the Lungs, Large Intestine, Pericardium, Sanjiao, and both the Heart and Small Intestine in the little finger. When your fingertips touch, there is a small yet distinct energetic impulse generated through those meridians, and as you can see, they largely coincide with the Yin organs influenced by

the region between the shoulder blades. The additional affected organs are the Yang partners of the Heart (the Small Intestine), the Pericardium (the Sanjiao), and the Lungs (the
Large Intestine).

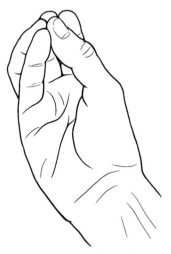

Figure 17.13 (Beak Hand)

Each finger also has a Five Element correspondence. From thumb to little finger,
these are Earth, Wood, Fire, Metal, and Water. The Beak Hand unifies the energies of
the Five Elements, balancing the body in a different way than the acupuncture end
points do. Since all of the Five Elements are represented here, this harmonizes their
energies throughout your entire body.

Once you are reasonably comfortable with the Side Channel Stance, shoulder
blade awareness and movement, and Beak Hands, you are ready to begin this Qigong
practice for the Heart. Don't worry if you are not "perfect" in these preparatory steps.

Physical Instruction

Begin by standing in a Side Channel Stance, facing forward and with weight distributed evenly between both legs. Raise your arms out to your sides, both palms facing outward with elbows slightly bent and their tips pointed toward the ground. Do your best to keep your shoulders relaxed, not hunched, and feel the weight of your arms gently pull your shoulder blades away from your spine. This is your starting posture.

You can begin the movement from either side of your body; it really makes no difference. For the sake of this description, we'll start by moving the body from the left to the right. Turn your head to face your left hand and focus your eyes on the tips of your left fingers (**Figure 17.14** on next page). Next, five things happen simultaneously:

1. Keeping your torso completely perpendicular to the ground (no leaning) and always facing straight forward (no turning or twisting at the waist or shoulders), shift your body weight entirely to your right leg. When all your weight is on your right leg, lift your left heel slightly off the ground (less than one inch) while keeping the ball of your left foot firmly in contact with the ground.

2. Gradually form a Beak Hand with your left hand while allowing your left elbow to sink closer to the ground, bending your arm about 70 percent of its full capacity to bend. This draws your left wrist closer to your left shoulder. Your wrist should stay at the same height throughout the bend of your left arm, somewhere between the height of the top of your shoulder and your shoulder's nest. Ideally, your wrist should comfortably bend enough so that the tips of your Beak Hand fingers point to the ground. If your wrists are too tight to allow this, it's okay if your beak fingers point outward. The fingers of your Beak Hand should only fully touch at the instant all your weight is shifted to your right leg.

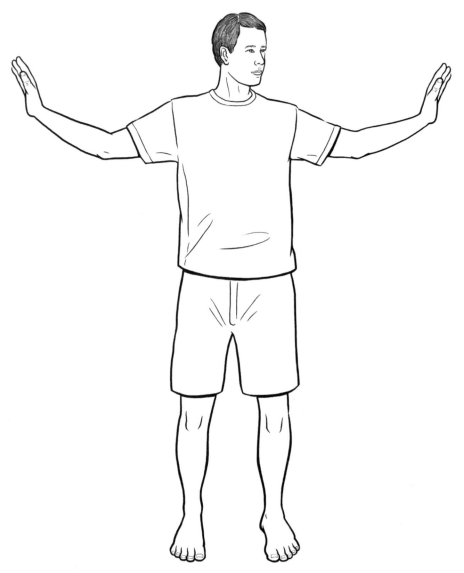

Figure 17.14 (Qigong for the Heart)

3. Your right arm extends slightly farther to the right, palm still facing outward. Your right elbow should not fully straighten but only straighten to about 70 percent of its full capacity.

4. While performing steps 2 and 3, your left shoulder blade should move as close to your spine as possible. Simultaneously, your right shoulder blade should move as far away from your spine as possible. In fact, the movements of each arm should feel as though they are initiated by the movements of the shoulder blades. This single part of the practice provides the greatest physical benefits of the entire movement, as it frees up all the muscles between the shoulder blades, allowing the heart to be innervated by both the nervous system and the acupoint energies located there.

5. As you shift your weight and move your shoulder blades, hands, and arms, turn your head from the left to the right. Your eyes should trace an imaginary line as your head turns, approximately twelve to eighteen inches in front of your body. The imaginary line should stay at the height level of your left fingertips, moving to the left shoulder's nest, heart, right shoulder's nest, and right fingertips. Your gaze ends at your right fingertips once your weight is fully shifted and your left hand has formed a Beak Hand.

Now you've completed one repetition (**Figure 17.15** on next page). From that position, repeat the movement in exactly the same way, this time moving from right to left. Place your left heel back on the ground, shift your weight fully from your right leg to your left, open your left Beak Hand while forming one with your right hand, move both shoulder blades to the left, turn your head left while tracing the imaginary line with your eyes back to your left fingertips, and raise your right heel slightly off the ground.

Alternating sides with each repetition, build yourself up to being able to do twenty repetitions, ten on each side, with no sense of strain or fatigue. Practice this for as long as you need in order to be sure you're following the physical instruction as closely as possible. This may take days or weeks.

Assuming an even number of repetitions, you'll do your last rep facing left. To end your practice session, bring your weight back to center and face your head forward so that your nose lines up over your navel while simultaneously opening your right Beak Hand and extending your right arm out to your side so that you are once again in your starting posture. At this point in your practice, you can end simply by allowing your arms to lower to your sides.

So far we've only addressed the physical movement. Once that becomes comfortable, you can then begin working on the breathing.

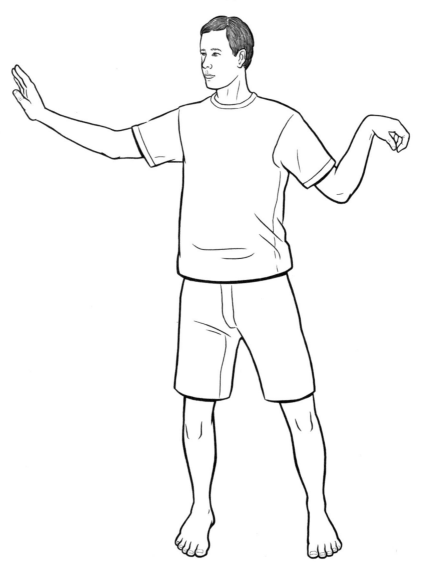

Figure 17.15 (Qigong for the Heart)

Breathing Instruction

Follow all the general breathing guidelines from Chapter 16. Once you are clear about that, add the breathing to this practice. Here's how.

Get in your starting posture, with your arms up and out to the sides of your body. Your gaze is on your left fingertips. As you shift your weight to the right, repeating all the five steps of the physical instructions, inhale into your belly through your nose. At the end of the turn to the right, at the instant your Beak Fingers touch, begin your exhalation again through your nose. Stay in that posture until you've completed your exhalation. If you're a complete beginner, these are the most important breathing aspects and all you need to practice at this point.

For additional benefit, the initial portion of the exhalation should have a bit more strength behind it, followed by a lingering, softer tail. The image you can use is that of an arrow being released by a drawn bow. The arrow initially leaves the bow propelled with apparent speed and power but then gradually arcs to the earth with a more gentle descent. Do your best to pattern your breath after that trajectory, being mindful to use no force or strain.

During the gentle arc of the trailing breath, feel your right arm continuing to extend very slightly and slowly. The physical movement at this point might be so slight as to seem invisible, but as long as you are exhaling, you want to feel your right arm continuing to slightly extend. Remember that you do not want your elbow to straighten fully. It's best to keep a 20–30 percent bend and a sense of elasticity in your arm even at its fullest extension. Ideally, you also want to move your left shoulder blade slightly closer to your spine, again without using force.

From that position, repeat the movement in exactly the same way in the opposite direction, inhaling as you move from right to left. Place your left heel back on the ground, shift your weight fully from your right leg to your left, open your left Beak Hand while forming one with your right hand, move both shoulder blades to the left, turn your head left while tracing the imaginary line with your eyes back to your left fingertips, and raise your right heel slightly off the ground. As soon as your Beak Fingers touch and your weight is fully shifted to the left, begin your exhalation as above.

Alternating sides with each repetition, build yourself up to being able to do twenty repetitions, ten on each side, with no sense of strain or fatigue. Practice this for as long as you need in order to be sure you're following the physical and breathing instruction as closely as possible. This may take days or weeks.

With the combined regulation of the body and breath, you are beginning to generate some Qi despite not directly focusing on that aspect yet, so a slightly different ending procedure will serve you better. Assuming an even number of repetitions, you'll do your last rep facing left. Now bring your weight back to the center, with your head facing forward so that your nose lines up over your navel. While centering your weight, simultaneously inhale and draw your left hand back into a Beak Hand so that you have two Beak Hands. On an exhalation, extend both arms out to your sides, with your palms open and facing outward. Complete the exhalation and then lower your arms, bringing your hands to your Dantian. Conclude your practice with Qi storage at the Dantian.

Mind/Qi Instruction

There is a saying used in both Chinese medicine and Qigong communities that "the Qi moves the body, but the mind moves the Qi." Until you become adept enough to clearly feel your Qi as a distinct quality, you'll use your mind to access it by placing your mental focus on the part of the body where you want to direct your Qi. In this Heart practice, you will also be placing some of your mental focus outside your body, moving Qi through the portion of your energy body that relates to and connects with the physical regions we're addressing.

There are a few Qi flows used in this practice. We'll include two here. For our purposes, the most important one to begin with involves pulling Qi in through the hand forming the beak and releasing it out of the open palm on the opposite side. This pulling and releasing will exactly coordinate with the physical movement and the breath, which is why you need to be comfortable with those before beginning this final piece. The movement and breath should be able to be performed with little or no distraction, so most of your attention can now be used to mentally guide your Qi.

Get in the starting posture as described above. You can begin the movement from either side of your body, but for consistency with the previous instructions, this description begins with your head facing left as you prepare to shift your weight to the right.

Place your mental focus at the tips of your left fingers. (You can select just one finger if that's easiest for you.) As you inhale and shift your weight to the right while forming a Beak Hand with your left hand, shift your mental focus to follow along with the rightward motion. Do your best to feel your point of focus move sequentially through your left hand and wrist, along the inner (Yin) surface of your forearm, elbow, upper arm, shoulder, and shoulder's nest and through your chest to your heart at about the same time you've inhaled half of your breath with your head facing straight forward and the time you are double weighted for the instant before your left heel raises.

As you continue your inhalation and shift to the right, focus your mind sequentially on your right shoulder's nest, shoulder, along the inner surface of your upper arm, elbow, lower arm, wrist, hand, and palm. At the instant your left hand has fully formed the Beak Hand, exhale and release the Qi that is present at your right palm, allowing your mind to move out beyond your palm and the tips of your right fingers. It doesn't have to move very far out; anywhere between six and eighteen inches is sufficient. With practice over time, feel for the energetic surge that happens at the instant your left fingertips touch, which travels along the same trajectory through which you just moved your mind. At that time you may also feel an energetic "bump" as the Qi moves through your heart, which has its own very strong energy field.

Because we've followed the inner Yin surfaces of the arms in this practice, we've activated all the Yin meridians of the arm, including the Heart, Pericardium, and Lungs. This dredges those channels, clearing energetic obstruction and allowing more Qi to flow through them unimpeded, while discharging any harmful pathogenic influences within the channels.

Repeat the exact same procedure as you move back to the left. The better you are able to coordinate your physical movement and breath with your mental focus, the more Qi you will be able to move. This can take some time (weeks or months) and will continue to improve the more you practice. From now on, always do twenty repetitions, ten on each side. If you want additional benefit, it's best to do another full set of twenty rather than five or ten more repetitions. You can do another set of twenty at a different time of the day if you'd prefer. Once this has become comfortable, you can add the final part of guiding your Qi.

Your head turns in coordination with your weight shift because you are using your eyes to trace the imaginary line between six and eighteen inches in front of you, along the same Qi trajectory your mind induced through your physical body. That imaginary line is actually the perimeter of your Qi body (your energy body), and your visual focus helps guide Qi through it as well. Now, as you shift your weight and pull Qi from the Beak Hand side and release it though the opposite open palm, you will simultaneously guide Qi through your Qi body, using visual focus to move your mind along that pathway outside your body.

Getting Qi to flow through your Qi body encourages deeper Qi flow within your physical body, amplifying the benefits of the arm Yin trajectory. It also clears the earliest stages of potential pathogenic invasion of the Heart through the Qi body before it can ever manifest physically. To take fullest advantage of this, after you are able to follow the perimeter of your Qi body in front of you, guided by your eyes, feel for Qi moving behind your body along the same trajectory. If you were to look down on your body, the external Qi pathway would look like a football shape from Beak Hand to open palm fingertips. With the combined regulation of the body, breath, and mind, you are generating Qi through the Yin meridians of your arms, through your heart, and more generally throughout your body.

After your last repetition, remember to store your Qi at your Dantian. Perform the same closing physical movements you did at the end of the breathing instructions, bringing your hands to your Dantian. Follow the instructions for storing Qi in the Dantian in Chapter 16.

If you are trying to heal a Heart problem, the best time to practice this exercise is between 11 a.m. and 1 p.m., when its energy is ascendant.

Qigong for the Kidneys

This simple Qigong is part of an Eight Extraordinary Meridians Qigong set. Chinese physicians who learn and practice this use Sword Fingers, where the thumb, ring, and little finger tips touch to form a circle while the index and middle fingers are extended. Since Sword Fingers requires more precision in tracing the selected meridian line with the extended index and middle fingers, we will use an open hand, which is easier and produces nearly as strong an effect. If you are an acupuncturist or otherwise sufficiently experienced in Chinese medicine or Qigong practices, you may substitute Sword Fingers for the open palm in the following instructions.

The open-palm version is used in Harmonizing the Taiji, a stand-alone Qigong practice having a few variations. This version addresses most aspects related to Kidney function. It traces the *Daimai*, one of the Eight Extraordinary Meridians (see **Figure 2.2**), and is sometimes included in other Qigong sets that focus on the Daimai or the Kidneys.

The Daimai intersects all twelve of the regular acupuncture meridians, providing a direct avenue of access for the Kidneys to support the rest of the body. Its name translates to "girdling vessel," since it girds each of the twelve meridians, holding them in place. It intersects the Dantian and the Mingmen, as well as the Kidneys themselves. The Dantian is the energy center that influences the physical health of the entire body, and the Mingmen, the "Life Gate Fire," is sometimes colloquially called "the rear Dantian" for its wide range of health benefits in ways related to both the Dantian and the Kidneys. The wider swath generated by using open palms also intersects the upper and middle portions of the Urinary Bladder, the Kidneys' paired Yang organ, for additional direct benefits. As the Daimai is used to treat a variety of gynecological concerns, this Qigong is beneficial in relieving the physical and emotional distresses that often accompany menstruation.

I once heard an anecdote about this Qigong. Among the survivors of a Himalayan plane crash, one passenger knew the practice and taught it to others who were willing to learn. It took weeks for them to be rescued. During that time, some of the survivors died, and many others suffered the effects of extreme hypothermia and frostbite. Among those practicing Qigong, there were no deaths and very few ill effects from the intense cold. While I consider this a credible account, I haven't been able to verify it with casual research, so you may want to take it with a grain of salt. However, considering the purpose of the practice, it's certainly plausible.

Physical Instruction

Stand in a Side Channel Stance. To begin, simply let your arms hang at your sides. The first thing to practice is to shift your weight toward the balls of your feet while remaining completely vertical—that is, without leaning forward. Your heels should remain in complete contact with the ground. Then shift your weight to your heels, without leaning backward. Your toes should remain in complete contact with the ground. Pay attention to how it feels to have your weight fully forward and fully backward. Shift forward and backward a number of times, for as long as it takes to be sure you have it.

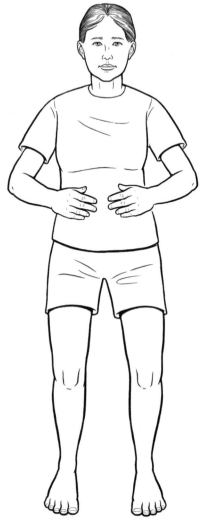

Figure 17.16 (Qigong for the Kidneys)

Next, place your arms in front of you, so that your palms are facing your body, at the most comfortable distance between six and eighteen inches from your body. The *Laogong* point at the center of your palms should be directed toward your Dantian, about two inches below your navel (**Figure 17.16**). Without shifting your weight, trace your Daimai with your palms, with your left hand moving to the left of your body and your right hand to the right. Try to maintain whatever distance from your body your palms began at. The Daimai rises a couple of inches as it rounds the top of the hips and then goes straight back to your spine, at about the height of your second lumbar vertebra, L2. Your kidneys are located two to three inches to either side of your spine, with the Mingmen between them and right on your spine at the height of L2. Keep Laogong facing toward your Daimai throughout this excursion. The fingertips of each hand should nearly touch as Laogong points to Mingmen.

It's important to keep your shoulders as relaxed as possible through this practice. Do your best to keep Laogong facing your body even behind your back (**Figure 17.17** on next page). If your shoulders are very tight or painful, you may not be able to do that. In that case, as soon as it becomes necessary, rotate your hands so that LI 4, *Hegu* (**Figure 17.18** on page 321), faces your Daimai, and continue on to Mingmen. After Laogong, Hegu is the most energetically sensitive point on your hands and will provide similar benefit. Then trace your Daimai back to the front of your body, all the way to your Dantian. If using Hegu at your back, rotate your hands as soon as possible so that Laogong faces your Daimai. Remember that the Daimai lowers about two inches as you pass over the crest of your hips moving forward. Repeat this a number of times until it becomes clear and comfortable. With enough repetitions, many shoulder restrictions free up, so you may find you can use Laogong throughout the exercise even if you weren't able to do so initially.

Next, combine the weight shift with the hand and arm movement. With hands in front of your Dantian, begin with your weight shifted forward. As your hands move rearward, gradually shift your weight toward your heels. Once your hands reach Mingmen, your weight should be fully on your heels. As your hands move forward, gradually shift your weight forward. When your hands reach your Dantian, your weight should once again be fully shifted to the balls of your feet. On your very last repetition, at this point bring your hands to your Dantian to gather Qi and shift your weight back to neutral at the center of your foot.

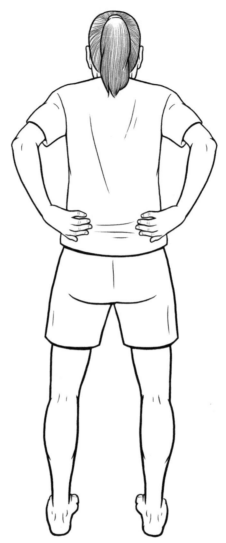

Figure 17.17 (Qigong for the Kidneys)

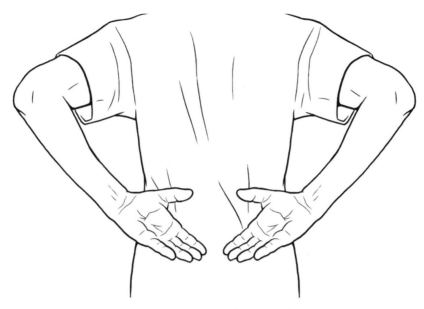

Figure 17.18 (Qigong for the Kidneys)

Breathing Instructions

Follow the general breathing guidelines in Chapter 16. With your hands in front of your Dantian, inhale fully without moving. Then exhale slowly and begin the movement, shifting your weight and arms rearward. Your exhalation should be complete by the time your palms face Mingmen. As you inhale, shift your weight and move your arms forward. Your inhalation should be complete by the time your palms face your Dantian.

If you are able to fill your belly with breath at each inhalation, you'll see that everything moves forward together on the inhalation—belly, hands, and weight—and everything moves rearward on the exhalation. Your belly retracts to its starting position on the exhalation, moving toward your spine.

Mind/Qi Instructions

There are ways Qi is moved purely biomechanically, meaning it happens more or less automatically if you follow the physical instructions well. When you shift your weight to the balls of your feet, you are stimulating *Yongquan*, or K 1, the first point of the Kidney meridian. Yongquan governs the rising of Qi. In fact, it is a particularly strong revival point used in acupuncture in cases of fainting, as it rapidly and strongly moves Qi up to the head to revive the patient. Here, because your hands trace the Daimai, most of that rising Qi gets shunted into the Daimai to be distributed to the kidneys, Mingmen, and Dantian.

When you shift your weight to your heels, you are stimulating the heel point called *Shimian*, colloquially known as "the insomnia point." Shimian governs descending Qi flows. It is used in acupuncture to draw excess Qi down from the head, one of the primary causes of insomnia. Here, most of the downward flow is initiated at the level of the Daimai and is used to release and drain pathogenic Qi that will be softened and dislodged by this practice.

Laogong (with or without Hegu) is used to sense and connect with the Qi of the Daimai, and by extension the Dantian, kidneys, and Mingmen. The instruction to place your hands six to eighteen inches from your body is because that is where you'll find the perimeter of your Qi body, also known as the etheric body. Because your hands are at the height of the Daimai, you'll be communicating with the part of the Daimai that extends through your Qi body, and that will connect you with the Daimai within your body.

The exact perimeter varies from person to person. It can vary in any individual daily, based upon the person's current state of health, how rested they are, how energized they may feel, and other factors, but you will almost always find it within that six-to-eighteen-inch range. You have to assess this by feel. Laogong is the most energetically sensitive spot on your hands, so focus your attention there and feel for some sense of connection, of contact with your Qi body. A number of sensations are possible, including a magnetic attraction or repulsion, an electrical tingling, a feeling like water or wind moving beneath your palm, changes in temperature, and others. If you are unable to feel your Qi body directly at this time, place your hands where they feel the most comfortable. It's likely that part of your feeling of comfort is due to your connecting with your Qi body.

After you've established your comfortable distance, move your hands around your Daimai as instructed above, while maintaining that sense of Qi connection at Laogong, however it feels to you. This may take some time to sense, so don't be discouraged if you don't get it right away. It may take days, weeks, or longer. Don't try to rush it.

Once you've accomplished that, the next step is to cup your palms slightly and feel for a drawing in at Laogong. You will not be trying to pull Qi into Laogong but be using Laogong to grab and pull Qi through your Daimai. (If you are using Sword Fingers, curve your index and middle fingers slightly to increase the pull of Qi along the Daimai.) At this point, vary the distance your hands are from your body and see if the sense of grabbing and pulling is stronger slightly closer or farther than where you began. Now when your hands circle your Daimai, feel for both the connection at Laogong and a similar sensation of something being pulled through your Daimai. The sensations will initially be strongest at your Dantian and Mingmen. Your kidneys will wake up next, and eventually you'll feel an even movement throughout your Daimai.

For our purposes, there's no need to mentally guide Qi up and down your legs. Simply allow the upward and downward flows to happen naturally through the alternating stimulation of Yongquan and Shimian.

After your last repetition, remember to store your Qi at your Dantian to close your session.

If you are trying to heal a Kidney or Urinary Bladder problem, the best time to practice this exercise is between 3 p.m. and 7 p.m., when the energy of those organs is ascendant.

Qigong for the Liver

This is another practice I learned from Master Hong Liu. Physically simpler than the Lung Qigong, it is an excellent stand-alone Qigong for the Liver and Gall Bladder.

Physical Instructions

Stand in a Side Channel Stance. Throughout this exercise, your eyes need to be kept wide open as though you were startled. If you experience any eye soreness or tearing, don't be alarmed. It's neither harmful nor an indication that you're doing something wrong. Since your Liver opens to your eyes, it can mean there is some weakness in either the Liver or in the eyes themselves. As you continue this practice over time and your Liver becomes healthier, your eyes will stop feeling sore or tearing.

Extend your arms in front of you, bend your elbows, point your elbow tips toward the ground (not out to the sides), and face your palms up and toward you at shoulder height, as though you were carrying a large bundle. This is your starting position.

Inhaling, draw your open hands toward your eyes. Make sure your elbows stay pointed toward the ground, and keep your shoulders relaxed. As your hands get closer to your face, focus your left eye on the center of your left palm, and your right eye on the center of your right palm (**Figure 17.19**). This can be challenging at first, and your eyes may feel crossed, but it will become easier and feel more natural with practice.

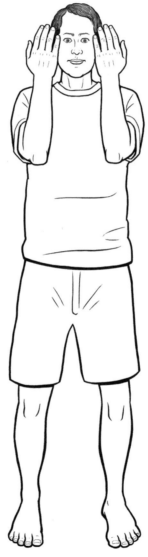

Figure 17.19 (Qigong for the Liver)

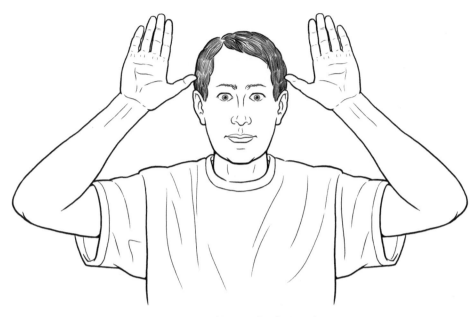

Figure 17.20 (Qigong for the Liver)

When your hands are just a few inches from your face, part them, and, while keeping your palms facing your head, circle your left hand to the left side of your head, and your right hand to the right side of your head. Once they reach your ears, draw your shoulder blades toward your spine while gradually rotating your hands until your palms face forward. Continue to move your hands slightly rearward and upward while rotating them, until they are just above your ears when your palms become fully forward. Extend your thumbs to touch the sides or your head, just behind the tops of each ear (**Figure 17.20**).

Keeping your palms forward and thumbs in contact with your head, trace a line with your thumb tips in a semicircle behind your ears until they are just behind the bottoms of your earlobes. That line is a portion of the Gall Bladder meridian, and the light touch helps stimulate Qi flow through it.

Moving your shoulder blades away from your spine, extend your arms straight in front of you, fingers fully extended upward with palms facing forward at eye height. As soon as your hands are far enough in front of you to see, focus your left eye on the center of the back of your left hand, and your right eye on the center of the back of your right hand. Keep your elbow tips pointed toward the ground throughout, arms parallel to the ground. Straighten your arms as much as you can without locking your elbows, as though you were pushing something away from you. You should feel some tension in your arms at this point, as the Qi gathers in your arms and hands.

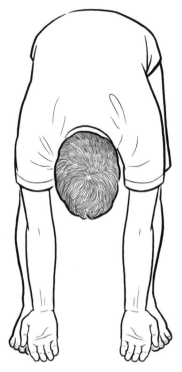

Figure 17.21 (Qigong for the Liver)

Exhaling, keep your arms extended and elbows not locked, with your wrists remaining bent as close to 90 degrees as possible, and bend forward from your waist. Bend until your palms are just a few inches above the floor, facing the ground. This forward bend gently pressurizes the liver and gall bladder, beginning an internal massage of those organs. In this bent position, circle your wrists, pointing the fingertips of each hand first outward and then down as though sliding them over the surface of a soccer ball, until your palms are facing forward and slightly upward, with the little fingers of each hand just an inch or so apart. Cup your palms as though you are trying to scoop water up from a pond. Relax your arms and hands, releasing any tension that may be present (**Figure 17.21**).

Inhale. Return to an upright position, keeping your palms cupped and arms extended with a slight bend in your elbows. This rising up opens your waist and decompresses your liver and gall bladder, bringing in fresh Qi and blood. When you are fully upright again, you should be in your starting position, ready to begin another repetition. Continue your inhalation through the beginning of your next repetition.

On your last repetition, as you bring your palms close to your eyes, roll your elbows out to the sides and trace parallel lines down the front of your body with each open palm, approximately below each eye. Your fingertips should be close but not touch. When your hands reach your navel, cross them over your Dantian for Qi storage.

Breathing Instructions

Follow the breathing pattern provided in the physical instructions above. There is only one full inhalation and exhalation through one repetition of this entire practice, which may be challenging for you at first. It will be most practical to learn the physical movements with no particular attention placed on your breathing—that is, just breathe normally, any way that is comfortable for you. That way you can practice as slowly as you need in order to learn it. Once the movement has been learned, then add the breathing component. When including the breathing, you will have to pace your movement to time it to a comfortable breath. If your breath is short, your movement will have to be relatively fast. Now you can work on gradually extending the length of a comfortable breath, which will allow you to slow your movement.

Include the breathing instructions from the general breathing guidelines in Chapter 16. On inhalations, direct your breath to your liver, as it will increase the massaging effect. On your exhalations, feel your liver relax and expand, releasing any toxic accumulation along with your breath.

Mind/Qi Instructions

The Liver opens to the eyes, and the eyes reflect the health of the Liver. The most common example is that of jaundice, where a liver disease will turn the whites of the eyes yellow. Using acupuncture, many eye problems are treated by needling points on the Liver and Gall Bladder meridians. Improving the health of those organs, in specific ways, can improve the health and functioning of the eyes. Using Qigong, you can directly treat the eyes and, through their internal connections, benefit the health of the Liver and Gall Bladder.

When you move your hands toward your eyes while inhaling, actively push Qi from the Laogong point at the center of your palms into your eyes, left palm to left eye, right palm to right eye. Use your inhalation to facilitate drawing Qi into your eyes, your breath and Qi both moving inward.

Circling your thumbs around the backs of your ears traces part of the Gall Bladder meridian, stimulating Qi flow to benefit the eyes, Liver, and Gall Bladder. While this happens biomechanically to some extent, your mental focus, assisted by the Qi you just pushed into your eyes, will tune you in to the Qi there and further amplify its flow, increasing the healing benefits.

Bending forward, you can feel your liver more easily due to the compression caused by the bend. Keep a portion of your mental focus on your Liver throughout the rest of this practice, no matter how many repetitions you do. That focus will keep Qi directed to your Liver and increase its healing. While exhaling on the bend, release any feeling of stuck or bound Qi, which in all cases is pathogenic.

The Gall Bladder meridian ends at the fourth toe, while the Liver meridian begins at the big toe. At the bottom of the bend, as you swirl your hands around the imaginary soccer ball, you are sweeping Qi from your outer toes toward your big toe and simultaneously scooping up Qi from the earth. As you rise up, bring Qi up your Liver meridian—you can just feel for it up the big toe side of your legs—while bringing Qi up directly in front of you in your cupped hands. Your inhalation facilitates that, drawing in Qi while you draw in breath.

After your last repetition, remember to store your Qi at your Dantian to close your session.

If you are trying to heal a Liver or Gall Bladder problem, the best time to practice this exercise is between 11 p.m. and 3 a.m., when the energy of those organs is ascendant.

Chapter 18

Prescriptions:
Restore and Maintain Inner Harmony

In this chapter, everything you've learned about natural healing is combined synergistically in a useful, practical way. Most Chinese doctors who practice numerous healing modalities have stated that people who are ill must combine many methods to restore the body to optimal balanced health, including acupuncture, herbs, massage, Qigong, and diet. Diseases originate from different causes, and while some have a rapid onset, most develop over time. When numerous modalities are applied in an integrated way, those diseases will be resolved most fully and in the shortest time possible. When those modalities are applied preventatively, a person will rarely become sick, will recover much faster when they do get sick, will minimize or eliminate many common age-related conditions, and will live a longer, healthier life.

Below you'll find conditions presented alphabetically for your convenience. In some cases, a few are grouped together under one primary heading, when the conditions are distinctly related in some way. For example, poor digestion, nausea, diarrhea, constipation, food poisoning, and abdominal distension and pain are all included under the heading "Digestive System Disorders."

Beneath the heading, you'll first see the appropriate Qigong exercise(s) to practice. Since each Qigong addresses a specific organ, you will immediately know which organs are most involved with the condition being treated. Remember that these Qigongs are named for their related Yin organ, but its Yang paired organ may be equally involved.

If more than one Qigong is recommended, you can either practice each Qigong every day—best if time permits—or you can alternate Qigongs on a daily basis.

It's a good idea to learn all the Qigongs as soon as possible. On their own they are very beneficial as daily practices to build health and energy. They take a little time to learn and then to acquire proficiency. Once learned, you will be able to draw on them as needed when working on a health challenge. As the old Chinese saying goes, "Don't wait until you are thirsty to begin digging a well."

Next, you'll find an acupressure prescription. The selected points are commonly used in acupuncture treatments. Modifications may be included to address related conditions that have unique characteristics. Recommendations are given for tonification and sedation techniques. Remember that harmonization techniques are always appropriate. Point locations are given in Chapter 13, and acupressure techniques are taught in Chapter 12.

Herbal patent formulas follow next. Sometimes a single patent is provided, and sometimes more than one is suggested. Unless otherwise stipulated, you can choose among any of the suggested patents, which can make it easier for you find a suitable one. Your personal circumstances may be different from those of someone else with similar symptoms. If you compare the recommended formulas, you will be able to select the best fit for you. The number that follows the patent name guides you to where the patent was introduced by the same number in Chapter 15, so you can easily review its actions and characteristics.

As different companies may include different quantities or concentrations of herbal ingredients per tablet or pill, follow the dosage recommendations they provide on their packaging materials. Typically, for the BB-sized tea pills, you'll take eight pills, three times per day. Some companies make larger herbal tablets, requiring three tablets three times per day. Remember that these are not synthetic drugs but actual herbs, so a larger quantity of pills is necessary to provide you with a sufficient amount of herbs.

Finally, you'll find dietary recommendations, divided into beneficial foods and specific food remedies. Include as many of the beneficial foods in your daily diet as possible. They are foods that are most readily available to Westerners. Other less familiar foods are used by the Chinese, and they routinely add some medicinal herbs in their stews, soups, and porridges. Those have been purposely omitted here, in order to make all of your food choices accessible.

The food remedies are recipes used to treat specific conditions. Remember that foods have the same qualities and characteristics as herbs, regarding taste, Qi, channels entered, and so on. Some foods, especially spices and herbs but also some beans, grains, and root vegetables, are used as medicinal substances. Most foods may be weaker than those used in Chinese herbology, but when consumed regularly they provide a beneficial cumulative effect. They are most effective when integrated with other treatment modalities.

Some foods are not considered to be healthy choices by contemporary Western standards. For example, some remedies call for large quantities of sugar. Sugar has medicinal properties that are beneficial in these instances, outside of the non-nutritional caloric and high carbohydrate content that makes it anathema to most health-conscious Westerners. Of course, a diabetic should still omit sugar, but anyone else trying to resolve a health challenge can safely include it for the relatively short period of time required. Similarly, tofu is made from soybeans, which are both estrogenergic and among the most prevalent of genetically modified foods. While the estrogen-like effects can be safely discounted in short-term use (except in cases of preexisting hormone-dependent cancers), genetically modified foods should always be avoided. Make sure you use verifiably organic soy products whenever possible. In fact, organic foods are generally the best to use regardless, since our food supply and many aspects of the foods themselves—lower and altered nutritional content as well as herbicide, pesticide, and industrial waste contamination—have been changed significantly since these food remedies were devised.

In a very few conditions, no foods are given. This is not an oversight. Food information for those conditions is either conflicting, very complicated, or missing from the literature.

You may find yourself drawn to only one approach, like Qigong, or possibly two, like herbs and diet. That's okay; you will get plenty of health improvements from just that. You do have to start somewhere, and you can't do it all at once. Pick the things that appeal to you most and build on that. Eventually combining all approaches in the integrated way shown here will give you the very best outcome, so try to include all as soon as you're able. Once you see how rewarding it is, it will be very easy to continue.

Start simply. Pick one condition to work on or the wellness self-care protocol at the end of this chapter, and familiarize yourself with each treatment aspect involved with that one condition. That's relatively easy to do, and the success you have there will encourage you to include more over time.

The following is a prescription index with integrated healing for common conditions.

Abscesses

Qigong

- Lung.
- Secondary: Spleen, Liver.

Acupoints

- For superficial abscess, face and skin: Lu 6, LI 4, LI 11, (LI 20 if not the site of an abscess), St 36, St 40, Sp 6, Sp 10, UB 40, GB 20. Tonify St 36 and Sp 6. Sedate all others.
- For breast abscesses, add: Ren 17, St 18, Liv 3. Sedate.
- With more Damp (swelling, blisters, oozing), add: Sp 9. Sedate.

Patent Remedy

- For oral or superficial abscesses: Superior Sore Throat Powder Spray (9).

Food Remedy

- For breast abscess: Grind a large handful of mung beans. A coffee grinder will work for this. Mix 2 tablespoons of the powder in a cup of warm water and drink the full cup. Do this twice a day.

Topical

- For Hot or Cold abscesses: Grate a sweet potato to get a quantity sufficient to cover the affected area and apply directly on the abscess or lesion. Leave in place for at least 20 minutes. Apply 2–3 times per day.
- For Cold abscesses only, appearing white with no redness or inflammation: Finely chop a raw scallion, mix it with an egg white, and apply directly on the lesion. Leave in place for as long as possible, and reapply every 4 hours.

Allergies

Qigong

- For airborne and skin allergies: Lung.
- For food allergies: Spleen and Liver.

Acupoints

- For airborne and skin allergies: Lu 7, LI 4, LI 20 Ren 17, SJ 5, Liv 3, GB 1, GB 20, UB 2. During active allergies, sedate all points. Without or between active allergic reaction, tonify all points.
- Food allergy: St 25, St 36, St 40, Sp 6, Liv 3, Liv 13, Ren 12. During active allergies, sedate all points. Without or between active allergic reaction, tonify all points.

Patent Remedy

- For airborne and skin allergies: Yin Qiao Jie Du Pian (1), Xiao Feng San (2), Xiao Yao Wan (24).
- For food allergy: Kang Ning Wan (Stomach Curing Pills, 14), Xiao Yao Wan (24).

Beneficial Foods

- Basil, bee pollen, bok choy, celery, honeycomb, kale, pearl barley, red onions, scallions, spearmint, spinach.

Arthritis

Most types of arthritis are caused by Wind and Damp obstructing the channels, often combined with Cold or Heat. This Wind invasion is characterized by pain that is intermittent or that appears in one part of the body, then disappears only to appear in another part of the body, as if being blown about by the wind. Damp is characterized by feelings of heaviness, either in the afflicted joints or throughout the body, with a dull ache and possible swelling. If Cold is present, the pain is sharp and in a fixed location, and the joints or entire body may feel cold. If Heat is present, the joints feel inflamed and may appear red and swollen. The entire body may also feel hot. All of these symptoms may be exacerbated in someone having a physical or constitutional weakness (Zhengqi) or a weak immune system (Weiqi).

Qigong

- Primary: Kidney.
- Secondary: Lung and Spleen.

Acupoints

Treatment must address three factors. First, Wind and Damp need to be expelled; then local obstructions, the painful joints, must be cleared; and finally, potential weaknesses must be strengthened.

- To clear Wind and Damp: Lu 7, GB 20, St 40, Sp 9, Sp 10. Sedate all.
    - With Heat, add: SJ 5, LI 11. Sedate all.
- To free up local obstruction: Select painful or tender points at the affected joint(s). For example, for wrist pain, you could choose among LI 5, SI 5, P 7, SJ 5, Lu 9, and H 5, H 6, or H 7. Sedate all. Refer to the illustrations in Chapter 13 or in Appendix 1 for points grouped by body region to get useful point ideas.
- To strengthen the body and enhance the pain-relieving benefits of the previous points: K3, Ren 4, UB 11, St 36, Sp 6, GB 34, GB 39. Tonify all.

Patent Remedy

- Du Huo Ji Sheng Wan (31)

Beneficial Foods

- For Wind Damp arthritis: Black beans, grains, grapes, green leafy vegetables, scallions. Add the foods beneficial for urinary pain and retention. Those are diuretic and will drain Damp.
- With Cold, add: Chicken, garlic, ginger, grapes, green onions, lamb, mustard greens, parsnip, pepper.
- With Heat, add: Cabbage, dandelion, mung beans, soybean sprouts, watermelon, and a wide variety of other fruits and vegetables.

- Freely include analgesic and anti-inflammatory foods from the bottom of the "Pain, Joints and Limbs" prescription.

Food Remedy

- Eggplant is a nightshade, and there is some controversy over whether nightshades increase the inflammation of arthritis. However, the eggplant *root* is exempt from such controversy and relieves arthritis pain. It is also energetically neutral, neither hot nor cold, and can be used in both Hot and Cold types of arthritis.
- If you can tolerate alcohol, put 3.5 ounces (about a ½ half cup) of eggplant root in a quart of rice wine, and let it soak for at least a week. Then drink 1 ounce twice a day. You can prepare more than one bottle at a time, since longer soaking is desirable. The alcohol provides a medicinal benefit as it invigorates the channels and moves the Qi, which assists in reducing pain.
- If you can't drink alcohol, low boil ½ ounce of eggplant root in 3 cups of water until it reduces to about 2 cups, in approximately 30–40 minutes. Drink 1 cup twice a day.

Breathing Disorders

Qigong

- Lung.
- Secondary: Kidney.

Acupoints

- In all cases: Ren 17, Ren 22.
- For Wind Cold (cough with some thin, whitish phlegm, short, rapid breathing, and symptoms of a common cold), add: Lu 7, LI 4. Sedate all.
- For Damp Heat (cough with thick, yellow phlegm, rapid, shallow breathing, coarse voice, feeling restless or agitated, feverish), add: Lu 5, St 40, Ren 12. Sedate all.
- For Lung and Kidney deficiency (weak cough with little or no phlegm, fatigue, weak voice, shortness of breath, especially with exertion): Lu 1, Lu 7, Lu 9, K 3, K 6, Ren 6, St 36, Sp 3, Sp 6. Tonify all.

- For emphysema, bronchitis, or pneumonia, choose the above points that best match presenting symptoms.

Patent Remedy

- For asthma, emphysema: Qing Qi Hua Tan Wan (11) for Spleen Deficiency with Phlegm, Ping Chuan Wan (12) for Kidneys Failing to Grasp Lung Qi.
- For bronchitis: Qing Qi Hua Tan Wan (11), Xiao Chai Hu Tang (28).
- For chronic pneumonia: Qing Qi Hua Tan Wan (11).

Beneficial Foods

- For asthma: Almonds, basil, carrots, daikon radish, figs, garlic, ginger, honey, kale, onions, pumpkin, sesame seeds, tangerine, walnuts.
- For bronchitis: Carrots, daikon radish, ginger, honey, pears, pumpkin, seaweed, sweet potatoes, walnuts, water chestnut.

Food Remedy

- For asthma: Drink 1 cup of fresh fig juice 3 times per day. You can make your own fig juice by putting 2 or 3 figs in a blender with some water, enough to make 1 cup.
- For bronchial asthma: Boil 7 ounces of tofu with 2 ounce of honey and 1 ounce of fresh radish with enough water to keep them covered. Allow this to simmer into a thick soup, and eat it over the course of 1 day. Frequently, symptoms may be relieved by the end of the first day. Repeat as needed.
- For bronchitis: Low boil 1 cup of fresh yellow chrysanthemum flowers in 4 cups of water for 40 minutes, until you have a thick tea. For added benefit, boil with 1½ inches of fresh ginger root, sliced thin. Add honey to taste, and drink throughout the day.
- For walking pneumonia:
    - Boil 2 cups of water and add 1 tablespoon blackstrap molasses. Allow to cool to room temperature and add 2 tablespoon freshly squeezed (not bottled) lemon juice. Drink 1 cup twice a day.

- Juice enough celery, oranges and parsley to extract 2 ounces of juice from each. Combine, and drink 6 ounces twice a day.
- For a serious cough from various types of Lung disease. The following was related to me by a noted Chinese doctor and Qigong master:

  Get a whole chicken. A one-year-old chicken is best for lung problems. If you can't get a verifiable one-year-old, it should be possible to make sure it is free range and organic. Next, get 14 ounces (400 grams) of fresh organic ginger root, sliced thin. Pluck the chicken feathers but leave the skin on—this is important. (In the United States, it's most common to get a cleaned and plucked chicken. Make sure the skin is still on.) Place the chicken and ginger in a large pot and add a lot of water, enough to completely cover them. Boil together for 1–2 hours. After 1–2 hours, drink the whole pot of broth while still very warm, but don't eat the chicken. (You can eat the chicken later if you want, but it's not part of this treatment.) The exact amount of liquid was not stipulated, but it will be at least a few cups.

  Before drinking the broth, take a hot shower to warm your body and open your pores. After drinking, take a sauna if possible or cover yourself with thick blankets to induce a sweat. Ginger is a hot substance, and it also releases the surface. When you drink it, it will dispel toxic Heat from your body. Chicken directs this action.

  This sweat will be sticky, primarily from the lungs, due to substantial and insubstantial Phlegm that may be found in different places throughout your body. This treatment is also good for Phlegm nodules, possibly including lipomas.

  This is a one-time treatment, but it may be repeated at intervals if needed. Reportedly, it has cured patients who have had asthma for more than ten years with only one treatment.
  - Variations for lung cancer: Replace chicken with crocodile meat, still using 14 ounces of ginger. Water turtle is also good for all kinds of cancer and for treating many lung diseases.
- For any Lung problem: Asian pears are ideal for any lung problem and especially good for dry symptoms. Cut the top off an Asian pear and core it. Fill the hollowed core with honey. While honey is best, sugar is okay. If you are coughing up

white phlegm, use white rock sugar. If yellow phlegm, use brown sugar. If possible, add ½ teaspoon of powdered *Chuan Bei Mu* (fritillaria bulb) for additional benefit, but this is not a requirement. Put the top of the pear back on, and then steam it for 1–2 hours. Its color should become very dark; then it is ready. Eat 2 every day, and doing so at Lung time (3 a.m. to 5 a.m.) is best. Otherwise eat 1 in the morning and 1 in the late afternoon or evening. This is said to benefit lung cancer. In the case of lung cancer, eat 2 every morning and 2 every evening.

Common Cold or Flu

Qigong

• Lung.

Acupoints

• Lu 7, LI 4, SJ 5, GB 20. Sedate all.
• With cough, add: Ren 17, 22, Lu 5. Sedate all.
• With fever, add: LI 11. Sedate.
• With nasal congestion, add: LI 20, St 3, Du 23. Sedate all.
• With headache, add: St 8, GB 14. Sedate all.

Patent Remedy

• For common cold and flu: Yin Qiao Jie Du Pian (1), Gan Mao Ling (4).
• With cough: Yin Qiao Jie Du Pian (1) or Gan Mao Ling (4), with Zhi Ke Chuan Bei Pi Pa Lu (7) or Lo Han Guo Zhi Ke Lu (8).
• With fever: Yin Qiao Jie Du Pian (1).
• With nasal congestion: Bi Yan Pian (3).
• With headache: Most colds commonly cause headaches. Some herbs in each of the above formulas intrinsically address that. For additional help, see the prescriptions under "Headache."
• With sore throat: Yin Qiao Jie Du Pian (1) with Lo Han Guo Zhi Ke Lu (8) or Superior Sore Throat Powder Spray (9).

Beneficial Foods

- For Wind Cold type: Basil, cinnamon, garlic, ginger, onions, parsnip, scallions, spearmint.
- For Wind Heat type: Apples, burdock root, cabbage, cilantro, chrysanthemum flowers, dandelion, pears, peppermint.

Food Remedy

- For Wind Cold type: Add ½ cup fresh cilantro, ½ cup scallions, and 1½ inch fresh ginger root, sliced thin, to a pot containing 3 cups of water. Low boil for 30 minutes, and drink the tea throughout the day. Repeat as necessary.
- For Wind Heat type: Low boil ½ cup each of fresh yellow chrysanthemum flowers and dandelion in 4 cups of water for 30 minutes. In the last 10 minutes, add 2 tablespoons peppermint leaves. Drink freely throughout the day, and repeat as necessary.

Digestive System Disorders

Qigong

- Spleen.
- A simple Qigong practice: Twiddle your thumbs, slowly to start, evenly, and with as precise a circular motion between your thumbs as you can. This aids digestion and aids thought processes and concentration as a secondary benefit, since the thumb area corresponds to the Spleen/Earth element.
- Exercise for constipation and diarrhea: For constipation, extend your arms forward, parallel to each other and to the ground, with your palms down. Put your mind on LI 4 and Lu 6. Then rapidly, forcefully, externally rotate your arms, so your palms face upward or slightly outward. Repeat 200–300 times, breathing naturally. This opens LI 4 and Lu 6. For a healthy, clear colon, this outward turning is best. For diarrhea, start with your palms facing up and turn them rapidly and forcefully inward. With no particular problem, rotate your arms and hands with equal force and intent in both directions. This will maintain balance and keep the meridians open.

Acupoints

- In the absence of digestive disorders, tonify these points regularly to improve digestive functions and build energy: Sp 6, St 36, Ren 6, Ren 12, LI 10.

- For poor appetite, nausea, abdominal gas, chronic diarrhea: St 25, St 36, Sp 3, Sp 4, P 6, Ren 12. Tonify all.

- For acute (rapid onset) diarrhea: St 25, St 36, Sp 9, LI 11, Ren 12. Sedate all.

- For constipation from excess (very infrequent bowel movements, abdominal fullness and swelling, heat sensations, thirst, bad breath): St 25, SJ 6, K6, LI 4, LI 11, Liv 3, Ren 12. Sedate all.

- For constipation from deficiency (dull or dry skin, lips, and hair, shortness of breath, tiring easily, aversion to cold, cold sensation in abdomen, possibly with pain): LI 10, Liv 13, St 25, St 36, Sp 3, SJ 6, K6. Tonify all.

- Simple constipation treatment: In this practice, LI 4 is paired with Lu 6, Kong Zui. *Kong* means an "opening" or "hole." *Zui* means "maximum" (or "collection"). One interpretation of this point's name is anus. Using sedation techniques, perform acupressure to both points.

Patent Remedy

Most of the digestive disorder symptoms are caused either by a Spleen Qi deficiency that generates Damp or by Damp from another source that impairs Spleen function. In either case, both the Spleen and Damp must be addressed, with the root cause taking greatest priority. If Damp is greater than Spleen deficiency, the patent formula Ping Wei Pian is the best choice. If Spleen Qi deficiency is greater than Damp, Liu Jun Zi Tang is the best choice. Xiang Sha Liu Jun Zi Tang is a pretty even balance between the two. Kang Ning Wan (Stomach Curing Pills) is almost universally effective in quickly relieving stomach distress, although the underlying cause may still need treatment.

- For poor appetite, poor digestion, diarrhea, nausea, abdominal gas, abdominal distension/discomfort: Ping Wei Pian (13), Liu Jun Zi Tang (11), Xiang Sha Liu Jun Zi Tang (18).

- For constipation: Kang Ning Wan (14).

- For food poisoning: Kang Ning Wan (14), Ban Xia Huo Po Tang (19).
- For stomach pain/distention/food stagnation: Bao He Wan (15).

Beneficial Foods

- For constipation: Apples, bananas, beets, bok choy, cabbage, cauliflower, chives, figs, honey, kale, onions, prunes, pears, spinach, sweet potatoes.

Food Remedy

- For constipation: In a juicer, juice 1 small or ½ large beet and 1/3 to ½ fresh head of cabbage. Add water to taste if you need to dilute it. Drink on an empty stomach.

There are many possible food remedies to address separate digestive or stomach disorders. The simplest is one that's effective in most cases:

- Cut a 1½- to 2-inch piece of fresh ginger root, slice it into many thin segments, and low boil it in 2–3 cups of water for 30 minutes. Sip the ginger tea until the distress has passed. It's okay to add a little honey to sweeten it. This often works for motion sickness and morning sickness as well.

Additional Note

Advice from Chinese folk wisdom: "Walk one hundred steps after each meal to assist digestion." The beginning of the Spleen and end of the Stomach meridians are in the legs, along with many of their most used acupoints, which may be the origin of this saying.

Dizziness

Qigong

- Liver.

Acupoints

- Du 20, Liv 2, Liv 3, GB 20, K 3, St 36, Sp 6. Harmonize all.

Patent

- Xiao Yao Wan (24), Si Wu Tang (38), Liu Wei Di Huang Wan (43).

Food Remedy

- Eat 1–2 handfuls of sunflower seeds. Chew thoroughly before swallowing. Follow with 1 teaspoon of honey and 1 cup of room-temperature water.
- As a tasty side dish, select a desired quantity of spinach, soak it in hot water for 3–4 minutes, season it with sesame oil, and enjoy.

Dry Hair, Nails, and Skin

Qigong

- Lung.
- Secondary: Kidney and Spleen.

Acupoints

- Lu 9, H 7, St 36, Sp 6, 10, K 6. Tonify all.

Patent Remedy

- Si Wu Tang (38), Shou Wu Zhi (39).

Beneficial Foods

- Generally nourishing Blood and Yin: Beef, cantaloupe, eggs, milk/dairy, ham, honey, lemons, soybeans or tofu, spinach, star fruit, sweet potatoes, walnuts, watermelon.

Eczema

Qigong

- Lungs.

Acupoints

- LI 4, LI 11, Du 20, Sp 10, St 36, UB 40, Liv 3. Sedate all.

Patent Remedy

• Xiao Feng San (2).

Beneficial Foods

• Adzuki beans, broccoli, corn silk, dandelion, mung beans, pearl barley, potatoes, seaweed, water chestnut, watermelon.

Food Remedy

• Crush a potato to make a paste. Apply directly to the affected areas, and change the dressing 2–3 times per day. It is reported that symptoms usually improve within 2–3 days.

Edema (Generalized)

Qigong

• Kidney, Lung.
• Secondary: Spleen.

Acupoints

• Lu 7, LI 4, 11, Sp 9. Sedate all.
• St 36, K 7, Ren 4. Tonify all.

Patent Remedy

• Wu Ling San (30). While effective for all types of fluid retentions and accumulation, the pills are milder than the raw herb formula. This makes them a safer choice for self-care, although it may take longer to see results.

Beneficial Foods

• Adzuki beans, apples, beef, carrots, chestnuts, celery, coconut, corn, corn silk tea, fava beans, garlic, ginger, mandarin orange, millet, oats, pearl barley, scallions, spinach, watermelon, wheat.

Food Remedy

- For general edema: Steam 1 pound of beef. While cooking the beef, soak 2 tablespoons of grated ginger root in 2 ounces of rice vinegar. When the beef is cooked, season with the ginger vinegar and eat on an empty stomach. Alternatively, stew the beef in water for 2 hours, adding enough water as needed to keep it covered, and drink the liquid.
- For edema in heart and kidney disease: Low boil 2½–3 ounces of fresh watermelon rind in 3 cups of water for 30 minutes. Divide the tea into 2 portions, and drink half in the morning, half in the evening.

Emotional Distress

Qigong

- For anger or depression: Liver.
- For anxiety: Heart.

Acupoints

- For anger: Liv 3, LI 4, 11, Du 20, GB 21, Yintang. Sedate all.
- For depression: Liv 3, 14, LI 4, K 1, H 5, P 6, GB 20, Yintang. Tonify all.
- For anxiety: H 6, H 7, Sp 6, Liv 3, Du 20, Ren 17, Ren 15, Yintang. Sedate or harmonize all.

Patent Remedy

- For anger/irritability or depression: Xiao Yao Wan (24).
- For anxiety: Gui Pi Wan (22), An Mian Pian (20), Tian Wang Bu Xing Dan (21), Ba Zhen Wan (34).

Eye/Vision Problems

Qigong

- Liver.

Acupoints

- For all eye problems: Liv 1, Liv 3, GB 1, GB 20, GB 37, LI 4, St 2, St 8, St 36, K 3, UB 1, UB 2, SJ 23, Du 23, Yintang. Harmonize all.

Patent Remedy

- For blurry or weak vision: Qi Ju Di Huang Wan (44).
- For cataracts: Ming Mu Di Huang Wan (45).
- For dry eyes: Qi Ju Di Huang Wan (44).
- For eye pressure: Ming Mu Di Huang Wan (45).
- For floaters/eye spots: Si Wu Tang (38).
- For glaucoma: Ming Mu Di Huang Wan (45), Long Dan Xie Gan Wan (26).
- For night blindness: Qi Ju Di Huang Wan (44).
- For red eyes: Ming Mu Di Huang Wan (45).

Beneficial Foods

- For cataracts: Black beans, carrots, cilantro, cloves, chrysanthemum, goji berries, spinach, sweet potatoes.
- For glaucoma and eye pressure: Beets, beet greens, black sesame seeds, carrots, chrysanthemum, goji berries, grapefruits, lemons, oranges, peppermint, spearmint.
- For night blindness: Carrots, goji berries, sweet potato.

Food Remedy

- For blurry vision: Collect 5 teaspoons of lemon seeds and let dry. Grind them into a fine powder, using either a food processor or coffee grinder. (Traditionally, a mortar and pestle were used.) Mix 1 teaspoon into a glass of warm water and drink once a day for 5 days.
- For cataracts: Cook ½ cup black beans until soft. Bake 1 small sweet potato and remove the skin. Steam a large handful each of goji berries and walnut pieces. Mash all the ingredients together with 1–2 teaspoons honey. Every day, eat 1 tablespoon twice a day, 30 minutes before or 1–2 hours after a meal. Continue for at least 1 month.
- For glaucoma: Low boil ½ cup of fresh yellow chrysanthemum flowers in 3 cups of water for 30 minutes. In the last 5 minutes, add 2 tablespoons peppermint leaves. Drink freely throughout the day, and repeat as necessary.

Fatigue

Qigong

- Spleen.
- Secondary: Kidney.

Acupoints

- St 36, St 40, Sp 6, Liv 13, K 3, K 7, Lu 9, LI 10, Ren 17, Du 20. Tonify all.

Patent Remedy

- Ba Zhen Wan (34). Depending on the presentation, you can add Si Jun Zi Tang (35), with more signs of Qi deficiency, or Si Wu Tang (38), with more signs of Blood deficiency.

Beneficial Foods

- Beef, brown rice, carrots, chestnuts, chicken, dairy, black or red dates, fish, ginger, green beans, hazelnuts, honey, lamb, onions, pork, rye, sesame seeds, shrimp, sweet potatoes, papaya, pumpkin, pumpkin seeds, walnuts.

Fever

Qigong

- Not recommended with active fever.

Acupoints

- LI 4, LI 11, Lu 10, GB 20, SJ 5. Sedate all.
- K 6. Tonify.

Patent Remedy

- With common cold or flu: Yin Qiao Jie Du Pian (1).

Beneficial Foods

- Apples, celery, chrysanthemum tea, cilantro, dandelion, lemons, marjoram, peppermint tea, mung beans, olives, pears, pumpkin, star fruit, tofu, watermelon.

Gall Bladder, Inflammation and Stones

Qigong

• Liver.

Acupoints

• GB 34, 39, 40, 41, Liv 13, 14. Sedate all.

• St 36. Tonify.

Patent Remedy

• Long Dan Xie Gan Wan (26).

Beneficial Foods

• For gallstones: See Urinary System Disorders. Add turmeric and ginger to reduce inflammation and pain.

Headache

Qigong

• For headache at the sides and top of head: Liver (Gall Bladder).

• For headache at the forehead: Spleen (Stomach).

• For headache at the base of the skull: Kidneys (Urinary Bladder).

• For headache due to a cold: Lungs. See also "Common Cold or Flu."

Acupoints

• GB 14, GB 20, GB 41, UB 2, UB 59, UB 60, UB 62, Liv 3, LI 4, ST 8, SJ 23, Du 20, Du 23. Sedate all.

• With Damp, add: St 40. Sedate all.

Patent Remedy

• For Liver Qi Stagnation: Xiao Yao Wan (24).

• For Spleen/Stomach Damp: Ping Wei Pian (13).

Beneficial Foods

• Chrysanthemum, ginger, peppermint, shiitake mushrooms, spinach.

Food Remedy

• While headaches arise from different sources and must accordingly be treated differently for best results, for most headaches from tension, stress, and emotional concerns, this tea is often effective: Bring 1½–2 cups of water to a boil, and add 2 tablespoons chrysanthemum flowers, 2 teaspoons loose green tea, and 1 teaspoon peppermint. Boil for 5 minutes only, strain the tea, and drink while warm. A little honey may be added to taste.

• For tension headaches: Boil ½ ounce of fresh basil in 3 cups of water for about 20 minutes. Then add 1 teaspoon each of peppermint and spearmint leaves, and boil for another 5 minutes. Turn off the heat, and add 2 tablespoons honey. Drink twice a day. Note: Basil is slightly warm, and spearmint is warm, but peppermint is cool and will balance their warming effects. Honey is neutral. This tea is suitable for headaches with either Cold or Heat signs, with or without a common cold.

Heart Conditions

Qigong

• Heart.

Acupoints

• H 3, H 7, P 6, Sp 3, 4, Liv 3, Ren 17, UB 60, K 3. Tonify all.

Patent Remedy

• For angina and chest pain: Dan Shen Yin (53).
• For palpitations: Gui Pi Wan (22).

Beneficial Foods

• For the Heart in general: Apples, bananas, bean sprouts, black sesame seeds, brown rice, celery, chicory, Chinese yams, coconut, ginger, goji berries, honey, hawthorn berries, onions, pearl barley, seaweed, shiitake mushrooms, wheat.

- Additional foods that help lower cholesterol: Eggplant, garlic, celery, tomatoes, kelp.

Hemorrhoids

Qigong

- Spleen, Kidney.

Acupoints

- UB 40, UB 57, Du 1, Sp 3, Sp 4, Sp 6, K 7. Tonify all.

Patent Remedy

- Bu Zhong Yi Qi Wan (36).

Beneficial Foods

- Banana, figs, prunes, Swiss chard, most vegetables and fruits.

Food Remedy

- Simmer a few leaves of mustard in 1–1½ cups water until it forms a pasty, thick liquid. Apply to the affected area while warm.
- Eat two bananas, with the peels on, early in the day before eating any other food. You can steam the bananas to soften the peel if you'd like, but this is not necessary. Use organic bananas and wash the skin thoroughly before consuming.

Hepatitis, Enlarged Liver

Qigong

- Liver.
- Secondary: Spleen.

Acupoints

- Liv 3, Liv 13, Liv 14, GB 34, Sp 9, 15. Sedate all.
- P 6. Tonify.

Patent Remedy

• Shu Gan Wan (25).

Beneficial Foods

Hepatitis is almost always a Damp Heat disease. Many of these foods are cooling and drain Damp Heat.

• Apples, adzuki beans, barley, beet greens, bok choy, buckwheat, grapes, carrot, carrot greens, celery, corn silk, cucumber, dandelion greens, day lilies, eggplant, fig leaves, hawthorn berries, millet, oranges, pears, pig gallbladder, pineapple, sprouted wheat, water chestnut, watermelon.

Food Remedy

• Boil 5 red dates, 1 small handful of peanuts, and 1 teaspoon rock sugar or brown sugar in 1½–2 cups of water. When the liquid is reduced by half to ¾–1 cup, drink it all, about 1 hour before bedtime.

• Make a tea from 1 small handful each of corn silk, beet greens, and dandelion greens. Low boil in 3 cups of water until it reduces to 2 cups. Drink 1 cup twice a day.

Hernia

Qigong

• Spleen, Liver.

Acupoints

• Liv 3, Liv 8, Sp 6, St 21, St 29, St 36, K 1, Du 20, Ren 6.

Patent Remedy

• Bu Zhong Yi Qi Wan (36).

Food Remedy

• Low boil 4 figs and 1 small handful each of fennel and orange seed in 3 cups of water, until reduced to 2 cups in about 30 minutes. Drink 1 cup twice a day. For additional benefit, grind 1 handful of coriander seeds to fine powder in a coffee grinder and stir 2 teaspoons into each cup of tea.

Herpes, Oral or Genital

Qigong

• Liver, Lung.

• Secondary: Spleen and Kidney.

Acupoints

• GB 20, LI 4, LI 11, LI 20, UB 40, St 36, Sp 6, Sp 9, Sp 10, K 10, K 13. Sedate all during an outbreak.

• LI 4, St 36, Sp 6, Liv 3, 8, K 3, SJ 5. Tonify all when dormant.

Patent Remedy

• Long Dan Xie Gan Wan (26).

Beneficial Foods

• Carrots, daikon radish, honeysuckle flower (tea), mung beans, peppermint.

Food Remedy

• Apply honey topically a few times a day to soothe and promote healing.

Hives

Qigong

• Lung.

Acupoints

• LI 4, LI 11, UB 40, Sp 6, Sp 10. Sedate all.

Patent Remedy

• Xiao Feng San (2).

Beneficial Foods

- Chrysanthemum tea, black beans, black dates, black sesame seeds, corn silk tea, ginger, hawthorn berries, licorice root, mung beans, papaya, pearl barley, peppermint, shiitake mushrooms.

High Blood Pressure

Qigong

- Liver, Heart.
- Secondary: Kidney.

Acupoints

- Liv 3, GB 14, GB 20, H 7, LI 4, LI 11, St 36. Sedate all.
- K 6, Sp 6, Sp 9. Tonify all.

Patent Remedy

- Dan Shen Yin (53), Bao He Wan (15).

Beneficial Foods

Some of these foods are diuretic, some directly lower blood pressure, and others lower cholesterol.

- Apples, asparagus, bamboo shoots, bananas, buckwheat, celery, corn, corn silk tea, eggplant, figs, garlic, hawthorn berries, honey, lemons, mushrooms, onion, papaya, pearl barley, spinach, tomatoes, water chestnut, watermelon.

Food Remedy

- Eat 1 onion each day.
- Eat 3 apples each day. (Apples appear to normalize blood pressure, whether high or low.)
- Make a thick soup with celery, onion, garlic, water chestnuts, and tomatoes. For added benefit, rinse some seaweed to remove the excess salt, and include that along with pearl barley and some seafood for protein. Make this one of your regular meals for lunch or dinner a few times each week.

Immune Support

Qigong

• Lung, Kidney, Spleen.

Acupoints

• Lu 9, LI 10, K 3, St 36, Sp 6, Ren 6. Tonify all.
• SJ 5. Sedate.

Patent Remedy

• Yu Ping Feng San (5), Shen Qi Da Bu Wan (37), Ba Zhen Wan (34).

Beneficial Foods

Since the immune system may be weak for different reasons, addressing the root cause will provide the best results. A strong body will generate a strong immune system. A common way to strengthen the body is to tonify both Qi and Blood, following the same strategy used in the formula Ba Zhen Wan.

• Some foods that generally tonify Qi include beef, cherries, chicken, dates, grapes, honey, most fish, royal jelly, shiitake mushrooms, squash, sweet potatoes, and white rice.
• Some foods that generally tonify Blood include beets, clams, eggs, goji berries, ham, liver (beef, pig, sheep, and goat), milk, octopus, and spinach.
• Since the Lungs influence Weiqi, or defensive Qi, which acts as the immune system's first line of defense, foods to support the Lungs will improve that aspect of immunity. Some of those foods include almonds, Asian pear, brown sugar, cheese, garlic, ginger, orange, papaya, peach, pearl barley, strawberries, walnuts, and watercress.

Insomnia

Qigong

• Heart.
• Secondary: Liver, Kidney, Spleen.

Acupoints

- H 7, Sp 6, K 3. Tonify all.
- Du 20, Yintang, Liv 3, LI 4, St 36, St 41. Sedate all.
- Optionally, harmonize all points in both groups.

Patent Remedy

- For general insomnia: Suan Zao Ren Tang (23), An Mian Pian (20).
- For Heart and Spleen: Gui Pi Wan (22).
- For Heart and Kidney: Tian Wang Bu Xing Dan (21).
- For Heart and Liver: An Mian Pian (20).

Beneficial Foods

- Cabbage, celery with beet greens, dates (red and black), mulberry tea, peanuts, wheat.

Food Remedy

- Low boil 10 black dates with 6 longan berries and 1 teaspoon honey in 2 cups of water. When the water is reduced to 1 cup, drink the tea about ½ hour before bedtime. You may need to continue this for a few nights before getting satisfactory results.

Men's Health

Qigong

- Kidney.
- Secondary: Spleen.
- Simple healing exercise for prostate, urinary bladder, reproductive organs, and rectum: Sit on the edge of a chair, heels together, toes pointing out at 180 degrees (or as close as possible.) Keep your body relaxed. If there's tension in your legs, that indicates a need to be more opened. Stay in this posture until you become comfortably fatigued. Then reverse your feet—toes in, heels out—as much as

possible. This helps heal or prevent problems with uterus or prostate. Switch back and forth between each position as you get tired or sore.

Acupoints

- For premature ejaculation: K 3, K 12, Sp 6, Ren 4, Ren 6; tonify all. Ren 1, H 7; sedate.
- For prostatitis: Ren 1, Ren 3, Sp 9, Sp 6, K 1, K 6, Liv 3, Liv 8. Harmonize all.
- For impotence: Ren 3, Ren 4, K 3, K 10, H 7, P 6, Sp 6, St 36. Tonify all.

Patent Remedy

- For premature ejaculation: Jin Gui Shen Qi Wan (40).
- For prostatitis: Ba Zheng Tang (29).
- For impotence: Jin Gui Shen Qi Wan (40), You Gui Wan (42), Shou Wu Zhi (39).

Beneficial Foods

- For premature ejaculation: Cherries, fava beans, raspberries.
  - With Cold/Kidney Yang Deficiency symptoms, add warming foods: Chicken (organic and grass fed—do not eat chicken treated with hormones, as those will cause or increase sexual problems), eggs, ginger, lamb, scallions, sesame seeds, walnuts.
- For enlarged prostate and general prostate health: Cherries, corn silk tea, figs, goji berries, mangoes, pumpkin seeds, saw palmetto, seaweed, sunflower seeds, tangerines. In the absence of prostate inflammation, burning urination, or pain, adding the foods for impotence will offer additional help.
- For impotence: Chives, eggs, ginger, goji berries, lamb, ginseng, kidney beans, sweet potatoes, scallions, sesame seeds, shrimp, walnuts.

Food Remedy

- For impotence: Eat 20 walnuts a day for 1 month.

Motion Sickness

Qigong

- Liver.

- Secondary: Spleen.

Acupoints

- Du 26, Ren 17, Ren 12, P 6, St 36, Liv 3, GB 20. Reduce all.

Patent Remedy

- Kang Ning Wan (14) with Xiao Yao Wan (24).

Food Remedy

- Low boil 1 ounce of sliced fresh ginger root in 4 cups of water for 30 minutes. Add 1–2 tablespoons of honey. This is best prepared before a trip if motion sickness is anticipated.

Pain, Joints and Limbs

Qigong

- Kidney, Spleen, Liver.

Acupoints

- K 3, K 7, K 10, UB 62, UB 60, UB 59, UB 57, UB40, UB 11, UB 10, Sp 21, Sp 10, Sp 6, Sp 4, St 41, St 36, St 35, Liv 3, Liv 8, Liv 7, GB 41, GB 40, GB 39, GB 34, GB 21, GB 20. Sedate all.

Most of these points are good for reducing general pain and inflammation, and all are good for local areas of pain. Choose from among them freely. With minor pain, just a few might be necessary. With more serious pain or pain throughout your body, select more or all. Use sedation techniques on all. For local pain in the hands, wrists, elbows, and shoulders, choose the sensitive points in those areas from the Hand Yin and Yang meridians (H, P, Lu, SI, SJ, LI).

Patent Remedy

- For bone spurs and back pain: Kang Gu Zheng Sheng Pian (32).
- For general joint and limb pain: Yan Hu Suo Zhi Tong Pian (49).
- For pain in limbs with swelling: Yi Yi Ren Tang (48).
- For upper body joint pain and arthritis: Chuan Bi Tang (54).
- For lower body joint pain and arthritis: Du Huo Ji Sheng Wan (31).
- For low back pain and weakness: Kang Gu Zheng Sheng Pian (32), Du Huo Ji Sheng Wan (31).

Beneficial Foods

Note that the foods in this pain category are not analgesics but are aimed at strengthening the weaknesses that are the root cause of the pain. For general pain from any source, it's fine to add a few common single herbs. These include turmeric and ginger, both of which are used in Chinese herbology and reduce inflammation and pain. Papaya is also used in Chinese medicine and contains the proteolytic enzyme papain, which helps reduce pain. Pineapple contains bromelain, another proteolytic enzyme. The African herb devil's claw is a potent pain reliever, working similarly as a COX-2 inhibitor without the dangerous side effects. White willow bark is a Native American remedy for pain and is the original source of aspirin (salicylic acid), in its safest natural form. Turmeric, ginger, papaya, and pineapple can all be added to or be eaten as foods. All, including the extracted papain and bromelain, can be taken in pill or capsule form, available in most drug and nutrition supplement stores. In that case, follow the instructions on each product's label.

- For joint pain, same as for Wind Damp arthritis. Add the appropriate food choices for Heat or Cold if they are present.
- For back pain with Cold: Chicken (organic and grass fed), eggs, ginger, lamb, lentils, scallions, sesame seeds, walnuts.
- For back pain with Heat: Most fresh fruits and vegetables, most beans.

Pain, General and Traumatic

Qigong

• Kidney, Liver, Spleen.

In the case of recent trauma, limit to only whichever Qigongs may be possible without increasing pain.

Acupoints

Choose from among the joint and limb pain points from under "Pain, Joints and Limbs," with these modifications:

• Do not put pressure directly on any acute injury. You can, however, treat the same body part on the uninjured side. For example, if you've injured your left knee, use acupoints GB 34, Liv 8, St 35, St 36, Sp 10, UB 40, and K 10 on your right knee. You can also select points above and below the injured knee on the left leg.

• During the acute phase of the injury, sedation techniques are still appropriate to reduce pain and inflammation. After the acute phase has passed, you need to tonify to heal injured tissue, rebuild energy, and generate blood. Tonify St 36, Sp 3, Sp 6, K 3, K 7, Ren 4, Ren 6. Sedation should still be used on any areas of lingering pain, to reduce Qi stagnation, Blood Stasis, and any other channel obstruction.

• For chronic pain conditions, follow the instructions in the preceding paragraph. That is, sedate any areas of chronic pain, and tonify St 36, Sp 3, Sp 6, K 3, K 7, Ren 4, and Ren 6 to strengthen and heal your body. Harmonize Liv 3 and LI 4 to smooth Qi systemically, reducing general pain, tension, and emotional distress.

Patent Remedy

• For abdominal Pain: Yan Hu Suo Zhi Tong Pian (49). Also see Digestive System Disorders.

• For general pain: Yan Hu Suo Zhi Tong Pian (49).

• With internal or external bleeding: Yunnan Te Chuan Tian Qi Pian (50), Yunnan Bai Yao (51).

• For pain from traumatic injury: Jin Gu Die Shang Wan (52), Yunnan Bai Yao (51).

Poor Memory

Qigong

• Heart, Kidney, Spleen.

Acupoints

• H 3, H 7, P 6, UB 10, Du 20. Harmonize all.
• K 1, K 6, Sp 6, St 36, Ren 4, Ren 6. Tonify all.

Patent Remedy

• Tian Wang Bu Xing Dan (21), Gui Pi Wan (22).

Urinary System Disorders

Qigong

• Kidney.

Acupoints

• K 3, K 6, K 10, K 13, Ren 1, Ren 3, Ren 6, Sp 6, Sp 9, Liv 3, Liv 8. Harmonize all.

Patent Remedy

• For urinary pain, frequency, retention: Ba Zheng Tang (29), Zhi Bai Di Huang Wan (46).
• For kidney stones/infection: Te Xiao Bai Shi Wan (33).

Beneficial Foods

• For urinary pain, difficulty, retention: Asian pear, black beans, cantaloupe, carrots, celery, chestnut, chickweed, corn, corn silk tea, cranberry juice (unsweetened), dandelion greens, eggplant, grapes, kidney beans, millet, mung beans, Napa cabbage, pearl barley, peanuts, peppermint tea, purslane, raspberries, spinach, squash, star fruit, strawberries, watermelon, wheat, white rice, walnut, watercress.

- For stones: Beet greens, broccoli, chestnut, chives, corn silk tea, cranberry juice (unsweetened), green tea, kale, pearl barley, peanuts, seaweed, walnut, water chestnut, watermelon (including rind).

Food Remedy

- For painful or burning urination:
  - Juice carrots and celery in a 3:2 ratio (approximately 5 ounces of carrot juice to 3 ounces of celery) and drink 8 ounces 3 times a day until the condition clears.
  - Drink corn silk tea throughout the day until the condition clears.
- For stones:
  - Grind 2–3 cups of shelled walnuts into a fine powder. Add an equal amount of brown sugar. Roast in sesame oil, taking care to let the walnut powder brown but not burn. Consume ¼ of the mixture 4 times throughout the day.
  - Add 2 teaspoons of uncooked ground walnut powder to each cup of corn silk tea, and drink 5 glasses daily.
  - Cut up four star fruits, place in a pot with 3 cups of water and 1 tablespoon of honey, and low boil for 1 hour. Drink the tea and eat the star fruit. Do this once a day.

Women's Health/Gynecology

Qigong

- Liver, Spleen, Kidney.

Acupoints

- For amenorrhea: Ren 3, St 29, Sp 10, Liv 3, LI 4; sedate or harmonize all. Sp 6, St 36; tonify or harmonize all.
- For dysmenorrhea: Ren 3, Sp 10, St 29, LI 4, Liv 3; sedate or harmonize all. Sp 6, St 36; tonify or harmonize all.

- For irregular menstruation, short cycles (consistently less than 28 days): LI 11, Ren 3, SP 10, Liv 3, K6; sedate or harmonize all. Sp 6, St 36; harmonize.
- For irregular menstruation, long cycles (consistently more than 28 days): Ren 4, Ren 6, Ren 12, Sp 6, St 36; tonify all. Liv 3, LI 4; harmonize.
- For irregular menstruation, variable cycles: Ren 6, Ren 17, Liv 3, Liv 14, LI 4, Sp 6; harmonize all. K 3, K 10, K 13; tonify or harmonize all.
- For premenstrual syndrome: Liv 3, Liv 14, LI 4, K 3, K 13, Sp 3, Sp 6, Ren 3, Du 20. Harmonize all.
- For morning sickness: P 6, Ren 12, Liv 3, Liv 13, St 36, Sp 4. Harmonize all.
- For menopausal hot flashes: Du 20, GB 21, Liv 14, LI 11, Ren 3; sedate all. K 6; tonify. Liv 3, LI 4; harmonize.

Patent Remedy

- For amenorrhea: Shou Wu Zhi (39).
- For dysmenorrhea: Yan Hu Suo Zhi Tong Pian (49), Yunnan Te Chuan Tian Qi Pian (50).
- For irregular menstruation: Ba Zhen Wan (34) for three weeks beginning at end of menses, followed by Xiao Yao Wan (24) or Dan Zhi Xiao Yao Wan (27) for one week, ending at beginning of menses.
- For premenstrual syndrome: Xiao Yao Wan (24), Dan Zhi Xiao Yao Wan (27).
- For morning sickness: Shang Xia Liu Jun Zi Tang (18), Ban Xia Huo Po Tang (19), or Shen Ling Bai Zhu Pian (16).
- For menopause/hot flashes: Dan Zhi Xiao Yao Wan (27), Da Bu Yin Wan (47).

Beneficial Foods

- For PMS: In the absence of Heat symptoms, include these foods in your diet about one week before menses begins. Ginger, green onions, fennel, spinach, walnuts, hawthorn berries, cinnamon, black pepper.

- For morning sickness: Brown sugar, ginger, lentils, millet.

- For menopause: Black beans, black dates, chrysanthemum flowers, cherries, goji berries, mulberries, soy beans, sweet potatoes, tofu, tomatoes.

Food Remedy

- Low boil 1 ounce of sliced fresh ginger root in 4 cups of water for 30 minutes. Add 3 ounces of brown sugar and simmer another 10 minutes. Sip throughout the morning as needed. While 3 ounces of brown sugar are used in the traditional remedy, 1–2 tablespoons of honey may be added to the ginger tea instead, with comparable results.

Wellness Self-Care Protocol

If you're in good health, here's a protocol you can use as preventive medicine, for health maintenance and improvement. Over time it will improve your energy, strengthen your immune system, clarify your mind, and balance your emotions. While this will help prevent the onset of illness, if you do become sick or injured, it's best to postpone this protocol while following the appropriate healing procedures in this chapter. Once you've recovered, resume your wellness self-care.

Qigong

- All. Practice each for about 5 minutes every day, or select a different one each day throughout the weekdays, practicing for about 20 minutes a day. On the weekends, select the ones you enjoy the most. If you want to practice longer, that's okay. Be sure to follow all the practice guidelines from Chapter 16.

Acupoints

- Du 20, GB 21, LI 10, Lu 9, Ren 6, Ren 4, St 36, Sp 6, K3, Liv 3. Harmonize all.

Patent Remedy

- Ba Zhen Wan (34).

- During demanding times when you may expend a lot of energy, consider adding Shen Qi Da Bu Wan (37).

- Older adults begin to experience a progressive decline in Yin somewhere between 50 and 60 years of age. A useful Yin-nourishing maintenance formula to add is Liu Wei Di Huang Wan (43). If you are older, feel chilled easily, and are sensitive to cold, instead of Liu Wei Di Huang Wan, select Jin Gui Shen Qi Wan (40). It includes Liu Wei Di Huang Wan to nourish Yin but adds some warming herbs that nourish Yang as well.

Concluding Remarks

As comprehensive as this book is, you may choose to work with it exclusively for a time, especially if you want to fully incorporate Chinese holistic healing practices in the integrated, personalized ways taught here. I hope it serves you well both in helping you accomplish your immediate health goals and as a useful, practical, and inspirational introduction to a much vaster world of possibilities for living a long, healthy, and balanced life.

Of course, no single book can provide you with everything you might want or need. For further resources, my first recommendation is *Chinese Healing Exercises: A Personalized Practice for Health & Longevity*. It's presented in a way that works synergistically with the Qigong, acupressure, herbs, and dietary practices you've learned here. The exercise prescriptions in that book can be simply and effectively added to the prescriptions in this book and can be used as a foundation for a daily wellness practice. It provides similar guidance in helping you choose the exercises that will work best for you, removing any guesswork for beginners while being open-ended enough for more experienced readers to freely select among the ones that suit them best.

Other resources include the books in the following bibliography and recommended reading sections. Some of those are technical, some are purely informational, and some offer guidance in related practices. Each will open many other avenues of exploration.

There are thousands of books and even more instructional sources on the Internet offering various types of self-help and healing techniques. If you look carefully, you'll find that a great many of them are derived from Chinese and other traditional sources, simplified and packaged to accommodate the fast-paced, time-restricted sensibilities of modern life. If you're drawn to any of those, try interpreting them through the perspective of Chinese holism. Remember that this book is intended to help you incorporate a paradigm of integrated natural holistic health. Be mindful of how other self-care practices and professional medical approaches might fit that paradigm when deciding whether or not to include them in your life. That may be the single most beneficial lesson you can take from this book, as it can inform most, or all, of your health and wellness choices moving forward.

Glossary of Western Drug Actions

Analgesic: Acting to relieve pain.

Androgenergic: Acting in ways similar to or stimulating the release of male hormones; promoting the development of male characteristics.

Antibiotic: A substance that destroys or inhibits the growth of microorganisms, primarily bacteria.

Anticholinergic: Blocking the action of the neurotransmitter acetylcholine; used to treat various conditions such as gastrointestinal cramps, muscle spasms, asthma, depression, and sleep disorders.

Anticoagulant: Inhibiting the coagulation of blood (blood thinner); primarily used to prevent blood clots.

Anticonvulsant: Inhibiting convulsions; a drug used to prevent or control convulsions and seizures.

Antidiarrheal: Controlling or counteracting diarrhea.

Antiemetic: Preventing or relieving nausea and vomiting.

Antifungal: A substance that destroys or inhibits the growth of fungi, such as ringworm, athlete's foot, candidiasis, and cryptococcal meningitis.

Antihypertensive: Reducing or controlling high blood pressure.

Anti-inflammatory: Reducing inflammation and many of its signs, such as swelling, tenderness, fever, and pain.

Antimicrobial: A substance that destroys or inhibits the growth of microbes and inhibits their pathogenic action. Antibiotics are one type of antimicrobial.

Antineoplastic: Inhibiting the growth and spread of tumors and malignant cells.

Antiparasitic: Acting against parasites, destroying them, or inhibiting their growth and reproduction.

Antipyretic: Used to reduce or prevent fever.

Antitussive: Used to prevent or relieve a cough.

Antiviral: A substance that kills viruses or suppresses their ability to replicate.

Astringent: Causing the tightening and contraction of body tissues, reducing bleeding from minor abrasions, diminishing mucus discharge, and holding in other body fluids.

Bronchodilator: A substance that relaxes the bronchial muscles, widening the bronchial air passageway to improve ventilation to the lungs and facilitate breathing.

Cardiotonic: Having a favorable, tonic effect on the heart, improving the strength of its contraction and overall functions.

Cathartic: A strong laxative, having a purging, cleansing effect through bowel evacuation.

Decongestant: A medication or treatment used to relieve nasal congestion.

Diaphoretic: Inducing profuse perspiration.

Diuretic: Causing increased urine production and flow.

Enzymatic: Related to or produced by an enzyme. As used in this book, primarily digestive enzymes to aid in digestive processes.

Expectorant: A substance that thins, drains, and clears mucus from the lungs, promoting its discharge as phlegm (sputum).

Hemostatic: Acting to reduce bleeding or hemorrhage; arresting the flow of blood within the vessels.

Hypnotic: Acting to induce sleep. Sometimes used in anesthesia, and related to sedatives.

Laxative: Tending to loosen and relax, to stimulate the evacuation of the bowels.

Prokinetic: Stimulating movement or motility, usually referring to gastrointestinal motility; increasing the frequency of contractions in the small intestine.

Sedative: Soothing, promoting calm, inducing sleep, and tranquilizing. Relieving stress, anxiety, and irritability.

Appendix 1

Point Location by Body Region

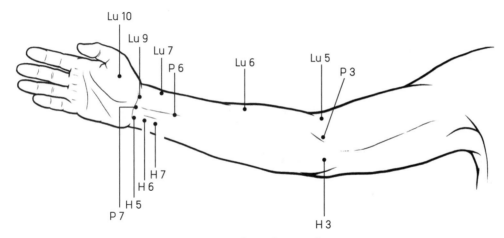

Figure A1 (Palm and Front of Arm)

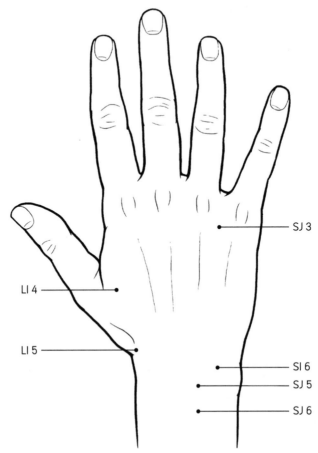

Figure A2 (Back of Hand)

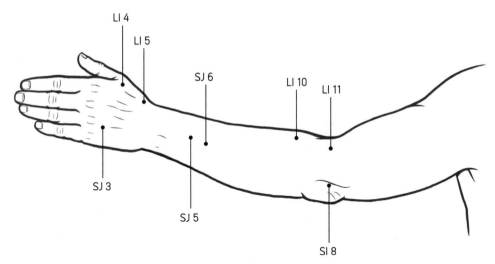

Figure A3 (Back of Hand and Arm)

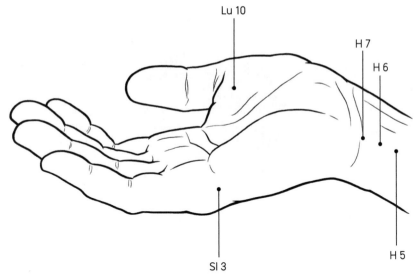

Figure A4 (Edge of Hand)

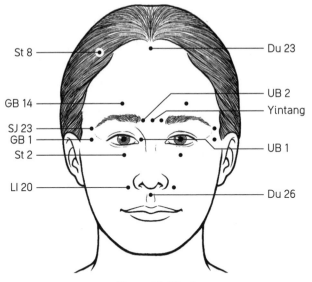

Figure A5 (Face)

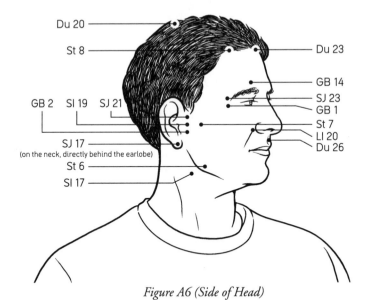

Figure A6 (Side of Head)

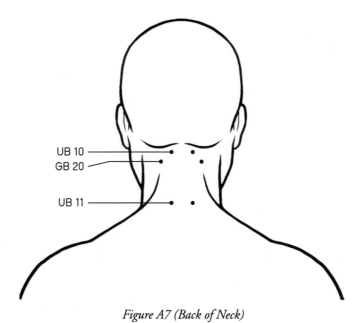

UB 10
GB 20
UB 11

Figure A7 (Back of Neck)

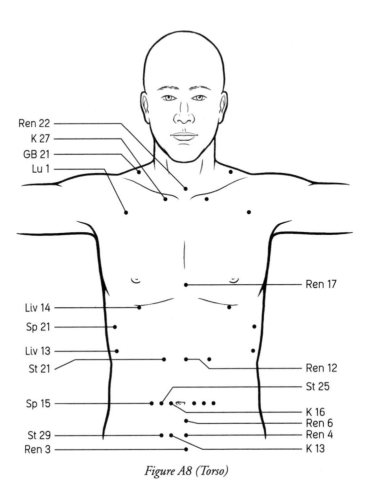

Ren 22
K 27
GB 21
Lu 1

Ren 17

Liv 14
Sp 21
Liv 13
St 21

Ren 12
St 25

Sp 15

K 16
Ren 6
Ren 4

St 29
Ren 3

K 13

Figure A8 (Torso)

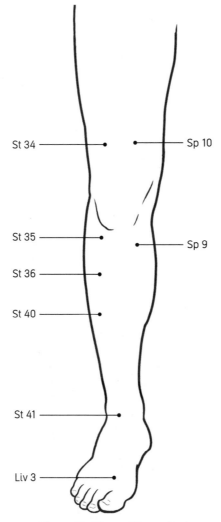

St 34 ——————•   • ——— Sp 10

St 35 ——————•   • ——— Sp 9

St 36 ——————•

St 40 ——————•

St 41 ——————•

Liv 3 ——————•

Figure A9 (Front of Lower Leg)

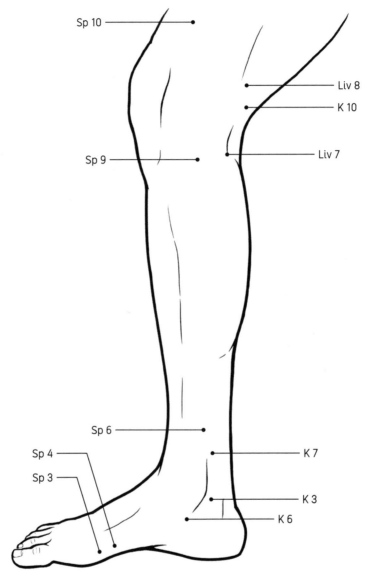

Figure A10 (Inside of Lower Leg)

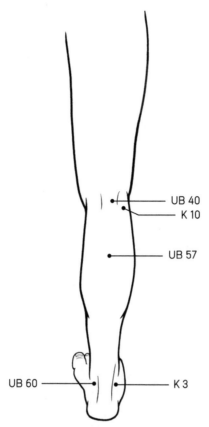

UB 40
K 10
UB 57
UB 60
K 3

Figure A11 (Back of Lower Leg)

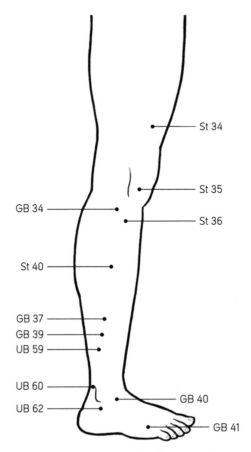

Figure A12 (Outside of Lower Leg)

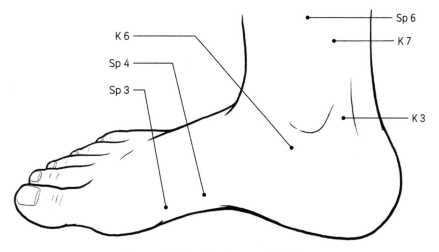

Figure A13 (Inside of Foot and Ankle)

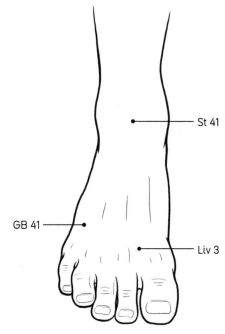

Figure A14 (Front and Top of Foot)

Appendix 2

Chapter Notes

Note 1.1

There is a type of Qi in the atmosphere, *Qingqi* or "clear Qi," that enters us with every breath we take, and through the function of the Lungs, it becomes a part of the Qi we use in our body.

Note 1.2

Some Chinese physicians use *infra*sound in medical devices intended to promote Qi flow.

Note 2.1

Classically, they are said to transport both Qi and blood in differing proportions. While that concept still exists and is taught today, it is rarely used in most contemporary clinical settings.

Note 5.1

The Chinese word for Heart is *Xin*. In other contexts, usually in intermediate to higher level Qigongs and in various meditation practices, Xin also may be interpreted as Heart-Mind, indicating the qualities of the Heart that are associated with mind, including emotions, consciousness, and spirit. While not often fully considered in contemporary clinical settings, these attributes are still observed and assessed by practitioners of classical Chinese medicine, usually from a Daoist perspective.

Note 5.2

Western medicine does not attribute most of these functions to the spleen. It is a perspective unique to Chinese medicine, but there are more similarities than you might think.

Most people don't know much about the spleen, so it can seem like a mysterious organ. Many even consider it expendable since it can be surgically removed without causing death or immediate, obvious complications. Here are the main things the spleen does according to Western medicine:

The spleen has numerous functions in regards to blood and immune system support. It acts as a blood filter, helping to purify blood. Part of that purification involves breaking down old or damaged red blood cells and recycling the component parts, including iron—the "hem-" in hemoglobin—into new, healthy red blood cells. The spleen is able to increase in size to store about a cup of blood in reserve. This reserve can be especially valuable in the case of traumatic blood loss. The spleen's reserve also contains about half of the body's monocytes, large white blood cells that promote tissue healing in any injured tissue, including the heart.

The spleen synthesizes antibodies, which are immune cells that assist in immune system functions. It removes antibody-coated bacteria and fights other bacteria that can cause pneumonia and meningitis. If the spleen is removed, the liver will take over some of its functions, but you will be more at risk for developing many types of infections, including the previously mentioned pneumonia and meningitis.

Chinese medicine does not distinguish between spleen and pancreas functions, considering them to be part of the same system. In fact, some schools of Chinese medicine refer to it as the spleen/pancreas. If we take into account the pancreas's primary roles of regulating blood sugar (which influences perceived energy levels) and the release of enzymes that assist in the digestion of protein, fats, and carbohydrates in the small intestine, we have a strong correlation between the Chinese and Western medical understanding of spleen functions. The interpretation of how those ends are achieved may be very different, but the end results are very similar.

To summarize the similarities, both East and West see the spleen (pancreas) as integral to the generation of blood, the digestion and assimilation of food, energy production, and tissue repair.

Note 5.3

There is a point on the low back, Du 4, which is called *Mingmen*. It is frequently needled or warmed with the herb moxa to tonify Kidney Yang and to treat various sexual, gynecological, and obstetric disorders and Kidney-related low back pain. More rarely, it is used to treat constitutional weakness believed to be associated with original Qi. That latter function, which does directly address the Mingmen, is not universally agreed upon.

Note 5.4

Western medicine has noted at least one correlation between kidneys and bone. In chronic kidney disease–mineral and bone disorder (CKD-MBD), the kidneys are known to be the source of this serious condition that causes systemic alterations in bone structure.

Note 6.1

Combining Eastern and Western perspectives, it's interesting to note that the Stomach's ascendant time of 7 a.m. to 9 a.m. makes it ideally suited to digest a protein-rich breakfast—stomach acids only break down proteins—while the Small Intestine time of 1 p.m. to 3 p.m. makes it suited to digest a fat- and carbohydrate-rich lunch. Fats and carbohydrates are only broken down by enzymes, bile, and other digestive fluids in the small intestine. This is another example of the importance of aligning lifestyle choices with the body's natural diurnal rhythms, in keeping with the organs' ascendant times.

Note 6.2

For comparison, if a person is suffering from a Cold condition, urine is clear and profuse. If there is excess Heat, often causing a burning sensation when urinating, the urine will be very dark yellow and scant. These indicators are used when applying Chinese diagnostic methods.

Note 6.3

The strong energetic link between the Sanjiao and Pericardium is most clearly demonstrated by the functions of a point on the Pericardium meridian: P 6, *Neiguan*, "Inner Pass." P 6 is the Luo connecting point with the Sanjiao and has a very wide range of clinical effects, benefitting almost all of the internal organs. This is due to the Sanjiao being the passageway through the entire body, harmonizing the functional activities of organs in all three Burners.

Note 11.1

Throughout history, needles have been made from bone, stone, and various metals, including silver and gold. Acupuncture needles are solid and very fine, slightly thicker than a human hair. Sloped back equally in all directions from its tip, the point is shaped more like a pine needle, and its insertion is more like parting the skin than like cutting through it.

Although some older traditional Chinese acupuncturists may autoclave their needles, sterilizing them for reuse in the same way surgical instruments are sterilized in hospitals, almost all acupuncturists in the United States use sterile, disposable, single-use needles, and many states require that by law. In this way, cross-infection from one patient to another is impossible.

Note 11.2

These days, people are inundated with a multitude of dietary advice, most aimed at weight loss and control, while others claim to be the best for overall health for everyone. Some of these include the Pritikin, Atkins, South Beach, and Zone diets, eating according to your blood type, veganism, and omnivore and Paleo diets. While it's impossible to comment on all of those in any meaningful way here, keep in mind that as with all health approaches, holistic or otherwise, there is no one way that is universally best for everyone.

Note 12.1

For example, in the point-strike martial art of *Dimmak*, strong targeted blows by a skilled martial artist can induce paralysis or cardiac or respiratory arrest by striking points on the arm alone.

Note 14.1

As an example of how symptoms may worsen, when using echinacea to treat a cold as mentioned in Chapter 14, you need to know it is a very cold herb, and can damage the

Spleen and Stomach if used for more than a few days. In the case of someone who may have a preexisting Spleen Qi or Yang deficiency, this could lead to severe diarrhea and abdominal cramping, causing dehydration, poor appetite, and poor nutrient absorption, with an accompanying worsening of health.

Note 14.2

While Western pharmacology does not make such distinctions, pharmaceuticals can be analyzed within this paradigm nonetheless. For example, when viewed through the lens of Chinese medicine, antibiotics as a class are uniformly cold to very cold, treating bacterial infections that almost always produce Heat signs, like fever, redness, and inflammation. The most common side effects of antibiotics are diarrhea, nausea, vomiting, abdominal cramping, loss of appetite, and, occasionally, white patches on the tongue. All of the digestive symptoms indicate injury to the Spleen and Stomach, which are easily damaged by cold substances. Cold substances are contraindicated in patients exhibiting symptoms of Spleen Qi or Yang deficiency. White patches on the tongue are one diagnostic indicator of internal Cold. Antibiotic effects and side-effect symptoms can be explained by Chinese medical analysis.

Note 14.3

Licorice root, or *Gan Cao*, is a sweet herb used to harmonize the effects of other herbs in a formula. My first herbs teacher likened it to a sweet "little sister" who can make a family feel peaceful and close when there might otherwise be some familial discord.

Bibliography

Becker, Robert O., and Gary Selden. *The Body Electric: Electromagnetism and the Foundation of Life.* New York: Quill, 1985.

Bensky, Dan, and Andrew Gamble. *Chinese Herbal Medicine: Materia Medica.* Seattle: Eastland Press, 1986.

Chang, Stephen T. *The Tao of Sexology: The Book of Infinite Wisdom.* San Francisco: Tao Publishing, 1986.

De Vernejoul, Pierre, Pierre Albarède, and Jean Claude Darras. "Nuclear Medicine and Acupuncture Message Transmission." *The Journal of Nuclear Medicine* 33, no. 3 (March 1, 1992): 409–12.

Ellis, Andrew W., Nigel Wiseman, and Ken Boss. *Grasping the Wind: An Exploration into the Meaning of Acupuncture Point Names.* Taos, NM: Paradigm Publications, 1989.

Fratkin, Jake. *Chinese Herbal Patent Formulas.* Boulder, CO: Shya Publications, 1990.

Hamilton, Marc T., Genevieve N. Healy, David W. Dunstan, Theodore W. Zderic, and Neville Owen. "Too Little Exercise and Too Much Sitting: Inactivity Physiology and the Need for New Recommendations on Sedentary Behavior." *Current Cardiovascular Risk Reports* 2, no. 4 (July 2008): 292–98. doi:10.1007/s12170-008-0054-8 PMCID: PMC3419586 NIHMSID: NIHMS182380.

Hui, Kathleen K. S., Jing Liu, and Kenneth K. Kwong. "Functional Mapping of the Human Brain during Acupuncture with Magnetic Resonance Imaging Somatosensory Cortex Activation." World Journal of Acupuncture-Moxibustion 7, no. 3 (1997): 44–49.

Kaptchuk, Ted. *The Web That Has No Weaver: Understanding Chinese Medicine.* New York: Congdon and Weed, Inc., 1983.

Lade, Arnie. *Acupuncture Points: Images & Functions.* Seattle: Eastland Press, 1989.

Lian, Yu-Lin, Chun Yang Chen, Michael Hammes, and Bernard C. Kolster. *The Seirin Pictorial Atlas of Acupuncture.* Cologne: Konemann Inc., 1999.

Liangyue, Deng, Gan Yijun, He Shuhui, Ji Xiaoping, Li Yang, Wang Rufen, Wang Wenjing, Wang Xuetai, Xu Hengzi, Xue Xiuling, and Yuan Jiuling. *Chinese Acupuncture and Moxibustion.* Beijing: Foreign Languages Press, 1987.

Maciocia, Giovanni. *The Foundations of Chinese Medicine: A Comprehensive Text for Acupuncturists and Herbalists.* London: Churchill Livingstone, 1989.

Osler, William. *Sir William Osler: Aphorisms from His Bedside Teachings and Writings.* New York: Henry Schuman, Inc., 1950.

Reid, Daniel P. *The Tao of Health, Sex, and Longevity: A Modern Practical Guide to the Ancient Way.* New York: Fireside Publishing, 1989.

Zhu, You-Ping. *Chinese Materia Medica: Chemistry, Pharmacology and Applications.* Boca Raton, FL: CRC Press, 1998.

Zhufan, Xie, and Huang Xiaokai. *Dictionary of Traditional Chinese Medicine.* Hong Kong: The Commercial Press, Ltd., 1984.

Recommended Reading

Benfield, Harriet, and Efrem Korngold. *Between Heaven and Earth: A Guide to Chinese Medicine.* New York: Ballantine Books, 1991.

Cardoza, Steven. *Chinese Healing Exercises: A Personalized Practice for Health & Longevity.* Woodbury, MN: Llewellyn Publications, 2013.

Chao-liang, Chang, Cao Qing-rong, and Li Bao-zhen. *Vegetables as Medicine: A Safe and Cheap Form of Traditional Chinese Food Therapy.* Subang Jaya, Malaysia: Pelanduk Publications, 1999

Frantzis, Bruce. *Dragon and Tiger Medical Qigong, Vol. 1: Develop Health and Energy in 7 Simple Movements.* Berkeley, CA: North Atlantic Books, 2010.

———. *Dragon and Tiger Medical Qigong, Vol. 2: Qi Cultivation Principles and Exercises.* Berkeley, CA: North Atlantic Books, 2014.

Liu, Hong. *Mastering Miracles: The Healing Art of Qigong as Taught by a Master.* New York: Warner Books, 1997.

Lu, Henry C. *Chinese System of Food Cures: Prevention & Remedies.* New York: Sterling Publishing Co., Inc., 1986.

Pei, Fang Jing. *Natural Remedies from the Chinese Cupboard: Healing Foods and Herbs.* Boulder, CO: Weatherhill, 1998.

Index

A

acquired essence, 76, 78, 81

acquired Qi, 89, 97

acupoint, 163, 189–192, 311

acupressure, 1, 6, 7, 149, 150, 156, 161, 164, 176, 177, 180, 183, 184, 189, 192, 195, 197, 199, 201, 203, 208, 211, 213, 216, 220, 223, 225, 227, 231, 233, 235, 284, 299, 330, 340, 365

acupuncture, 1, 6, 7, 13–16, 26, 28, 29, 31–34, 37, 61, 74, 96, 116, 151, 161–170, 173, 177, 178, 180, 183, 193, 195, 205, 210, 214, 218, 221, 222, 228, 236, 237, 241, 299, 300, 307, 308, 317, 322, 327, 329, 330, 386

allopathic, 12, 52, 239

anger, 9, 65, 67, 69, 70, 102, 105, 112, 142, 143, 190, 267, 344

ascendant (time), 54, 55, 57, 62, 65, 68, 71, 75, 88–90, 92, 93, 95, 170, 283, 284, 299, 305, 316, 323, 328, 385

B

Beak Hands, 307–309, 311, 313–316

bitter, 57, 91, 121, 180, 240, 246, 247

C

channel, 6–8, 28, 32, 61, 63, 108, 133, 138, 141, 163, 167, 169, 174, 178, 202, 204–206, 210, 224–229, 241, 247, 248, 261, 268, 273, 275, 280, 298, 305, 315, 331, 333, 335, 358

Chong, 29, 31, 143, 144, 221, 230

Cold, 41–45, 64, 75, 101, 105, 107–109, 120, 135–141, 146–147, 154–158, 168, 206, 232, 243, 246–250, 252, 255, 261–262, 265, 275, 332–335, 339, 348, 355, 357, 385

Cun, 185–187, 196, 198, 200, 202, 204–207, 209–212, 215, 217, 218, 221, 222, 224, 226, 228–230, 233, 234, 236, 237

D

Daimai, 29, 30, 317, 319, 322, 323

Damp, 9, 10, 64, 71, 72, 74, 101–109, 120, 139, 144, 145, 155, 157–159, 163, 165, 166, 202, 205–209, 229–232, 235–237, 240, 243, 245, 247–249, 261, 263–265, 267–269, 273, 275, 332–335, 340, 347, 350, 357

Dantian, 3, 29, 80, 129, 285, 286, 299, 305, 314, 316–319, 321–323, 327, 328

deficiency, deficient, 4, 21, 41, 43–45, 47, 58, 59, 64, 66, 67, 69, 70, 72, 73, 81, 83–85, 108, 112, 116–119, 129, 132, 135–139, 141, 142, 144–147, 155–159, 163, 165, 173, 199, 206, 209, 219, 246, 251–256, 262, 263, 270, 273, 335, 336, 340, 346, 355, 387

Dryness, 59, 62, 85, 101–104, 109, 120, 158

E

Eight Principles, 41, 135

ejaculation, 83, 126–128, 145, 146, 208, 236, 254, 355

electroacupuncture, 7, 163, 168

endorphins, 169

excess, 7, 41, 43–45, 64, 66, 67, 69, 72, 106, 118, 122, 124, 132, 135–138, 143–146, 155–160, 163, 180, 221, 247, 322, 340, 352, 385

External Pathogenic Factors (EPFs), 100, 101, 103, 180

Extraordinary Fu Organs, 51

Extraordinary Meridians, Extraordinary Vessels, 29, 278, 316, 317

F

fear, 9, 75, 84–86, 102, 114–116

Fire, 37–40, 57, 61, 70, 76, 80, 81, 87, 95, 100, 101, 103, 104, 106, 109, 134, 137, 144, 146, 244, 248, 267, 273, 290, 308, 317

Five Element, 57, 61, 62, 65, 71, 75, 82, 87, 113, 133, 134, 139, 143, 240, 290, 308

Five Flavors, Five Tastes, 119, 134, 180

Four Level, 42, 43, 133, 139

fright, 75, 84, 85, 102, 114, 115

Fu, 51

G

Gall Bladder, 27–29, 31, 32, 46, 51, 68, 87, 90–92, 96, 153, 157, 193, 196, 203, 226, 227, 229, 230, 232, 240, 267, 323, 325, 328, 347

grief, 9, 62, 64, 65, 67, 102, 112, 113

Guqi, 3, 71, 72

H

harmonize, harmonizing (techniques), 66, 83, 124, 163, 178, 191–192, 200, 204–209, 221–223, 230, 232, 237, 240, 258, 263, 265–267, 304, 309, 317, 330, 341, 344, 354, 355, 358–362, 386, 387

Heart, 27, 51–52, 54, 55, 57–61, 63, 66–68, 72–74, 82, 87, 89, 90, 95, 96, 105, 106, 108, 111–113, 115, 121–123, 125, 132, 139–142, 147, 153, 155–157, 159, 162, 195, 210–212, 222, 223, 240, 241, 248, 253, 254, 255, 260, 265, 266, 273, 275, 290, 305–312, 314–316, 348, 352–354, 359, 383

holism, holistic, 1–3, 10–12, 16, 23, 36, 37, 52–55, 99, 102, 103, 133, 149, 151, 161, 176, 179–181, 239, 240, 284, 365, 366, 386

homeostasis, 11, 12, 133

hormone(s), 14, 16, 47, 77, 99, 126, 129, 169, 331, 355, 367

Horse Stance, 300, 301, 303, 304

Hun, 65, 70

I

integration, integrated (practices), 1, 2, 5, 6, 13–16, 149, 151, 161, 163, 180, 284, 329, 331, 332, 365, 366

Internal Pathogenic Factors (IPFs), 100, 102–103, 111–115

J

Jing, 3, 13, 51, 75–85, 125–127, 129, 130, 132, 146, 169, 215, 228, 270, 271

Jingluo, Jingluoqi, 28

Jingqi, 3, 77

joy, 9, 57, 59, 60, 102, 111, 113, 121, 126

K

Kidney(s), 3, 27, 31, 46, 51, 52, 54, 61, 63, 70, 74, 75–86, 90, 93–94, 95, 97, 108–110, 114–115, 120–126, 129, 132, 145–147, 153, 155–157, 159, 195, 208, 219–222, 232, 236, 237, 240, 253, 256, 263, 265, 268, 269, 271–273,

290, 316–321, 322, 323, 334, 335, 336, 342, 343, 346, 349, 351, 353, 354, 355, 356, 358–360, 385

Kwa, 279, 280, 298, 299

L

Large Intestine, 27, 28, 33, 51, 87, 89, 90, 92, 93, 113, 153, 195, 200, 201, 221, 240, 289, 290, 298, 299, 307, 308

Liver, 3, 27, 28, 51–53, 65–70, 85, 90, 91, 96, 102–106, 111, 112, 117, 121, 124, 125, 129, 130, 132, 134, 138, 142–144, 153, 155–157, 193, 196, 203, 208, 219, 222, 224, 227–233, 240, 247, 253–256, 265–268, 270, 272, 273, 275, 290, 323–328, 332, 333, 341, 344, 347, 349–354, 356, 358, 360

Lower Jiao (Burner), 51, 61, 94–96, 132, 205, 267

Lungs, 28, 51, 52, 55, 58, 61–65, 67, 70, 72, 73, 82, 83, 92–96, 109, 112, 113, 120, 121, 125, 133, 140–141, 153, 157, 159, 162, 164, 165, 196, 197, 199, 202, 222, 240, 241, 248, 260, 262, 263, 289–299, 306–308, 315, 333, 335, 338, 342, 343, 347, 351, 353, 383

Luo, 28, 88, 385

M

meridian(s), 6, 7, 25–29, 31–34, 42, 46, 51, 58, 61, 63, 65, 69, 72, 74, 75, 88, 94, 95, 97, 104, 107, 115, 135, 136, 143, 144, 157, 161–163, 168–170, 189–196, 198, 210, 211, 214, 215, 217, 218, 221, 232, 234, 278, 283, 289, 290, 298, 299, 307, 315–317, 322, 325, 328, 339, 341, 356, 385

Middle Jiao (Burner), 96, 132, 204, 249, 263, 270, 275

Mingmen, 3, 76, 80, 110, 146, 317, 319, 321–323, 385

moxibustion, 7, 37, 162, 168

N

neurotransmitters, 169

nutrition, 8, 16, 42, 67, 75, 97, 118, 130, 141, 144, 252, 253, 357

O

Organ System(s), 3, 7, 28, 52, 66, 111, 140, 152, 179, 284

P

patterns of disharmony, 100, 103, 117–119, 130, 131, 133, 134, 139, 146, 161, 260

Pericardium, 25, 27, 33, 51, 61, 94, 95, 158, 195, 222, 223, 290, 306–308, 315, 385

pinyin, 3, 259

Po, 62, 64, 65, 70, 249, 255, 260, 265, 275, 341, 361

postnatal Jing. *See* acquired essence

postnatal Qi, 72

pregnancy, 10, 129, 130, 152, 155, 195, 205, 209, 210, 218, 221, 222, 228, 236, 237, 260, 267, 268, 274, 275

prenatal essence, 76, 78–80

psychospiritual aspects, 54, 60, 64, 70, 74, 86

pulse diagnosis, 140, 153

Q

Qigong, 1, 3, 6, 7, 9, 11, 14, 15, 28, 55, 61, 62, 64, 72, 79, 80, 116, 119, 124, 127, 149, 150, 160, 161, 163, 164, 176–180, 277, 278, 281–284, 286, 287, 289–297, 299, 300, 302–306, 309, 310, 312, 314, 316–318, 320, 321, 323–326, 328–335, 337–339, 341–344, 346–354, 356, 358–360, 362, 365

Qingqi, 62, 64, 283, 383

S

sadness, 62, 64, 67, 102, 112, 113

salty, 75, 120, 121, 180, 240

Sanjiao, 27, 51, 61, 87, 94–97, 133, 196, 224, 225, 290, 307, 308, 385, 386

sedate, sedation (techniques), 159, 163, 168, 177, 178, 190–192, 248, 253, 255, 256, 330, 332–335, 338, 340, 342–344, 346, 347, 349, 351–356, 358, 360, 361, 368, 369

sex, 10, 47, 48, 79, 83, 84, 125–130, 287

Shen, 57, 60, 111, 151, 212, 218, 252, 254, 264, 270, 271, 274, 275, 348, 352, 353, 355, 361–363

Shimian, 294, 299, 322, 323

side channel(s), 278, 280, 305

Side Channel Stance, 278, 280, 281, 291, 306, 309, 317, 323

Six Stage, 133, 134, 139

Small Intestine, 27, 51, 67, 87, 88, 89–90, 92, 93, 110, 153, 195, 212–214, 240, 290, 307, 308, 385

sour, 65, 121, 180, 240, 254, 255, 266

spicy, 62, 120, 121, 180, 240, 241, 243, 249, 250

Spleen, 3, 4, 27, 46, 51, 52, 58, 62, 64, 67, 71–75, 76, 77, 81, 82, 88, 89, 91, 92, 96, 106–108, 111, 112, 114, 117–120, 122–125, 129, 130, 132, 134, 139, 141, 143–145, 147, 153, 155, 157, 162, 165, 195, 206–209, 222, 230, 232, 237, 240, 241, 248–251, 253, 255, 263–272, 290, 299–305, 332–334, 336, 339–343, 346, 347, 349–351, 353, 354, 356, 358–360, 384, 387

Stomach, 27, 32, 46, 51, 67, 72–73, 81, 82, 87, 88–89, 91, 96, 110, 112, 118, 120–123, 129, 141, 143, 153, 157–159, 165, 193, 195, 200–208, 217, 221–223, 232, 237, 240–

241, 248, 250, 254, 263–265, 299–305, 333, 340, 341, 344, 347, 385, 387

Summer Heat, 101, 105, 106, 217, 243, 245

sweet, 71, 73, 119, 121, 180, 240, 250, 252, 253, 255, 332, 336, 341, 342, 345, 346, 353, 355, 362, 387

Sword Fingers, 316, 323

T

Taiji, 1, 3, 6–8, 14, 15, 35–37, 39, 41, 47, 48, 77, 79, 116, 124, 133, 161, 164, 176, 179, 180, 278, 300, 307, 317

tongue diagnosis, 10, 29, 57, 58, 92, 105, 106, 140–147, 151, 157–160, 212, 387

tonify, tonification (techniques), 65, 80, 119, 163, 177, 178, 189–192, 196, 199, 207, 221, 232, 236, 237, 240, 252, 253, 261–271, 273, 330, 332–335, 340, 342–344, 346–349, 351–355, 358–361, 385

Traditional Chinese Medicine (TCM), 77, 78, 133–135, 139, 193

Triple Burner. *See* Sanjiao

Tuina, 3, 6, 7, 14, 161, 176, 177

U

Upper Jiao (Burner), 95, 113, 132, 306

Urinary Bladder, 25, 27, 31, 51, 63, 65, 83, 87, 90, 93–94, 96, 153, 169, 193, 195, 215, 216, 232, 235, 240, 268, 269, 317, 323, 347

V

virtue, 54, 57, 62, 65, 71, 75

vitamin, 8, 119, 175, 176, 253, 269

W

Waiqi, 3, 178

Weiqi, 42, 63, 96, 119, 120, 140, 141, 221, 261, 270, 334, 353

Wind, 65, 100–107, 111, 112, 117, 133, 137, 140, 141, 144, 154, 158, 193, 198–200, 202, 204, 206, 212, 214, 215, 217–219, 225–231, 233, 234, 241, 243, 247, 256, 260–262, 264, 268, 272, 273, 275, 322, 333–335, 339, 357

worry, 71, 74, 102, 114, 144, 309

X

Xin, 61, 71, 260, 275, 383

Xue, 28, 42, 209, 221

Y

Yang, 3, 13, 25, 27–31, 33–49, 51–53, 61, 68, 70, 71, 73, 74, 76, 77, 79–84, 87, 88, 90, 91, 93, 94, 96, 103–107, 109, 110, 117, 120, 121, 127–129, 132, 133, 135–139, 142, 144–146, 153, 157, 158, 162, 163, 168, 173, 181, 190, 200, 213, 218, 219, 221, 222, 228, 229, 236, 241, 243, 253, 254, 256, 260, 268, 270, 271, 283, 308, 317, 329, 355, 356, 363, 385, 387

Yang Qiao, 29

Yang Wei, 29, 31

Yin, 3, 13, 25, 27–31, 33–49, 51–54, 57–59, 63–65, 70, 72, 76, 77, 79–85, 87–94, 96, 105–107, 109, 110, 117, 120, 123, 127–129, 132, 133, 135–142, 147, 153, 155, 157–159, 163, 173, 181, 190, 196, 197, 199, 207, 209, 212, 219–221, 235, 240, 243, 245–247, 249, 251, 253–256, 260, 262, 265, 266, 270–274, 290, 298, 299, 307, 315, 316, 329, 333, 338, 342, 346, 348, 352, 356, 361, 363

Yin-Yang theory, 4, 25, 28, 38–40, 45–48, 59, 136
Yin Qiao, 29, 260, 333, 338, 346
Yin Wei, 29
Ying, 42, 202, 245
Yuan Jing. *See* prenatal essence
Yongquan, 292, 299, 321–323

Z

Zang, 51, 57
Zangfu, 51, 63, 95, 133–135, 139
Zhengqi, 28, 334
Zhenqi, 28
Zongqi, 62, 63, 72

To Write to the Author

If you wish to contact the author or would like more information about this book, please write to the author in care of Llewellyn Worldwide, and we will forward your request. Both the author and the publisher appreciate hearing from you and learning of your enjoyment of this book and how it has helped you. Llewellyn Worldwide cannot guarantee that every letter written to the author can be answered, but all will be forwarded. Please write to:

Steven Cardoza
℅ Llewellyn Worldwide
2143 Wooddale Drive
Woodbury, MN 55125-2989

Please enclose a self-addressed stamped envelope for reply,
or $1.00 to cover costs. If outside the USA, enclose
an international postal reply coupon.

Many of Llewellyn's authors have websites with additional information and resources. For more information, please visit our website at www.llewellyn.com.

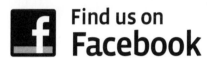
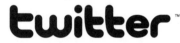

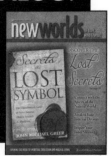

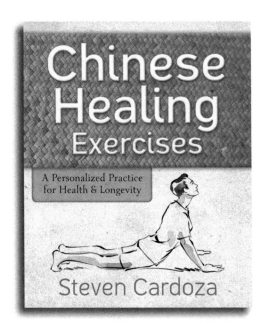

Chinese Healing Exercises

Exercises

A Personalized Practice
for Health & Longevity

Steven Cardoza

Chinese Healing Exercises
A Personalized Practice for Health & Longevity
STEVEN CARDOZA

Reduce pain, increase energy, stave off disease, reverse the signs of aging, and lengthen your life with simple Chinese healing exercises.

Based on acupressure, Taiji, Qigong, Daoist yoga, and other traditional Chinese health practices, these 88 exercises can be done by anyone of any age. Arranged into chapters devoted to specific parts of the body, each exercise includes illustrations, easy-to-follow instructions, and physical and energetic benefits. In simple language, Steven Cardoza, a Chinese medical physician, introduces the concept of *qi* and how each exercise regulates this vital life energy and influences our physical and emotional health. This book features an appendix of specific exercises that relieve aches and pains, allergies, digestive disorders, insomnia, stress, and other common health concerns. Also included is a glossary of terms to deepen your understanding of these beneficial Chinese practices.

978-0-7387-3754-6, 312 pp., 7 ½ x 9 ¹/₈ $21.99

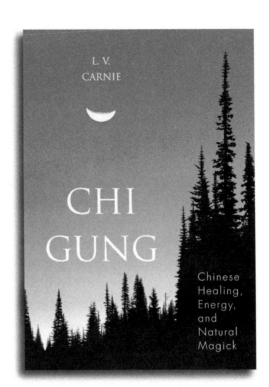

L. V.
CARNIE

CHI
GUNG

Chinese
Healing,
Energy,
and
Natural
Magick

Chi Gung
Chinese Healing, Energy and Natural Magick
L.V. CARNIE

You possess the ability to tap a bottomless well of physical and psychic energy (called *chi* in Chinese). With it you can harness the magickal power of the universe. How do you do it? By learning the ancient Chinese art of breath, posture, and sensory awareness as explained in *Chi Gung* by L.V. Carnie.

As you learn this system to direct your flow of chi, you will be able to achieve ultimate health and things you have only dreamed of:

Look and feel younger • Add healthy years to your life • Progress faster in martial arts training • Develop different types of psychic ability: heal at a distance, talk with spirits, move objects with your mind • Increase your fitness level • Help damaged tissue heal more quickly • Improve sexual performance • Learn to control your body temperature • Bond with your pets or with animals in the wild

Chi Gung is filled with simple but effective exercises for mind, body, and spirit that will open your flow of chi as they open you to a whole new world of possibilities. No other chi gung self-help book covers such a broad range of material or presents the actual training techniques for mastering the more advanced skills.

978-56718-113-5, 288 pp., 7 x 10   **$21.99**

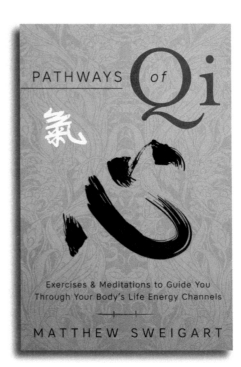

PATHWAYS of Qi

Exercises & Meditations to Guide You
Through Your Body's Life Energy Channels

MATTHEW SWEIGART

Pathways of Qi

Exercises & Meditations to Guide You
Through Your Body's Life Energy Channels

Matthew Sweigart

Nurture the flow of Qi energy in your body for a life of vibrancy, balance, and wellness. In *Pathways of Qi*, Chinese Medicine expert Matthew Sweigart shows how to use touch therapy, meditations, and gentle Qigong exercises to clear away blockages and open up to energetic nourishment.

Based on ancient wisdom traditions, these hands-on assessment and treatment techniques have been cultivated to heal the body, mind, emotions, and spirit. Explore the channels of energy in the body—known in Chinese Medicine as the meridians—and for each one, discover the limb position, yin/yang properties, corresponding elements, functions, affirmations, and more. With illustrations to help you master the physical postures and gestures, *Pathways of Qi* will guide you through gentle practices for a life of improved awareness, connection, and health.

978-0-7387-4822-1, 336 pp., 6 x 9   **$22.99**

To order, call 1-877-NEW-WRLD
Prices subject to change without notice
Order at Llewellyn.com 24 hours a day, 7 days a week!

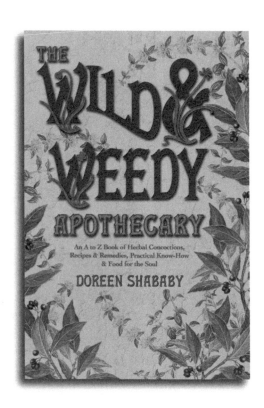

THE Wild & Weedy APOTHECARY

An A to Z Book of Herbal Concoctions,
Recipes & Remedies, Practical Know-How
& Food for the Soul

DOREEN SHABABY

The Wild & Weedy Apothecary
An A to Z Book of Herbal Concoctions, Recipes & Remedies, Practical Know-How & Food for the Soul
Doreen Shababy

Just outside your doorstep or kitchen window, hidden beneath a tall pine tree or twining through porch latticework, a wild and weedy apothecary waits to be discovered.

Herbalist Doreen Shababy shares her deep, abiding love for the earth and its gifts in this collection of herbal wisdom that represents a lifetime of work in the forest, field, and kitchen. This herbalism guidebook is jam-packed with dozens of tasty recipes and natural remedies, including Glorious Garlic and Artichoke Dip, Sunny Oatmeal Crepes, Candied Catnip Leaves, Lavender Lemonade, Roseberry Tea, Garlic Tonic, Parsnip Hair Conditioner, and Dream Charms made with Mugwort.

A sampling of the herbal lore, legend, and instruction found within these pages:

The difference between sweet-faced flowers and flowers with attitude • How to assemble a well-stocked pantry • The importance of gratitude • Plant-spirit communication basics • How to use local wild herbs • How to make poultices, teas, tinctures, balms, and extracts

978-0-7387-1907-8, 384 pp., 6 x 9   **$19.99**
